MW00800881

CONTENTS

VEGETABLE & VEGETARIAN RECIPES

Smoked Pumpkin Soup

Servings: 6
Cooking Time: 1 Hour And 33 Minutes
Ingredients:
- 5 pounds pumpkin, seeded and sliced
- 3 tablespoons butter
- 1 onion, diced
- 2 cloves garlic, minced
- 1 tablespoon brown sugar
- 1 teaspoon paprika
- ¼ teaspoon ground cinnamon
- ¼ teaspoon ground nutmeg
- ½ cup apple cider
- 5 cups broth
- ½ cup cream

Directions:
1. Fire the Traeger Grill to 180F. Use desired wood pellets when cooking. Close the lid and preheat for 15 minutes.
2. Place the pumpkin on the grill grate and smoke for an hour or until tender. Allow to cool.
3. Melt the butter in a large saucepan over medium heat and sauté the onion and garlic for 3 minutes. Stir in the rest of the ingredients including the smoked pumpkin. Cook for another 30 minutes.
4. Transfer to a blender and pulse until smooth.
Nutrition Info: Calories per serving: 246; Protein: 8.8g; Carbs: 32.2g; Fat: 11.4g Sugar: 15.5g

Grilled Potato Salad

Servings: 8
Cooking Time: 10 Minutes
Ingredients:
- 1 ½ pound fingerling potatoes, halved lengthwise
- 1 small jalapeno, sliced
- 10 scallions
- 2 teaspoons salt
- 2 tablespoons rice vinegar
- 2 teaspoons lemon juice
- 2/3 cup olive oil, divided

Directions:
1. Switch on the Traeger grill, fill the grill hopper with pecan flavored wood pellets, power the grill on by using the control panel, select 'smoke' on the temperature dial, or set the temperature to 450 degrees F and let it preheat for a minimum of 5 minutes.
2. Meanwhile, prepare scallions, and for this, brush them with some oil.
3. When the grill has preheated, open the lid, place scallions on the grill grate, shut the grill and smoke for 3 minutes until lightly charred.
4. Then transfer scallions to a cutting board, let them cool for 5 minutes, then cut into slices and set aside until required.
5. Brush potatoes with some oil, season with some salt and black pepper, place potatoes on the grill grate, shut the grill and smoke for 5 minutes until thoroughly cooked.
6. Then take a large bowl, pour in remaining oil, add salt, lemon juice, and vinegar and stir until combined.
7. Add grilled scallion and potatoes, toss until well mixed, taste to adjust seasoning and then serve.
Nutrition Info: Calories: 223.7 Cal ;Fat: 12 g ;Carbs: 27 g ;Protein: 1.9 g ;Fiber: 3.3 g

Wood Pellet Grilled Mexican Street Corn

Servings: 6
Cooking Time: 25 Minutes
Ingredients:
- 6 ears of corn on the cob, shucked
- 1 tbsp olive oil
- Kosher salt and pepper to taste
- 1/4 cup mayo
- 1/4 cup sour cream
- 1 tbsp garlic paste
- 1/2 tbsp chili powder
- Pinch of ground red pepper
- 1/2 cup cotija cheese, crumbled
- 1/4 cup cilantro, chopped
- 6 lime wedges

Directions:
1. Brush the corn with oil and sprinkle with salt.
2. Place the corn on a wood pellet grill set at 350°F. Cook for 25 minutes as you turn it occasionally.
3. Meanwhile mix mayo, cream, garlic, chili, and red pepper until well combined.
4. When the corn is cooked remove from the grill, let it rest for some minutes then brush with the mayo mixture.
5. Sprinkle cotija cheese, more chili powder, and cilantro. Serve with lime wedges. Enjoy.
Nutrition Info: Calories 144, Total fat 5g, Saturated fat 2g, Total Carbs 10g, Net Carbs 10g, Protein 0g, Sugar 0g, Fiber 0g, Sodium: 136mg, Potassium 173mg

Zucchini With Red Potatoes

Servings: 4

Cooking Time: 4 Hours
Ingredients:
- 2 zucchinis, sliced in 3/4-inch-thick disks
- 1 red pepper, cut into strips
- 2 yellow squash, sliced in 3/4-inch-thick disks
- 1 medium red onion, cut into wedges
- 6 small red potatoes, cut into chunks
- Balsamic Vinaigrette:
- 1/3 cup extra virgin olive oil
- 1/4 teaspoon salt
- 1/4 cup balsamic vinegar
- 2 tsp Dijon mustard
- 1/8 teaspoon pepper

Directions:
1. For Vinaigrette: Take a medium-sized bowl and blend together olive oil, Dijon mustard, salt, pepper, and balsamic vinegar.
2. Place all the veggies into a large bowl and pour the vinaigrette mixture over it and evenly toss.
3. Put the vegetable in a pan and then smoke for 4 hours at a temperature of 225°F.
4. Serve and enjoy the food.
Nutrition Info: Calories: 381 Cal Fat: 17.6 g Carbohydrates: 49 g   Protein: 6.7 g Fiber: 6.5 g

Roasted Root Vegetables

Servings: 6
Cooking Time: 45 Minutes
Ingredients:
- 1 large red onion, peeled
- 1 bunch of red beets, trimmed, peeled
- 1 large yam, peeled
- 1 bunch of golden beets, trimmed, peeled
- 1 large parsnips, peeled
- 1 butternut squash, peeled
- 1 large carrot, peeled
- 6 garlic cloves, peeled
- 3 tablespoons thyme leaves
- Salt as needed
- 1 cinnamon stick
- Ground black pepper as needed
- 3 tablespoons olive oil
- 2 tablespoons honey

Directions:
1. Switch on the Traeger grill, fill the grill hopper with hickory flavored wood pellets, power the grill on by using the control panel, select 'smoke' on the temperature dial, or set the temperature to 450 degrees F and let it preheat for a minimum of 15 minutes.
2. Meanwhile, cut all the vegetables into ½-inch pieces, place them in a large bowl, add garlic, thyme, and cinnamon, drizzle with oil and toss until mixed.

3. Take a large cookie sheet, line it with foil, spread with vegetables, and then season with salt and black pepper.
4. When the grill has preheated, open the lid, place prepared cookie sheet on the grill grate, shut the grill and smoke for 45 minutes until tender.
5. When done, transfer vegetables to a dish, drizzle with honey, and then serve.
Nutrition Info: Calories: 164 Cal ;Fat: 4 g ;Carbs: 31.7 g ;Protein: 2.7 g ;Fiber: 6.4 g

Smoked Potato Salad

Servings: 4
Cooking Time: 40 Minutes
Ingredients:
- 2 lb. potatoes
- 2 tablespoons olive oil
- 2 cups mayonnaise
- 1 tablespoon white wine vinegar
- 1 tablespoon dry mustard
- 1/2 onion, chopped
- 2 celery stalks, chopped
- Salt and pepper to taste

Directions:
1. Coat the potatoes with oil.
2. Smoke the potatoes in the Traeger wood pellet grill at 180 degrees F for 20 minutes.
3. Increase temperature to 450 degrees F and cook for 20 more minutes.
4. Transfer to a bowl and let cool.
5. Peel potatoes.
6. Slice into cubes.
7. Refrigerate for 30 minutes.
8. Stir in the rest of the ingredients.
9. Tips: You can also add chopped hard-boiled eggs to the mixture.

Grilled Ratatouille Salad

Servings: 6
Cooking Time: 25 Minutes
Ingredients:
- 1 Whole sweet potatoes
- 1 Whole red onion, diced
- 1 Whole zucchini
- 1 Whole Squash
- 1 Large Tomato, diced
- As Needed vegetable oil
- As Needed salt and pepper

Directions:
1. Preheat grill to high setting with the lid closed for 10-15 minutes.
2. Slice all vegetables to a ¼ inch thickness.

3. Lightly brush each vegetable with oil and season with Traeger's Veggie Shake or salt and pepper.
4. Place sweet potato, onion, zucchini, and squash on grill grate and grill for 20 minutes or until tender, turn halfway through.
5. Add tomato slices to the grill during the last 5 minutes of cooking time.
6. For presentation, alternate vegetables while layering them vertically. Enjoy!

Smoked Stuffed Mushrooms

Servings: 12
Cooking Time: 1 Hour 15 Minutes
Ingredients:
- 12-16 white mushrooms, large, cleaned and stems removed
- 1/2 cup parmesan cheese
- 1/2 cup bread crumbs, Italian
- 2 minced garlic cloves
- 2 tbsp fresh parsley, chopped
- 1/4 -1/3 cup olive oil
- Salt and pepper to taste

Directions:
1. Preheat your Traeger 375F.
2. Remove mushroom very bottom stem then dice the rest into small pieces.
3. Combine mushroom stems, parmesan cheese, bread crumbs, garlic, parsley, 3 tbsp oil, pepper, and salt in a bowl, large. Combine until moist.
4. Layer mushrooms in a pan, disposable, then fill them with the mixture until heaping. Drizzle with more oil.
5. Place the pan on the Traeger grill.
6. Smoke for about 1 hour 20 minutes until filling browns and mushrooms become tender.
7. Remove from Traeger and serve.
8. Enjoy!

Nutrition Info: Calories 74, Total fat 6.1g, Saturated fat 1g, Total carbs 4.1g, Net carbs 3.7g, Protein 1.6g, Sugars 0.6g, Fiber 0.4g, Sodium 57mg, Potassium 72mg

Wood Pellet Grilled Vegetables

Servings: 8
Cooking Time: 15 Minutes
Ingredients:
- 1 veggie tray
- 1/4 cup vegetable oil
- 2 tbsp veggie seasoning

Directions:
1. Preheat the wood pellet grill to 375°F
2. Toss the vegetables in oil then place on a sheet pan.

3. Sprinkle with veggie seasoning then place on the hot grill.
4. Grill for 15 minutes or until the veggies are cooked.
5. Let rest then serve. Enjoy.
Nutrition Info: Calories 44, Total fat 5g, Saturated fat 0g, Total Carbs 1g, Net Carbs 1g, Protein 0g, Sugar 0g, Fiber 0g, Sodium: 36mg, Potassium 10mg

Stuffed Grilled Zucchini

Servings: 4
Cooking Time: 10 Minutes
Ingredients:
- 4 zucchini, medium
- 5 tbsp olive oil, divided
- 2 tbsp red onion, finely chopped
- 1/4 tbsp garlic, minced
- 1/2 cup bread crumbs, dry
- 1/2 cup shredded mozzarella cheese, part-skim
- 1/2 tbsp salt
- 1 tbsp fresh mint, minced
- 3 tbsp parmesan cheese, grated

Directions:
1. Halve zucchini lengthwise and scoop pulp ou. Leave 1/4 -inch shell. Now brush using 2 tbsp oil, set aside, and chop the pulp.
2. Saute onion and pulp in a skillet, large, then add garlic and cook for about 1 minute.
3. Add bread crumbs and cook while stirring for about 2 minutes until golden brown.
4. Remove everything from heat then stir in mozzarella cheese, salt, and mint. Scoop into the zucchini shells and splash with parmesan cheese.
5. Preheat your Traeger to 375F.
6. Place stuffed zucchini on the Traeger grill and grill while covered for about 8-10 minutes until tender.
7. Serve warm and enjoy.
Nutrition Info: Calories 186, Total fat 10g, Saturated fat 3g, Total carbs 17g, Net carbs 14g, Protein 9g, Sugars 4g, Fiber 3g, Sodium 553mg, Potassium 237mg

Sweet Potato Fries

Servings: 4
Cooking Time: 40 Minutes
Ingredients:
- 3 sweet potatoes, sliced into strips
- 4 tablespoons olive oil
- 2 tablespoons fresh rosemary, chopped
- Salt and pepper to taste

Directions:

1. Set the Traeger wood pellet grill to 450 degrees F.
2. Preheat it for 10 minutes.
3. Spread the sweet potato strips in the baking pan.
4. Toss in olive oil and sprinkle with rosemary, salt and pepper.
5. Cook for 15 minutes.
6. Flip and cook for another 15 minutes.
7. Flip and cook for 10 more minutes.
8. Tips: Soak sweet potatoes in water before cooking to prevent browning.

Roasted Spicy Tomatoes

Servings: 4
Cooking Time: 1 Hour And 30 Minutes
Ingredients:
- 2 lb. large tomatoes, sliced in half
- Olive oil
- 2 tablespoons garlic, chopped
- 3 tablespoons parsley, chopped
- Salt and pepper to taste
- Hot pepper sauce

Directions:
1. Set the temperature to 400 degrees F.
2. Preheat it for 15 minutes while the lid is closed.
3. Add tomatoes to a baking pan.
4. Drizzle with oil and sprinkle with garlic, parsley, salt and pepper.
5. Roast for 1 hour and 30 minutes.
6. Drizzle with hot pepper sauce and serve.
7. Tips: You can also puree the roasted tomatoes and use as sauce for pasta or as dip for chips.

Smoked 3-bean Salad

Servings: 6
Cooking Time: 20 Minutes
Ingredients:
- 1 can Great Northern Beans, rinsed and drained
- 1 can Red Kidney Beans, rinsed and drained
- 1 pound fresh green beans, trimmed
- 2 tablespoons olive oil
- Salt and pepper to taste
- 1 shallot, sliced thinly
- 2 tablespoons red wine vinegar
- 1 teaspoon Dijon mustard

Directions:
1. Fire the Traeger Grill to 500F. Use desired wood pellets when cooking. Close the lid and preheat for 15 minutes.
2. Place the beans in a sheet tray and drizzle with olive oil. Season with salt and pepper to taste.

3. Place in the grill and cook for 20 minutes. Make sure to shake the tray for even cooking.
4. Once cooked, remove the beans and place in a bowl. Allow to cool first.
5. Add the shallots and the rest of the ingredients. Season with more salt and pepper if desired. Toss to coat the beans with the seasoning.
Nutrition Info: Calories per serving: 179; Protein: 8.2 g; Carbs: 23.5g; Fat: 6.5g Sugar: 2.2g

Baked Parmesan Mushrooms

Servings: 8
Cooking Time: 15 Minutes
Ingredients:
- 8 mushroom caps
- 1/2 cup Parmesan cheese, grated
- 1/2 teaspoon garlic salt
- 1/4 cup mayonnaise
- Pinch paprika
- Hot sauce

Directions:
1. Place mushroom caps in a baking pan.
2. Mix the remaining ingredients in a bowl.
3. Scoop the mixture onto the mushroom.
4. Place the baking pan on the grill.
5. Cook in the Traeger wood pellet grill at 350 degrees F for 15 minutes while the lid is closed.
6. Tips: You can also add chopped sausage to the mixture.

Wood Pellet Grilled Zucchini Squash Spears

Servings: 5
Cooking Time: 10 Minutes
Ingredients:
- 4 zucchini, cleaned and ends cut
- 2 tbsp olive oil
- 1 tbsp sherry vinegar
- 2 thyme, leaves pulled
- Salt and pepper to taste

Directions:
1. Cut the zucchini into halves then cut each half thirds.
2. Add the rest of the ingredients in a ziplock bag with the zucchini pieces. Toss to mix well.
3. Preheat the wood pellet temperature to 350°F with the lid closed for 15 minutes.
4. Remove the zucchini from the bag and place them on the grill grate with the cut side down.
5. Cook for 4 minutes per side or until the zucchini are tender.

6. Remove from grill and serve with thyme leaves. Enjoy.

Nutrition Info: Calories 74, Total fat 5.4g, Saturated fat 0.5g, Total Carbs 6.1g, Net Carbs 3.8g, Protein 2.6g, Sugar 3.9g, Fiber 2.3g, Sodium: 302mg, Potassium 599mg

Broccoli-cauliflower Salad

Servings: 4
Cooking Time: 25 Minutes
Ingredients:
- 1½ cups mayonnaise
- ½ cup sour cream
- ¼ cup sugar
- 1 bunch broccoli, cut into small pieces
- 1 head cauliflower, cut into small pieces
- 1 small red onion, chopped
- 6 slices bacon, cooked and crumbled (precooked bacon works well)
- 1 cup shredded Cheddar cheese

Directions:
1. In a small bowl, whisk together the mayonnaise, sour cream, and sugar to make a dressing.
2. In a large bowl, combine the broccoli, cauliflower, onion, bacon, and Cheddar cheese.
3. Pour the dressing over the vegetable mixture and toss well to coat.
4. Serve the salad chilled.

Grilled Romaine Caesar Salad

Servings: 6
Cooking Time: 5 Minutes
Ingredients:
- ¼ cup extra virgin olive oil
- 2 cloves garlic, minced
- 1 teaspoon Dijon mustard
- 1 cup mayonnaise
- Salt and pepper to taste
- 2 head Romaine lettuce
- ¼ cup parmesan cheese
- Croutons, optional

Directions:
1. In a small bowl, combine the olive oil, garlic, mustard, and mayonnaise. Season with salt and pepper to taste. Mix and set aside.
2. Cut the Romaine in half lengthwise leaving the ends intact so that it does not come apart.
3. Fire the Traeger Grill to 400F. Use desired wood pellets when cooking. Close the lid and preheat for 15 minutes.
4. Brush the Romaine lettuce with oil and place cut side down on the grill grate. Cook for 5 minutes.

5. Once cooked, chop the lettuce and place on a bowl. Toss with the salad dressing, parmesan cheese, and croutons.

Nutrition Info: Calories per serving: 235 ; Protein: 7.5g; Carbs: 19.4 g; Fat: 9.7g Sugar: 8.3g

Roasted Okra

Servings: 4
Cooking Time: 30 Minutes
Ingredients:
- Nonstick cooking spray or butter, for greasing
- 1 pound whole okra
- 2 tablespoons extra-virgin olive oil
- 2 teaspoons seasoned salt
- 2 teaspoons freshly ground black pepper

Directions:
1. Supply your smoker with wood pellets and follow the manufacturer's specific start-up procedure. Preheat, with the lid closed, to 400°F. Alternatively, preheat your oven to 400°F.
2. Line a shallow rimmed baking pan with aluminum foil and coat with cooking spray.
3. Arrange the okra on the pan in a single layer. Drizzle with the olive oil, turning to coat. Season on all sides with the salt and pepper.
4. Place the baking pan on the grill grate, close the lid, and smoke for 30 minutes, or until crisp and slightly charred. Alternatively, roast in the oven for 30 minutes.
5. Serve hot.

Grilled Cherry Tomato Skewers

Servings: 4
Cooking Time: 50 Minutes
Ingredients:
- 24 cherry tomatoes
- 1/4 cup olive oil
- 3tbsp balsamic vinegar
- 4garlic cloves, minced
- 1tbsp fresh thyme, finely chopped
- 1tsp kosher salt
- 1tsp ground black pepper
- 2tbsp chives, finely chopped

Directions:
1. Preheat pellet grill to 425°F.
2. In a medium-sized bowl, mix olive oil, balsamic vinegar, garlic, and thyme. Add tomatoes and toss to coat.
3. Let tomatoes sit in the marinade at room temperature for about 30 minutes.
4. Remove tomatoes from marinade and thread 4 tomatoes per skewer.

5.   Season both sides of each skewer with kosher salt and ground pepper.
6.   Place on grill grate and grill for about 3 minutes on each side, or until each side is slightly charred.
7.   Remove from grill and allow to rest for about 5 minutes. Garnish with chives, then serve and enjoy!
Nutrition Info: Calories: 228 Fat: 10 g Cholesterol: 70 mg Carbohydrate: 7 g Fiber: 2 g Sugar: 3 g Protein: 27 g

Grilled Artichokes

Servings: 6
Cooking Time: 15 Minutes
Ingredients:
- 3 large artichokes, blanched and halved
- 3 + 3 tablespoons olive oil
- Salt and pepper to taste
- 1 cup mayonnaise
- 1 cup yogurt
- 2 tablespoons parsley, chopped
- 2 tablespoons capers
- Lemon juice to taste

Directions:
1.   Fire the Traeger Grill to 500F. Use desired wood pellets when cooking. Close the lid and preheat for 15 minutes.
2.   Brush the artichokes with 3 tablespoons of olive oil. Season with salt and pepper to taste.
3.   Place on the grill grate and cook for 15 minutes.
4.   Allow to cool before slicing.
5.   Once cooled, slice the artichokes and place in a bowl.
6.   In another bowl, mix together the mayonnaise, yogurt, parsley, capers, and lemon juice. Season with salt and pepper to taste. Mix until well-combined.
7.   Pour sauce over the artichokes.
8.   Toss to coat.
Nutrition Info: Calories per serving: 257; Protein: 6.7g; Carbs: 13.2 g; Fat: 20.9g Sugar: 3.7g

Caldereta Stew

Servings: 12
Cooking Time: 4 Hours
Ingredients:
- 2lb. chuck roast, sliced into cubes
- 2tablespoons olive oil
- 1carrot, sliced into cubes
- 2potatoes, sliced into cubes
- 4garlic cloves, chopped
- 2tablespoons tomato paste
- 2cups tomato sauce
- 2red bell peppers, sliced into strips

- 2green bell peppers, sliced into strips
- 2cups of water
- 1/2 cup cheddar cheese, grated
- 1/4 cup liver spread
- Salt to taste

Directions:
1.   Put the beef in a cast iron pan.
2.   Place this in the smoking cabinet.
3.   Open the side dampers and sear slide.
4.   Set the temperature to 375 degrees F.
5.   Smoke the beef for 1 hour and 30 minutes.
6.   Flip the beef and smoke for another 1 hour and 30 minutes.
7.   Add a Dutch oven on top of the grill.
8.   Pour in the olive oil.
9.   Add the carrots and potatoes.
10. Cook for 5 minutes.
11. Stir in the garlic and cook for 1 minute.
12. Transfer the beef to the Dutch oven.
13. Stir in the tomato paste, tomato sauce, bell peppers, and water.
14. Bring to a boil.
15. Reduce temperature to 275 degrees F.
16. Simmer for 1 hour.
17. Add the cheese and liver.
18. Season with the salt.
Nutrition Info: Calories: 191.1 Fat: 9.3 g Cholesterol: 34 mg Carbohydrates: 15.4 g Fiber: 1.8 g Sugars: 1.3 g Protein: 11.3 g

Southern Slaw

Servings: 10
Cooking Time: 1 Hour And 10 Minutes
Ingredients:
- 1 head cabbage, shredded
- ¼ cup white vinegar
- ¼ cup sugar
- 1 teaspoon paprika
- ½ teaspoon salt
- ½ teaspoon freshly ground black pepper
- 1 cup heavy (whipping) cream

Directions:
1.   Place the shredded cabbage in a large bowl.
2.   In a small bowl, combine the vinegar, sugar, paprika, salt, and pepper.
3.   Pour the vinegar mixture over the cabbage and mix well.
4.   Fold in the heavy cream and refrigerate for at least 1 hour before serving.

Garlic And Rosemary Potato Wedges

Servings: 4
Cooking Time: 1 Hour 30 Minutes

Ingredients:
- 4-6 large russet potatoes, cut into wedges
- ¼ cup olive oil
- 2garlic cloves, minced
- 2tablespoons rosemary leaves, chopped
- 2teaspoon salt
- 1teaspoon fresh ground black pepper
- 1teaspoon sugar
- 1teaspoon onion powder

Directions:
1. Preheat your smoker to 250 degrees Fahrenheit using maple wood
2. Take a large bowl and add potatoes and olive oil
3. Toss well
4. Take another small bowl and stir garlic, salt, rosemary, pepper, sugar, onion powder
5. Sprinkle the mix on all sides of the potato wedge
6. Transfer the seasoned wedge to your smoker rack and smoke for 1 and a ½ hours
7. Serve and enjoy!

Nutrition Info: Calories: 291 Fats: 10g Carbs: 46g Fiber: 2g

Vegetable Skewers

Servings: 4
Cooking Time: 20 Minutes
Ingredients:
- 2 cups whole white mushrooms
- 2 large yellow squash, peeled, chopped
- 1 cup chopped pineapple
- 1 cup chopped red pepper
- 1 cup halved strawberries
- 2 large zucchini, chopped
- For the Dressing:
- 2 lemons, juiced
- ½ teaspoon ground black pepper
- 1/2 teaspoon sea salt
- 1 teaspoon red chili powder
- 1 tablespoon maple syrup
- 1 tablespoon orange zest
- 2 tablespoons apple cider vinegar
- 1/4 cup olive oil

Directions:
1. Switch on the Traeger grill, fill the grill hopper with flavored wood pellets, power the grill on by using the control panel, select 'smoke' on the temperature dial, or set the temperature to 450 degrees F and let it preheat for a minimum of 5 minutes.
2. Meanwhile, prepared thread vegetables and fruits on skewers alternately and then brush skewers with oil.
3. When the grill has preheated, open the lid, place vegetable skewers on the grill grate, shut the grill,

and smoke for 20 minutes until tender and lightly charred.
4. Meanwhile, prepare the dressing and for this, take a small bowl, place all of its ingredients in it and then whisk until combined.
5. When done, transfer skewers to a dish, top with prepared dressing and then serve.

Nutrition Info: Calories: 130 Cal ;Fat: 2 g ;Carbs: 20 g ;Protein: 2 g ;Fiber: 0.3 g

Roasted Sheet Pan Vegetables

Servings: 6
Cooking Time: 20 Minutes
Ingredients:
- 1 small purple cauliflower, cut into florets
- 1 small yellow cauliflower, cut into florets
- 4 cups butternut squash
- 2 cups mushroom, fresh
- 3 tablespoons extra virgin olive oil
- 2 teaspoons salt
- 2 teaspoons black pepper

Directions:
1. Fire the Traeger Grill to 350F. Use desired wood pellets when cooking. Close the lid and preheat for 15 minutes.
2. Place the vegetables in a baking tray and season with olive oil, salt, and pepper. Toss to coat all vegetables.
3. Place in the grill and cook for 20 minutes. Make sure to shake the tray halfway through the cooking time for even cooking.

Nutrition Info: Calories per serving: 101; Protein: 3.8g; Carbs: 16.9g; Fat: 3.5g Sugar: 4.4g

Smoked Tomato And Mozzarella Dip

Servings: 4
Cooking Time: 1 Hour
Ingredients:
- 8ounces smoked mozzarella cheese, shredded
- 8ounces Colby cheese, shredded
- ½ cup parmesan cheese, grated
- 1cup sour cream
- 1cup sun-dried tomatoes
- 1and ½ teaspoon salt
- 1teaspoon fresh ground pepper
- 1teaspoon dried basil
- 1teaspoon dried oregano
- 1teaspoon red pepper flakes
- 1garlic clove, minced
- ½ teaspoon onion powder
- French toast, serving

Directions:

1. Preheat your smoker to 275 degrees Fahrenheit using your preferred wood
2. Take a large bowl and stir in the cheeses, tomatoes, pepper, salt, basil, oregano, red pepper flakes, garlic, onion powder and mix well
3. Transfer the mix to a small metal pan and transfer to a smoker
4. Smoke for 1 hour
5. Serve with toasted French bread
6. Enjoy!

Nutrition Info: Calories: 174 Fats: 11g Carbs: 15g Fiber: 2g

3. Tear four squares of aluminum foil large enough to completely cover an ear of corn.
4. In a medium bowl, combine the sour cream, mayonnaise, and cilantro. Slather the mixture all over the ears of corn.
5. Wrap each ear of corn in a piece of foil, sealing tightly. Place on the grill, close the lid, and smoke for 12 to 14 minutes.
6. Remove the corn from the foil and place in a shallow baking dish. Top with chipotle butter, the Parmesan cheese, and more chopped cilantro.
7. Serve immediately.

Smoked Watermelon

Servings: 5
Cooking Time: 45-90 Minutes
Ingredients:
- 1 small seedless watermelon
- Balsamic vinegar
- Wooden skewers

Directions:
1. Slice ends of small seedless watermelons
2. Slice the watermelon in 1-inch cubes. Put the cubes in a container and drizzle vinegar on the cubes of watermelon.
3. Preheat the smoker to 225°F. Add wood chips and water to the smoker before starting preheating.
4. Place the cubes on the skewers.
5. Place the skewers on the smoker rack for 50 minutes.
6. Cook
7. Remove the skewers.
8. Serve!

Nutrition Info: Calories: 20 Cal Fat: 0 g Carbohydrates: 4 g   Protein: 1 g Fiber: 0.2 g

Mexican Street Corn With Chipotle Butter

Servings: 4
Cooking Time: 12 To 14 Minutes
Ingredients:
- 4 ears corn
- ½ cup sour cream
- ½ cup mayonnaise
- ¼ cup chopped fresh cilantro, plus more for garnish
- Chipotle Butter, for topping
- 1 cup grated Parmesan cheese

Directions:
1. Supply your smoker with wood pellets and follow the manufacturer's specific start-up procedure. Preheat, with the lid closed, to 450°F.
2. Shuck the corn, removing the silks and cutting off the cores.

Smoked Eggs

Servings: 12
Cooking Time: 30 Minutes
Ingredients:
- 12 hardboiled eggs, peeled and rinsed

Directions:
1. Supply your smoker with wood pellets and follow the manufacturer's specific start-up procedure. Preheat the grill, with the lid closed, to 120°F.
2. Place the eggs directly on the grill grate and smoke for 30 minutes. They will begin to take on a slight brown sheen.
3. Remove the eggs and refrigerate for at least 30 minutes before serving. Refrigerate any leftovers in an airtight container for 1 or 2 weeks.

Grilled Baby Carrots And Fennel With Romesco

Servings: 8 To 12
Cooking Time: 45 Minutes
Ingredients:
- 1 Pound Slender Rainbow Carrots
- 2 Whole Fennel, bulb
- 2 Tablespoon extra-virgin olive oil
- 1 Teaspoon salt
- 2 Tablespoon extra-virgin olive oil
- To Taste salt
- 1 Tablespoon fresh thyme

Directions:
1. When ready to cook, set temperature to High and preheat, lid closed for 15 minutes. For optimal results, set to 500°F if available.
2. Trim the carrot tops to 1". Peel the carrots and halve any larger ones so they are all about 1/2" thick. Cut the fennel bulbs lengthwise into 1/2" thick slices.
3. Place the fennel and potato slices in a large mixing bowl. Drizzle with 2 Tbsp of the olive oil and a teaspoon of salt.
4. Toss to coat the vegetables evenly with the oil.

5. Place the carrots on a sheet pan. Drizzle with the additional 2 Tbsp of olive oil and a generous pinch of salt. Brush the olive oil over the carrots to distribute evenly.
6. Add the potatoes and fennel slices to the sheet pan. Nestle a few sprigs of herbs into the vegetables as well.
7. Place the pan directly on the grill grate and cook, stirring occasionally until the vegetables are browned and softened, about 35-45 minutes.
8. Allow to cool and serve with the Smoked Romesco Sauce. Enjoy!

Coconut Bacon

Servings: 2
Cooking Time: 30 Minutes
Ingredients:
- 3 1/2 cups flaked coconut
- 1 tbsp pure maple syrup
- 1 tbsp water
- 2 tbsp liquid smoke
- 1 tbsp soy sauce
- 1 tsp smoked paprika (optional)

Directions:
1. Preheat the smoker at 325°F.
2. Take a large mixing bowl and combine liquid smoke, maple syrup, soy sauce, and water.
3. Pour flaked coconut over the mixture. Add it to a cooking sheet.
4. Place in the middle rack of the smoker.
5. Smoke it for 30 minutes and every 7-8 minutes, keep flipping the sides.
6. Serve and enjoy.

Nutrition Info: Calories: 1244 Cal Fat: 100 g Carbohydrates: 70 g Protein: 16 g Fiber: 2 g

Butter Braised Green Beans

Servings: 6
Cooking Time: 20 Minutes
Ingredients:
- 24 ounces Green Beans, trimmed
- 8 tablespoons butter, melted
- Salt and pepper to taste

Directions:
1. Fire the Traeger Grill to 500F. Use desired wood pellets when cooking. Close the lid and preheat for 15 minutes.
2. Place all ingredients in a bowl and toss to coat the beans with the seasoning.
3. Place the seasoned beans in a sheet tray.
4. Cook in the grill for 20 minutes.

Nutrition Info: Calories per serving: 164; Protein: 1.6g; Carbs: 5.6 g; Fat: 15.8g Sugar: 1.3g

Bacon-wrapped Jalapeño Poppers

Servings: 8 To 12
Cooking Time: 40 Minutes
Ingredients:
- 12 large jalapeño peppers
- 8 oz cream cheese, softened
- 1cup pepper jack cheese, shredded
- Juice of 1 lemon1/2 tsp garlic powder
- 1/4 tsp kosher salt
- 1/4 tsp ground black pepper
- 12 bacon slices, cut in half

Directions:
1. Preheat pellet grill to 400°F.
2. Slice jalapeños in half lengthwise. Remove seeds and scrape sides with a spoon to remove the membrane.
3. In a medium bowl, mix cream cheese, pepper jack cheese, garlic powder, salt, and pepper until thoroughly combined.
4. Use a spoon or knife to place the cream cheese mixture into each jalapeño half. Make sure not to fill over the sides of the jalapeño half.
5. Wrap each cheese-filled pepper with a half slice of bacon. If you can't get a secure wrap, then hold bacon and pepper together with a toothpick.
6. Place assembled poppers on the grill and cook for 15-20 minutes or until bacon is crispy.
7. Remove from grill, allow to cool, then serve and enjoy!

Nutrition Info: Calories: 78.8 Fat: 7.2 g Cholesterol: 19.2 mg Carbohydrate: 1 g Fiber: 0.2 g Sugar: 0.7 g Protein: 2.5 g

Corn Chowder

Servings: 3 To 4
Cooking Time: 35 Minutes
Ingredients:
- 1/4 tsp. Cajun Seasoning
- 2tbsp. Butter, unsalted
- 2tbsp. Parsley, fresh and minced
- 1Onion quartered
- 1/2 cup Celery Stalks, diced
- 1/4 tsp. Sea Salt
- 2Garlic cloves
- 1/4 cup Heavy Cream
- 1/2 cup Carrot, diced
- 3cups Corn Kernels, frozen
- 2-1/2 cups Vegetable Broth
- 1/4 tsp. Black Pepper, grounded
- 1Red Potato, chopped

Directions:

1. To start with, keep butter, onion, and garlic in the pitcher of the blender.
2. After that, press the 'saute' button.
3. Next, stir in all the remaining ingredients to the pitcher and select the 'hearty soup' button.
4. Once the program gets over, transfer the soup to serving bowls and serve immediately.
5. Garnish with parsley leaves.

Nutrition Info: Calories: 499 Fat: 40 g Total Carbs: 32 g Fiber: 2.5 g Sugar: 7.3 g Protein: 6.8 g Cholesterol: 120 mg

Grilled Zucchini Squash Spears

Servings: 4
Cooking Time: 10 Minutes
Ingredients:
- 4 zucchini, medium
- 2 tbsp olive oil
- 1 tbsp sherry vinegar
- 2 thyme, leaves pulled
- Salt to taste
- Pepper to taste

Directions:
1. Clean zucchini, cut ends off, half each lengthwise, and cut each half into thirds.
2. Combine all the other ingredients in a zip lock bag, medium, then add spears.
3. Toss well and mix to coat the zucchini.
4. Preheat Traeger to 350F with the lid closed for about 15 minutes.
5. Remove spears from the zip lock bag and place them directly on your grill grate with the cut side down.
6. Cook for about 3-4 minutes until zucchini is tender and grill marks show.
7. Remove them from the grill and enjoy.

Nutrition Info: Calories 93, Total fat 7.4g, Saturated fat 1.1g, Total carbs 7.1g, Net carbs 4.9g, Protein 2.4g, Sugars 3.4g, Fiber 2.2g, Sodium 59mg, Potassium 515mg

Whole Roasted Cauliflower With Garlic Parmesan Butter

Servings: 5
Cooking Time: 45 Minutes
Ingredients:
- 1/4 cup olive oil
- Salt and pepper to taste
- 1 cauliflower, fresh
- 1/2 cup butter, melted
- 1/4 cup parmesan cheese, grated
- 2 garlic cloves, minced

- 1/2 tbsp parsley, chopped

Directions:
1. Preheat the wood pellet grill with the lid closed for 15 minutes.
2. Meanwhile, brush the cauliflower with oil then season with salt and pepper.
3. Place the cauliflower in a cast iron and place it on a grill grate.
4. Cook for 45 minutes or until the cauliflower is golden brown and tender.
5. Meanwhile, mix butter, cheese, garlic, and parsley in a mixing bowl.
6. In the last 20 minutes of cooking, add the butter mixture.
7. Remove the cauliflower from the grill and top with more cheese and parsley if you desire. Enjoy.

Nutrition Info: Calories 156, Total fat 11.1g, Saturated fat 3.4g, Total Carbs 8.8g, Net Carbs 5.1g, Protein 8.2g, Sugar 0g, Fiber 3.7g, Sodium: 316mg, Potassium 468.2mg

Smoked Pickles

Servings: 6
Cooking Time: 15 Minutes
Ingredients:
- 1-quart water
- ¼ cup sugar
- ½ quart white vinegar
- ½ cup salt
- ½ teaspoon peppercorns
- 1 ½ teaspoons celery seeds
- 1 ½ teaspoons coriander seeds
- 1 teaspoon mustard seeds
- 8 cloves of garlic, minced
- 1 bunch dill weed
- 12 small cucumbers

Directions:
1. Place the water, sugar, vinegar, salt, and peppercorns in a saucepan. Bring to a boil over medium flame.
2. Transfer to a bowl and allow to cool. Add in the rest of the ingredients.
3. Allow the cucumber to soak in the brine for at least 3 days.
4. When ready to cook, fire the Traeger Grill to 500F. Use desired wood pellets when cooking. Close the lid and preheat for 15 minutes.
5. Pat dry the cucumber with paper towel and place on the grill grate. Smoke for 15 minutes.

Nutrition Info: Calories per serving: 67; Protein: 2.4g; Carbs: 12.9g; Fat: 1.1g Sugar:8.5 g

Vegetable Sandwich

Servings: 4
Cooking Time: 45 Minutes
Ingredients:
- For the Smoked Hummus:
- 1 1/2 cups cooked chickpeas
- 1 tablespoon minced garlic
- 1 teaspoon salt
- 4 tablespoons lemon juice
- 2 tablespoon olive oil
- 1/3 cup tahini
- For the Vegetables:
- 2 large portobello mushrooms
- 1 small eggplant, destemmed, sliced into strips
- 1 teaspoon salt
- 1 small zucchini, trimmed, sliced into strips
- ½ teaspoon ground black pepper
- 1 small yellow squash, peeled, sliced into strips
- ¼ cup olive oil
- For the Cheese:
- 1 lemon, juiced
- ½ teaspoon minced garlic
- ¼ teaspoon ground black pepper
- ¼ teaspoon salt
- 1/2 cup ricotta cheese
- To Assemble:
- 1 bunch basil, leaves chopped
- 2 heirloom tomatoes, sliced
- 4 ciabatta buns, halved

Directions:
1. Switch on the Traeger grill, fill the grill hopper with pecan flavored wood pellets, power the grill on by using the control panel, select 'smoke' on the temperature dial, or set the temperature to 180 degrees F and let it preheat for a minimum of 15 minutes.
2. Meanwhile, prepare the hummus, and for this, take a sheet tray and spread chickpeas on it.
3. When the grill has preheated, open the lid, place sheet tray on the grill grate, shut the grill and smoke for 20 minutes.
4. When done, transfer chickpeas to a food processor, add remaining ingredients for the hummus in it, and pulse for 2 minutes until smooth, set aside until required.
5. Change the smoking temperature to 500 degrees F, shut with lid, and let it preheat for 10 minutes.
6. Meanwhile, prepare vegetables and for this, take a large bowl, place all the vegetables in it, add salt and black pepper, drizzle with oil and lemon juice and toss until coated.
7. Place vegetables on the grill grate, shut with lid and then smoke for eggplant, zucchini, and squash for 15 minutes and mushrooms for 25 minutes.

8. Meanwhile, prepare the cheese and for this, take a small bowl, place all of its ingredients in it and stir until well combined.
9. Assemble the sandwich for this, cut buns in half lengthwise, spread prepared hummus on one side, spread cheese on the other side, then stuff with grilled vegetables and top with tomatoes and basil.
10. Serve straight away.
Nutrition Info: Calories: 560 Cal ;Fat: 40 g ;Carbs: 45 g ;Protein: 8.3 g ;Fiber: 6.8 g

Smoked Deviled Eggs

Servings: 4 To 6
Cooking Time: 50 Minutes
Ingredients:
- 6 large eggs
- 1slice bacon
- 1/4 cup mayonnaise
- 1tsp Dijon mustard
- 1tsp apple cider vinegar
- 1/4 tsp paprika
- Pinch of kosher salt
- 1tbsp chives, chopped

Directions:
1. Preheat pellet grill to 180°F and turn smoke setting on, if applicable.
2. Bring a pot of water to a boil. Add eggs and hard boil eggs for about 12 minutes.
3. Remove eggs from pot and place them into an ice-water bath. Once eggs have cooled completely, peel them and slice in half lengthwise.
4. Place sliced eggs on grill, yolk side up. Smoke for 30 to 45 minutes, depending on how much smoky flavor you want.
5. While eggs smoke, cook bacon until it's crispy.
6. Remove eggs from the grill and allow to cool on a plate.
7. Remove the yolks and place all of them in a small bowl. Place the egg whites on a plate.
8. Mash yolks with a fork and add mayonnaise, mustard, apple cider vinegar, paprika, and salt. Stir until combined.
9. Spoon a scoop of yolk mixture back into each egg white.
10. Sprinkle paprika, chives, and crispy bacon bits to garnish. Serve and enjoy!
Nutrition Info: Calories: 140 Fat: 12 g Cholesterol: 190 mg Carbohydrate: 1 g Fiber: 0 Sugar: 0 Protein: 6 g

Scampi Spaghetti Squash

Servings: 4
Cooking Time: 40 Minutes

Ingredients:
- 1 spaghetti squash
- 2 tablespoons extra-virgin olive oil
- 1 teaspoon salt
- 1 teaspoon freshly ground black pepper
- 2 teaspoons garlic powder
- 4 tablespoons (½ stick) unsalted butter
- ½ cup white wine
- 1 tablespoon minced garlic
- 2 teaspoons chopped fresh parsley
- 1 teaspoon red pepper flakes
- ½ teaspoon salt
- ½ teaspoon freshly ground black pepper

Directions:
1. For the squash:
2. Supply your smoker with wood pellets and follow the manufacturer's specific start-up procedure. Preheat, with the lid closed, to 375°F.
3. Cut off both ends of the squash, then cut it in half lengthwise. Scoop out and discard the seeds.
4. Rub the squash flesh well with the olive oil and sprinkle on the salt, pepper, and garlic powder.
5. Place the squash cut-side up on the grill grate, close the lid, and smoke for 40 minutes, or until tender
6. For the sauce:
7. On the stove top, in a medium saucepan over medium heat, combine the butter, white wine, minced garlic, parsley, red pepper flakes, salt, and pepper, and cook for about 5 minutes, or until heated through. Reduce the heat to low and keep the sauce warm.
8. Remove the squash from the grill and let cool slightly before shredding the flesh with a fork; discard the skin.
9. Stir the shredded squash into the garlic-wine butter sauce and serve immediately.

Bunny Dogs With Sweet And Spicy Jalapeño Relish

Servings: 8
Cooking Time: 35 To 40 Minutes
Ingredients:
- 8 hot dog-size carrots, peeled
- ¼ cup honey
- ¼ cup yellow mustard
- Nonstick cooking spray or butter, for greasing
- Salt
- Freshly ground black pepper
- 8 hot dog buns
- Sweet and Spicy Jalapeño Relish

Directions:
1. Prepare the carrots by removing the stems and slicing in half lengthwise.

2. In a small bowl, whisk together the honey and mustard.
3. Supply your smoker with wood pellets and follow the manufacturer's specific start-up procedure. Preheat, with the lid closed, to 375°F.
4. Line a baking sheet with aluminum foil and coat with cooking spray.
5. Brush the carrots on both sides with the honey mustard and season with salt and pepper; put on the baking sheet.
6. Place the baking sheet on the grill grate, close the lid, and smoke for 35 to 40 minutes, or until tender and starting to brown.
7. To serve, lightly toast the hot dog buns on the grill and top each with two slices of carrot and some relish.

Ramen Soup

Servings: 2
Cooking Time: 35 Minutes
Ingredients:
- 4cups Chicken Stock
- 1tbsp. Extra Virgin Olive Oil
- 2Baby Bok Choy Head, leaves torn
- 1Shallot, chopped into 1-inch piece
- 3oz. Ramen, dried
- 4Garlic cloves
- 1tsp. Sesame Oil, toasted
- 2tsp. Ginger, fresh
- One bunch of Green Onion, sliced thinly
- 1cup Chicken, cooked and cut into 1-inch cubes

Directions:
1. First, keep the olive oil, shallot, garlic, and ginger in the blender pitcher.
2. After that, press the 'saute' button.
3. Next, stir in the chicken, green onions, chicken stock, and sesame oil into it.
4. Now, select the 'hearty soup' button.
5. Then, three minutes before the program ends, spoon in the ramen noodles and baby bok choy.
6. Check the chicken's internal temperature and ensure it is 165 ° F and if it is, then transfer the soup to the serving bowls.
7. Serve immediately and enjoy it.
Nutrition Info: Calories: 190 Fat: 8g Total Carbs: 25g Fiber: 1 g Sugar: 0.5 g Protein: 3 g Cholesterol: 2.5 mg

Grilled Sugar Snap Peas

Servings: 4
Cooking Time: 10 Minutes
Ingredients:
- 2-pound sugar snap peas, ends trimmed
- ½ teaspoon garlic powder

- 1 teaspoon salt
- 2/3 teaspoon ground black pepper
- 2 tablespoons olive oil

Directions:
1. Switch on the Traeger grill, fill the grill hopper with apple-flavored wood pellets, power the grill on by using the control panel, select 'smoke' on the temperature dial, or set the temperature to 450 degrees F and let it preheat for a minimum of 15 minutes.
2. Meanwhile, take a medium bowl, place peas in it, add garlic powder and oil, season with salt and black pepper, toss until mixed and then spread on the sheet pan.
3. When the grill has preheated, open the lid, place the prepared sheet pan on the grill grate, shut the grill and smoke for 10 minutes until slightly charred.
4. Serve straight away.

Nutrition Info: Calories: 91 Cal ;Fat: 5 g ;Carbs: 9 g ;Protein: 4 g ;Fiber: 3 g

Crispy Maple Bacon Brussels Sprouts

Servings: 6
Cooking Time: 1 Hour
Ingredients:
- 1lb brussels sprouts, trimmed and quartered
- 6 slices thick-cut bacon
- 3tbsp maple syrup
- 1tsp olive oil
- 1/2 tsp kosher salt
- 1/2 tsp ground black pepper

Directions:
1. Preheat pellet grill to 425°F.
2. Cut bacon into 1/2 inch thick slices.
3. Place brussels sprouts in a single layer in the cast iron skillet. Drizzle with olive oil and maple syrup, then toss to coat. Sprinkle bacon slices on top then season with kosher salt and black pepper.
4. Place skillet in the pellet grill and roast for about 40 to 45 minutes, or until the brussels sprouts are caramelized and brown.
5. Remove skillet from grill and allow brussels sprouts to cool for about 5 to 10 minutes. Serve and enjoy!

Nutrition Info: Calories: 175.3 Fat: 12.1 g Cholesterol: 6.6 mg Carbohydrate: 13.6 g Fiber: 2.9 g Sugar: 7.6 g Protein: 4.8 g

Bacon-wrapped Jalapeno Poppers

Servings: 6
Cooking Time: 20 Minutes
Ingredients:
- 6 jalapenos, Fresh

- 1/2 cup shredded cheddar cheese
- 4 oz soft cream cheese
- 1-1/2 tbsp Traeger veggie rub
- 12 bacon slices, thin cut

Directions:
1. Preheat your Traeger grill to 375F.
2. Halve the jalapenos lengthwise then scrape membrane and seeds using a spoon. rinse them and set aside.
3. Meanwhile, combine cheddar cheese, cream cheese, and veggie rub in a bowl, medium stirring until incorporated fully.
4. Fill the jalapenos with your cheese mixture then wrap each half with a bacon slice.
5. Place on your grill and grill for about 15-20 minutes until bacon becomes crispy and peppers are soft.
6. Serve and enjoy.

Nutrition Info: Calories 329, Total fat 25.7g, Saturated fat 11.4g, Total carbs 5g, Net carbs 4.6g, Protein 18.1g, Sugars 0.6g, Fiber 0.4g, Sodium 1667mg, Potassium 277mg

Smokey Roasted Cauliflower

Servings: 4 To 6
Cooking Time: 1 Hour 20 Minutes
Ingredients:
- 1head cauliflower
- cup parmesan cheese
- Spice Ingredients:
- 1tbsp olive oil
- 2cloves garlic, chopped
- 1tsp kosher salt
- 1tsp smoked paprika

Directions:
1. Preheat pellet grill to 180°F. If applicable, set smoke setting to high.
2. Cut cauliflower into bite-size flowerets and place in a grill basket. Place basket on the grill grate and smoke for an hour.
3. Mix spice Ingredients In a small bowl while the cauliflower is smoking. Remove cauliflower from the grill after an hour and let cool.
4. Change grill temperature to 425°F. After the cauliflower has cooled, put cauliflower in a resealable bag, and pour marinade in the bag. Toss to combine in the bag.
5. Place cauliflower back in a grill basket and return to grill. Roast in the grill basket for 10-12 minutes or until the outsides begin to get crispy and golden brown.
6. Remove from grill and transfer to a serving dish. Sprinkle parmesan cheese over the cauliflower and rest for a few minutes so the cheese can melt. Serve and enjoy!

Nutrition Info: Calories: 70 Fat: 35 g Cholesterol: 0 Carbohydrate: 7 g Fiber: 3 g Sugar: 3 g Protein: 3 g

Wood Pellet Smoked Vegetables

Servings: 6
Cooking Time: 15 Minutes
Ingredients:
- 1 ear corn, fresh, husks and silk strands removed
- 1yellow squash, sliced
- 1 red onion, cut into wedges
- 1 green pepper, cut into strips
- 1 red pepper, cut into strips
- 1 yellow pepper, cut into strips
- 1 cup mushrooms, halved
- 2 tbsp oil
- 2 tbsp chicken seasoning

Directions:
1. Soak the pecan wood pellets in water for an hour. Remove the pellets from water and fill the smoker box with the wet pellets.
2. Place the smoker box under the grill and close the lid. Heat the grill on high heat for 10 minutes or until smoke starts coming out from the wood chips.
3. Meanwhile, toss the veggies in oil and seasonings then transfer them into a grill basket.
4. Grill for 10 minutes while turning occasionally. Serve and enjoy.

Nutrition Info: Calories 97, Total fat 5g, Saturated fat 2g, Total Carbs 11g, Net Carbs 8g, Protein 2g, Sugar 1g, Fiber 3g, Sodium: 251mg, Potassium 171mg

Smoked Hummus

Servings: 6
Cooking Time: 20 Minutes
Ingredients:
- 1 ½ cups chickpeas, rinsed and drained
- ¼ cup tahini
- 1 tablespoon garlic, minced
- 2 tablespoons extra virgin olive oil
- 1 teaspoon salt
- 4 tablespoons lemon juice

Directions:
1. Fire the Traeger Grill to 350F. Use desired wood pellets when cooking. Close the lid and preheat for 15 minutes.
2. Spread the chickpeas on a sheet tray and place on the grill grate. Smoke for 20 minutes.
3. Let the chickpeas cool at room temperature.

4. Place smoked chickpeas in a blender or food processor. Add in the rest of the ingredients. Pulse until smooth.
5. Serve with roasted vegetables if desired.
Nutrition Info: Calories per serving: 271; Protein: 12.1g; Carbs: 34.8g; Fat: 10.4g Sugar: 5.7g

Salt-crusted Baked Potatoes

Servings: 6
Cooking Time: 40 Minutes
Ingredients:
- 6 russet potatoes, scrubbed and dried
- 3 tablespoons oil
- 1 tablespoons salt
- Butter as needed
- Sour cream as needed

Directions:
1. Fire the Traeger Grill to 400F. Use desired wood pellets when cooking. Close the lid and preheat for 15 minutes.
2. In a large bowl, coat the potatoes with oil and salt. Place seasoned potatoes on a baking tray.
3. Place the tray with potatoes on the grill grate.
4. Close the lid and grill for 40 minutes.
5. Serve with butter and sour cream.
Nutrition Info: Calories per serving: 363; Protein: 8g; Carbs: 66.8g; Fat: 8.6g Sugar: 2.3g

Kale Chips

Servings: 6
Cooking Time: 20 Minutes
Ingredients:
- 2 bunches of kale, stems removed
- ½ teaspoon of sea salt
- 4 tablespoons olive oil

Directions:
1. Switch on the Traeger grill, fill the grill hopper with apple-flavored wood pellets, power the grill on by using the control panel, select 'smoke' on the temperature dial, or set the temperature to 250 degrees F and let it preheat for a minimum of 15 minutes.
2. Meanwhile, rinse the kale leaves, pat dry, spread the kale on a sheet tray, drizzle with oil, season with salt and toss until well coated.
3. When the grill has preheated, open the lid, place sheet tray on the grill grate, shut the grill and smoke for 20 minutes until crisp.
4. Serve straight away.
Nutrition Info: Calories: 110 Cal ;Fat: 5 g ;Carbs: 15.8 g ;Protein: 5.3 g ;Fiber: 5.6 g

Grilled Corn With Honey Butter

Servings: 6
Cooking Time: 10 Minutes
Ingredients:
- 6 pieces corn, husked
- 2 tablespoons olive oil
- Salt and pepper to taste
- ½ cup butter, room temperature
- ½ cup honey

Directions:
1. Fire the Traeger Grill to 350F. Use desired wood pellets when cooking. Close the lid and preheat for 15 minutes.
2. Brush the corn with oil and season with salt and pepper to taste.
3. Place the corn on the grill grate and cook for 10 minutes. Make sure to flip the corn halfway through the cooking time for even cooking.
4. Meanwhile, mix the butter and honey on a small bowl. Set aside.
5. Once the corn is cooked, remove from the grill and brush with the honey butter sauce.

Nutrition Info: Calories per serving: 387; Protein: 5g; Carbs: 51.2g; Fat: 21.6g Sugar: 28.2g

Grilled Zucchini Squash

Servings: 6
Cooking Time: 10 Minutes
Ingredients:
- 3 medium zucchinis, sliced into ¼ inch thick lengthwise
- 2 tablespoons olive oil
- 1 tablespoon sherry vinegar
- 2 thyme leaves, pulled
- Salt and pepper to taste

Directions:
1. Fire the Traeger Grill to 350F. Use desired wood pellets when cooking. Close the lid and preheat for 15 minutes.
2. Place zucchini in a bowl and all ingredients. Gently massage the zucchini slices to coat with the seasoning.
3. Place the zucchini on the grill grate and cook for 5 minutes on each side.

Nutrition Info: Calories per serving: 44; Protein: 0.3 g; Carbs: 0.9 g; Fat: 4g Sugar: 0.1g

Potato Fries With Chipotle Peppers

Servings: 4
Cooking Time: 30 Minutes
Ingredients:
- 4 potatoes, sliced into strips
- 3 tablespoons olive oil
- Salt and pepper to taste
- 1 cup mayonnaise
- 2 chipotle peppers in adobo sauce
- 2 tablespoons lime juice

Directions:
1. Set the Traeger wood pellet grill to high.
2. Preheat it for 15 minutes while the lid is closed.
3. Coat the potato strips with oil.
4. Sprinkle with salt and pepper.
5. Put a baking pan on the grate.
6. Transfer potato strips to the pan.
7. Cook potatoes until crispy.
8. Mix the remaining ingredients.
9. Pulse in a food processor until pureed.
10. Serve potato fries with chipotle dip.
11. Tips: You can also use sweet potatoes instead of potatoes.

Wood Pellet Bacon Wrapped Jalapeno Poppers

Servings: 6
Cooking Time: 20 Minutes
Ingredients:
- 6 jalapenos, fresh
- 4 oz cream cheese
- 1/2 cup cheddar cheese, shredded
- 1 tbsp vegetable rub
- 12 slices cut bacon

Directions:
1. Preheat the wood pellet smoker and grill to375°F.
2. Slice the jalapenos lengthwise and scrape the seed and membrane. Rinse them with water and set aside.
3. In a mixing bowl, mix cream cheese, cheddar cheese, vegetable rub until well mixed.
4. Fill the jalapeno halves with the mixture then wrap with the bacon pieces.
5. Smoke for 20 minutes or until the bacon crispy.
6. Serve and enjoy.

Nutrition Info: Calories 1830, Total fat 11g, Saturated fat 6g, Total Carbs 5g, Net Carbs 4g, Protein 6g, Sugar 4g, Fiber 1g

Sweet Potato Chips

Servings: 3
Cooking Time: 35 To 45 Minutes
Ingredients:
- 2 sweet potatoes
- 1 quart warm water
- 1 tablespoon cornstarch, plus 2 teaspoons

- ¼ cup extra-virgin olive oil
- 1 tablespoon salt
- 1 tablespoon packed brown sugar
- 1 teaspoon ground cinnamon
- 1 teaspoon freshly ground black pepper
- ½ teaspoon cayenne pepper

Directions:
1. Using a mandolin, thinly slice the sweet potatoes.
2. Pour the warm water into a large bowl and add 1 tablespoon of cornstarch and the potato slices. Let soak for 15 to 20 minutes.
3. Supply your smoker with wood pellets and follow the manufacturer's specific start-up procedure. Preheat, with the lid closed, to 375°F.
4. Drain the potato slices, then arrange in a single layer on a perforated pizza pan or a baking sheet lined with aluminum foil. Brush the potato slices on both sides with the olive oil.
5. In a small bowl, whisk together the salt, brown sugar, cinnamon, black pepper, cayenne pepper, and the remaining 2 teaspoons of cornstarch. Sprinkle this seasoning blend on both sides of the potatoes.
6. Place the pan or baking sheet on the grill grate, close the lid, and smoke for 35 to 45 minutes, flipping after 20 minutes, until the chips curl up and become crispy.
7. Store in an airtight container.

Georgia Sweet Onion Bake

Servings: 6
Cooking Time: 1 Hour
Ingredients:
- Nonstick cooking spray or butter, for greasing
- 4 large Vidalia or other sweet onions
- 8 tablespoons (1 stick) unsalted butter, melted
- 4 chicken bouillon cubes
- 1 cup grated Parmesan cheese

Directions:
1. Supply your smoker with wood pellets and follow the manufacturer's specific start-up procedure. Preheat, with the lid closed, to 350°F.
2. Coat a high-sided baking pan with cooking spray or butter.
3. Peel the onions and cut into quarters, separating into individual petals.
4. Spread the onions out in the prepared pan and pour the melted butter over them.
5. Crush the bouillon cubes and sprinkle over the buttery onion pieces, then top with the cheese.
6. Transfer the pan to the grill, close the lid, and smoke for 30 minutes.
7. Remove the pan from the grill, cover tightly with aluminum foil, and poke several holes all over to vent.
8. Place the pan back on the grill, close the lid, and smoke for an additional 30 to 45 minutes.

9. Uncover the onions, stir, and serve hot.

Traeger Fries With Chipotle Ketchup

Servings: 6
Cooking Time: 10 Minutes
Ingredients:
- 6 Yukon Gold potatoes, scrubbed and cut into thick strips
- 1 tablespoon Traeger Beef Rub
- 1 tablespoon extra-virgin olive oil
- 1 teaspoon onion powder
- 1 teaspoon garlic powder
- ½ cup chipotle peppers, chopped
- 1 cup ketchup
- 1 tablespoon sugar
- 1 tablespoon cumin
- 1 tablespoon chili powder
- 1 whole lime
- 2 tablespoons butter

Directions:
1. Place the potatoes in a bowl and stir in the Traeger Beef Rub, olive oil, onion powder, and garlic powder. Toss to coat the potatoes with the spices.
2. Fire the Traeger Grill to 500F. Use desired wood pellets when cooking. Close the lid and preheat for 15 minutes.
3. Place the potatoes on a baking sheet lined with foil.
4. Place on the grill grate and cook for 10 minutes.
5. Meanwhile, place the rest of the ingredients in a small bowl and mix until well-combined.
6. Serve the fries with the chipotle ketchup sauce.

Nutrition Info: Calories per serving: 387 ;
Protein: 8.6g; Carbs: 79.3g; Fat: 5.6g Sugar: 13.7g

Grilled Corn On The Cob With Parmesan And Garlic

Servings: 6
Cooking Time: 30 Minutes
Ingredients:
- 4 tablespoons butter, melted
- 2 cloves of garlic, minced
- Salt and pepper to taste
- 8 corns, unhusked
- ½ cup parmesan cheese, grated
- 1 tablespoon parsley chopped

Directions:
1. Fire the Traeger Grill to 450F. Use desired wood pellets when cooking. Close the lid and preheat for 15 minutes.
2. Place butter, garlic, salt, and pepper in a bowl and mix until well combined.

3. Peel the corn husk but do not detach the husk from the corn. Remove the silk. Brush the corn with the garlic butter mixture and close the husks.
4. Place the corn on the grill grate and cook for 30 minutes turning the corn every 5 minutes for even cooking.
Nutrition Info: Calories per serving: 272; Protein: 8.8g; Carbs: 38.5g; Fat: 12.3g Sugar: 6.6g

Roasted Hasselback Potatoes

Servings: 6
Cooking Time: 30 Minutes
Ingredients:
- 6 large russet potatoes
- 1-pound bacon
- ½ cup butter
- Salt to taste
- 1 cup cheddar cheese
- 3 whole scallions, chopped

Directions:
1. Fire the Traeger Grill to 350F. Use desired wood pellets when cooking. Close the lid and preheat for 15 minutes.
2. Place two wooden spoons on either side of the potato and slice the potato into thin strips without completely cutting through the potato.
3. Chop the bacon into small pieces and place in between the cracks or slices of the potatoes.
4. Place potatoes in a cast iron skillet. Top the potatoes with butter, salt, and cheddar cheese.
5. Place the skillet on the grill grate and cook for 30 minutes. Make sure to baste the potatoes with melted cheese 10 minutes before the cooking time ends.
Nutrition Info: Calories per serving: 662; Protein: 16.1g; Carbs: 71.5g; Fat: 38g Sugar: 2.3g

Grilled Zucchini

Servings: 6
Cooking Time: 10 Minutes
Ingredients:
- 4 medium zucchini
- 2 tablespoons olive oil
- 1 tablespoon sherry vinegar
- 2 sprigs of thyme, leaves chopped
- ½ teaspoon salt
- 1/3 teaspoon ground black pepper

Directions:
1. Switch on the Traeger grill, fill the grill hopper with oak flavored wood pellets, power the grill on by using the control panel, select 'smoke' on the temperature dial, or set the temperature to 350

degrees F and let it preheat for a minimum of 5 minutes.
2. Meanwhile, cut the ends of each zucchini, cut each in half and then into thirds and place in a plastic bag.
3. Add remaining ingredients, seal the bag, and shake well to coat zucchini pieces.
4. When the grill has preheated, open the lid, place zucchini on the grill grate, shut the grill and smoke for 4 minutes per side.
5. When done, transfer zucchini to a dish, garnish with more thyme and then serve.
Nutrition Info: Calories: 74 Cal ;Fat: 5.4 g ;Carbs: 6.1 g ;Protein: 2.6 g ;Fiber: 2.3 g

Green Beans With Bacon

Servings: 6
Cooking Time: 20 Minutes
Ingredients:
- 4 strips of bacon, chopped
- 1 1/2 pound green beans, ends trimmed
- 1 teaspoon minced garlic
- 1 teaspoon salt
- 4 tablespoons olive oil

Directions:
1. Switch on the Traeger grill, fill the grill hopper with flavored wood pellets, power the grill on by using the control panel, select 'smoke' on the temperature dial, or set the temperature to 450 degrees F and let it preheat for a minimum of 15 minutes.
2. Meanwhile, take a sheet tray, place all the ingredients in it and toss until mixed.
3. When the grill has preheated, open the lid, place prepared sheet tray on the grill grate, shut the grill and smoke for 20 minutes until lightly browned and cooked.
4. When done, transfer green beans to a dish and then serve.
Nutrition Info: Calories: 93 Cal ;Fat: 4.6 g ;Carbs: 8.2 g ;Protein: 5.9 g ;Fiber: 2.9 g

Cauliflower With Parmesan And Butter

Servings: 4
Cooking Time: 45 Minutes
Ingredients:
- 1 medium head of cauliflower
- 1 teaspoon minced garlic
- 1 teaspoon salt
- ½ teaspoon ground black pepper
- 1/4 cup olive oil
- 1/2 cup melted butter, unsalted
- 1/2 tablespoon chopped parsley

- 1/4 cup shredded parmesan cheese

Directions:

1.   Switch on the Traeger grill, fill the grill hopper with flavored wood pellets, power the grill on by using the control panel, select 'smoke' on the temperature dial, or set the temperature to 450 degrees F and let it preheat for a minimum of 15 minutes.

2.   Meanwhile, brush the cauliflower head with oil, season with salt and black pepper and then place in a skillet pan.

3.   When the grill has preheated, open the lid, place prepared skillet pan on the grill grate, shut the grill and smoke for 45 minutes until golden brown and the center has turned tender.

4.   Meanwhile, take a small bowl, place melted butter in it, and then stir in garlic, parsley, and cheese until combined.

5.   Baste cheese mixture frequently in the last 20 minutes of cooking and, when done, remove the pan from heat and garnish cauliflower with parsley.

6.   Cut it into slices and then serve.

Nutrition Info: Calories: 128 Cal ;Fat: 7.6 g ;Carbs: 10.8 g ;Protein: 7.4 g ;Fiber: 5 g

Smoked Brussels Sprouts

Servings: 6
Cooking Time: 45 Minutes
Ingredients:

- 1-1/2 pounds Brussels sprouts
- 2 cloves of garlic minced
- 2 tbsp extra virgin olive oil
- Sea salt and cracked black pepper

Directions:

1.   Rinse sprouts

2.   Remove the outer leaves and brown bottoms off the sprouts.

3.   Place sprouts in a large bowl then coat with olive oil.

4.   Add a coat of garlic, salt, and pepper and transfer them to the pan.

5.   Add to the top rack of the smoker with water and woodchips.

6.   Smoke for 45 minutes or until reaches 250°F temperature.

7.   Serve

Nutrition Info: Calories: 84 Cal Fat: 4.9 g Carbohydrates: 7.2 g   Protein: 2.6 g Fiber: 2.9 g

Garlic And Herb Smoke Potato

Servings: 6
Cooking Time: 2 Hours
Ingredients:

- 1.5 pounds bag of Gemstone Potatoes
- 1/4 cup Parmesan, fresh grated
- For the Marinade
- 2 tbsp olive oil
- 6 garlic cloves, freshly chopped
- 1/2 tsp dried oregano
- 1/2 tsp dried basil
- 1/2 tsp dried dill
- 1/2 tsp salt
- 1/2 tsp dried Italian seasoning
- 1/4 tsp ground pepper

Directions:

1.   Preheat the smoker to 225°F.

2.   Wash the potatoes thoroughly and add them to a sealable plastic bag.

3.   Add garlic cloves, basil, salt, Italian seasoning, dill, oregano, and olive oil to the zip lock bag. Shake.

4.   Place in the fridge for 2 hours to marinate.

5.   Next, take an Aluminum foil and put 2 tbsp of water along with the coated potatoes. Fold the foil so that the potatoes are sealed in

6.   Place in the preheated smoker.

7.   Smoke for 2 hours

8.   Remove the foil and pour the potatoes into a bowl.

9.   Serve with grated Parmesan cheese.

Nutrition Info: Calories: 146 Cal Fat: 6 g Carbohydrates: 19 g   Protein: 4 g Fiber: 2.1 g

Feisty Roasted Cauliflower

Servings: 4
Cooking Time: 10 Minutes
Ingredients:

- 1cauliflower head, cut into florets
- 1tablespoon oil
- 1cup parmesan, grated
- 2garlic cloves, crushed
- ½ teaspoon pepper
- ½ teaspoon salt
- ¼ teaspoon paprika

Directions:

1.   Preheat your Smoker to 180 degrees F

2.   Transfer florets to smoker and smoke for 1 hour

3.   Take a bowl and add all ingredients except cheese

4.   Once smoking is done, remove florets

5.   Increase temperature to 450 degrees F, brush florets with the brush and transfer to grill

6.   Smoke for 10 minutes more

7.   Sprinkle cheese on top and let them sit (Lid closed) until cheese melts

8.   Serve and enjoy!

Nutrition Info: Calories: 45 Fats: 2g Carbs: 7g Fiber: 1g

Smoked Balsamic Potatoes And Carrots

Servings: 6
Cooking Time: 10 Minutes
Ingredients:
- 2 large carrots, peeled and chopped roughly
- 2 large Yukon Gold potatoes, peeled and wedged
- 5 tablespoons olive oil
- 5 tablespoons balsamic vinegar
- Salt and pepper to taste

Directions:
1. Fire the Traeger Grill to 400F. Use desired wood pellets when cooking. Close the lid and preheat for 15 minutes.
2. Place all ingredients in a bowl and toss to coat the vegetables with the seasoning.
3. Place on a baking tray lined with foil.
4. Place on the grill grate and close the lid. Cook for 30 minutes.

Nutrition Info: Calories per serving: 219; Protein: 2.9g; Carbs: 27g; Fat: 11.4g Sugar:4.5 g

Baked Sweet And Savory Yams

Servings: 6
Cooking Time: 55 Minutes
Ingredients:
- 3 pounds yams, scrubbed
- 3 tablespoons extra virgin olive oil
- Honey to taste
- Goat cheese as needed
- ½ cup brown sugar
- ½ cup pecans, chopped

Directions:
1. Fire the Traeger Grill to 350F. Use desired wood pellets when cooking. Close the lid and preheat for 15 minutes.
2. Poke holes on the yams using a fork. Wrap yams in foil and place on the grill grate. Cook for 45 minutes until tender.
3. Remove the yams from the grill and allow to cool. Once cooled, peel the yam and slice to ¼" rounds.
4. Place on a parchment-lined baking tray and brush with olive oil. Drizzle with honey, cheese, brown sugar, and pecans.
5. Place in the grill and cook for another 10 minutes.

Nutrition Info: Calories per serving: 421; Protein: 4.3g; Carbs: 82.4g; Fat: 9.3g Sugar:19.3 g

Apple Veggie Burger

Servings: 6
Cooking Time: 35 Minutes
Ingredients:
- 3 tbsp ground flax or ground chia
- 1/3 cup of warm water
- 1/2 cups rolled oats
- 1 cup chickpeas, drained and rinsed
- 1 tsp cumin
- 1/2 cup onion
- 1 tsp dried basil
- 2 granny smith apples
- 1/3 cup parsley or cilantro, chopped
- 2 tbsp soy sauce
- 2 tsp liquid smoke
- 2 cloves garlic, minced
- 1 tsp chili powder
- 1/4 tsp black pepper

Directions:
1. Preheat the smoker to 225°F while adding wood chips and water to it.
2. In a separate bowl, add chickpeas and mash. Mix together the remaining ingredients along with the dipped flax seeds.
3. Form patties from this mixture.
4. Put the patties on the rack of the smoker and smoke them for 20 minutes on each side.
5. When brown, take them out, and serve.

Nutrition Info: Calories: 241 Cal Fat: 5 g Carbohydrates: 40 g Protein: 9 g Fiber: 10.3 g

Wood Pellet Grilled Asparagus And Honey Glazed Carrots

Servings: 5
Cooking Time: 35 Minutes
Ingredients:
- 1 bunch asparagus, trimmed ends
- 1 lb carrots, peeled
- 2 tbsp olive oil
- Sea salt to taste
- 2 tbsp honey
- Lemon zest

Directions:
1. Sprinkle the asparagus with oil and sea salt. Drizzle the carrots with honey and salt.
2. Preheat the wood pellet to 165°F wit the lid closed for 15 minutes.
3. Place the carrots in the wood pellet and cook for 15 minutes. Add asparagus and cook for 20 more minutes or until cooked through.
4. Top the carrots and asparagus with lemon zest. Enjoy.

Nutrition Info: Calories 1680, Total fat 30g, Saturated fat 2g, Total Carbs 10g, Net Carbs 10g, Protein 4g, Sugar 0g, Fiber 0g, Sodium: 514mg, Potassium 0mg

Traeger Smoked Mushrooms

Servings: 2
Cooking Time: 45 Minutes
Ingredients:
- 4 cups whole baby portobello, cleaned
- 1 tbsp canola oil
- 1 tbsp onion powder
- 1 tbsp garlic, granulated
- 1 tbsp salt
- 1 tbsp pepper

Directions:
1. Place all the ingredients in a bowl, mix, and combine.
2. Set your Traeger to 180F.
3. Place the mushrooms on the grill directly and smoke for about 30 minutes.
4. Increase heat to high and cook the mushroom for another 15 minutes.
5. Serve warm and enjoy!

Nutrition Info: Calories 118, Total fat 7.6g, Saturated fat 0.6g, Total carbs 10.8g, Net carbs 8.3g, Protein 5.4g, Sugars 3.7g, Fiber 2.5g, Sodium 3500mg, Potassium 536mg

Roasted Vegetable Medley

Servings: 4 To 6
Cooking Time: 50 Minutes
Ingredients:
- 2medium potatoes, cut to 1 inch wedges
- 2red bell peppers, cut into 1 inch cubes
- 1small butternut squash, peeled and cubed to 1 inch cube
- 1red onion, cut to 1 inch cubes
- 1cup broccoli, trimmed
- 2tbsp olive oil
- 1tbsp balsamic vinegar
- 1tbsp fresh rosemary, minced
- 1tbsp fresh thyme, minced
- 1tsp kosher salt
- 1tsp ground black pepper

Directions:
1. Preheat pellet grill to 425°F.
2. In a large bowl, combine potatoes, peppers, squash, and onion.
3. In a small bowl, whisk together olive oil, balsamic vinegar, rosemary, thyme, salt, and pepper.

4. Pour marinade over vegetables and toss to coat. Allow resting for about 15 minutes.
5. Place marinated vegetables into a grill basket, and place a grill basket on the grill grate. Cook for about 30-40 minutes, occasionally tossing in the grill basket.
6. Remove veggies from grill and transfer to a serving dish. Allow to cool for 5 minutes, then serve and enjoy!

Nutrition Info: Calories: 158.6 Fat: 7.4 g Cholesterol: 0 Carbohydrate: 22 g Fiber: 7.2 g Sugar: 3.1 g Protein: 5.2 g

Grilled Baby Carrots And Fennel

Servings: 8
Cooking Time: 30 Minutes
Ingredients:
- 1-pound slender rainbow carrots, washed and peeled
- 2 whole fennel bulbs, chopped
- 2 tablespoons extra virgin olive oil
- 1 teaspoon salt
- Salt to taste

Directions:
1. Fire the Traeger Grill to 500F. Use desired wood pellets when cooking. Close the lid and preheat for 15 minutes.
2. Place all ingredients in a sheet tray and toss to coat with oil and seasoning.
3. Place on the grill grate and cook for 30 minutes.

Nutrition Info: Calories per serving:52 ; Protein: 1.2g; Carbs: 8.9g; Fat: 1.7g Sugar: 4.3g

Zucchini Soup

Servings: 4
Cooking Time: 35 Minutes
Ingredients:
- 2tbsp. Olive Oil
- 1lb. Zucchini, chopped coarsely
- 1Onion quartered
- 8 oz. Watercress, chopped
- Salt and Black Pepper, as needed
- Pinch of Saffron
- 3cups Chicken Broth
- 1tbsp. Heavy Cream

Directions:
1. First, place olive oil and onion in the blender pitcher and press the 'saute' button.
2. Once sautéed, add all the remaining ingredients to it.
3. Now, press the 'smooth soup' button.
4. Finally, transfer the soup to the serving bowls and serve immediately.

Nutrition Info: Calories: 249 Fat: 20 g Total Carbs: 15 g Fiber: 4.1 g Sugar: 10 g Protein: 4.9 g Cholesterol: 15 mg

Twice-smoked Potatoes

Servings: 16
Cooking Time: 1 Hour 35 Minutes
Ingredients:
- 8 Idaho, Russet, or Yukon Gold potatoes
- 1 (12-ounce) can evaporated milk, heated
- 1 cup (2 sticks) butter, melted
- ½ cup sour cream, at room temperature
- 1 cup grated Parmesan cheese
- ½ pound bacon, cooked and crumbled
- ¼ cup chopped scallions
- Salt
- Freshly ground black pepper
- 1 cup shredded Cheddar cheese

Directions:
1. Supply your smoker with wood pellets and follow the manufacturer's specific start-up procedure. Preheat, with the lid closed, to 400°F.
2. Poke the potatoes all over with a fork. Arrange them directly on the grill grate, close the lid, and smoke for 1 hour and 15 minutes, or until cooked through and they have some give when pinched.
3. Let the potatoes cool for 10 minutes, then cut in half lengthwise.
4. Into a medium bowl, scoop out the potato flesh, leaving ¼ inch in the shells; place the shells on a baking sheet.
5. Using an electric mixer on medium speed, beat the potatoes, milk, butter, and sour cream until smooth.
6. Stir in the Parmesan cheese, bacon, and scallions, and season with salt and pepper.
7. Generously stuff each shell with the potato mixture and top with Cheddar cheese.
8. Place the baking sheet on the grill grate, close the lid, and smoke for 20 minutes, or until the cheese is melted.

Smoked Cherry Tomatoes

Servings: 8-10
Cooking Time: 1 ½ Hours
Ingredients:
- 2 pints of tomatoes

Directions:
1. Preheat the electric smoker to 225°F while adding wood chips and water to the smoker.
2. Clean the tomatoes with clean water and dry them off properly.

3. Place the tomatoes on the pan and place the pan in the smoker.
4. Smoke for 90 minutes while adding water and wood chips to the smoker.
Nutrition Info: Calories: 16 Cal Fat: 0 g Carbohydrates: 3 g Protein: 1 g Fiber: 1 g

Vegan Smoked Carrot Dogs

Servings: 2
Cooking Time: 35 Minutes
Ingredients:
- 4 carrots, thick
- 2 tbsp avocado oil
- 1/2 tbsp garlic powder
- 1 tbsp liquid smoke
- Pepper to taste
- Kosher salt to taste

Directions:
1. Preheat your Traeger to 425F then line a parchment paper on a baking sheet.
2. Peel the carrots to resemble a hot dog. Round the edges when peeling.
3. Whisk together oil, garlic powder, liquid smoke, pepper and salt in a bowl, small.
4. Now place carrots on the baking sheet and pour the mixture over. Roll your carrots in the mixture to massage seasoning and oil into them. Use fingertips.
5. Roast the carrots in the Traeger until fork tender for about 35 minutes. Brush the carrots using the marinade mixture every 5 minutes.
6. Remove and place into hot dog buns then top with hot dog toppings of your choice.
7. Serve and enjoy!
Nutrition Info: Calories 76, Total fat 1.8g, Saturated 0.4g, Total 14.4g, Net carbs 10.6g, Protein 1.5g, Sugar 6.6g, Fiber 3.8g, Sodium 163mg, Potassium 458mg

Cajun Style Grilled Corn

Servings: 4
Cooking Time: 25 Minutes
Ingredients:
- 4 ears corn, with husks
- 1tsp dried oregano
- 1tsp paprika
- 1tsp garlic powder
- 1tsp onion powder
- 1/2 tsp kosher salt
- 1/2 tsp ground black pepper
- 1/4 tsp dried thyme
- 1/4 tsp cayenne pepper
- 2tsp butter, melted

Directions:

1. Preheat pellet grill to 375°F.
2. Peel husks back but do not remove. Scrub and remove silks.
3. Mix oregano, paprika, garlic powder, onion powder, salt, pepper, thyme, and cayenne in a small bowl.
4. Brush melted butter over corn.
5. Rub seasoning mixture over each ear of corn. Pull husks up and place corn on grill grates. Grill for about 12-15 minutes, turning occasionally.
6. Remove from grill and allow to cool for about 5 minutes. Remove husks, then serve and enjoy!
Nutrition Info: Calories: 278 Fat: 17.4 g Cholesterol: 40.7 mg Carbohydrate: 30.6 g Fiber: 4.5 g Sugar: 4.6 g Protein: 5.4 g

2. Splash the asparagus with oil and generously with a splash of salt.
3. Drizzle carrots generously with honey and splash lightly with salt.
4. Preheat your Traeger to 350F with the lid closed for about 15 minutes.
5. Place the carrots first on the grill and cook for about 10-15 minutes.
6. Now place asparagus on the grill and cook both for about 15-20 minutes or until done to your liking.
7. Top with lemon zest and enjoy.
Nutrition Info: Calories 184, Total fat 7.3g, Saturated fat 1.1g, Total carbs 28.6g, Net carbs 21g, Protein 6g, Sugars 18.5g, Fiber 7.6g, Sodium 142mg, Potassium 826mg

Smoked Healthy Cabbage

Servings: 5
Cooking Time: 2 Hours
Ingredients:
- 1head cabbage, cored
- 4tablespoons butter
- 2tablespoons rendered bacon fat
- 1chicken bouillon cube
- 1teaspoon fresh ground black pepper
- 1garlic clove, minced

Directions:
1. Preheat your smoker to 240 degrees Fahrenheit using your preferred wood
2. Fill the hole of your cored cabbage with butter, bouillon cube, bacon fat, pepper and garlic
3. Wrap the cabbage in foil about two-thirds of the way up
4. Make sure to leave the top open
5. Transfer to your smoker rack and smoke for 2 hours
6. Unwrap and enjoy!
Nutrition Info: Calories: 231 Fats: 10g Carbs: 26g Fiber: 1g

Grilled Asparagus & Honey-glazed Carrots

Servings: 4
Cooking Time: 35 Minutes
Ingredients:
- 1 bunch asparagus, woody ends removed
- 2 tbsp olive oil
- 1 lb peeled carrots
- 2 tbsp honey
- Sea salt to taste
- Lemon zest to taste

Directions:
1. Rinse the vegetables under cold water.

Chicken Tortilla Soup

Servings: 4
Cooking Time: 35 Minutes
Ingredients:
- 1/2 cup Black Beans, canned
- 1Jalapeno Pepper, halved and seeds removed
- 1-1/2 cup Chicken Stock
- 2Carrots, sliced into ¼-inch pieces
- 1/2 of 1 Onion, peeled and halved
- 1/2 cup Corn
- 3 Garlic cloves
- 14-1/2 oz. Fire Roasted Tomatoes
- 1/4 cup Cilantro Leaves
- 10 oz. Chicken Breast, diced into ½ inch
- For the seasoning mix:
- 1/4 tsp. Chipotle
- 1tsp. Cuminutes
- 1/2 tsp. Sea Salt
- 1/2 tsp. Smoked Paprika

Directions:
1. Place pepper, carrots, onion, garlic cloves, and cilantro in the blender pitcher.
2. Pulse the mixture for 3 minutes and then pour the chicken stock to it.
3. Pulse again for another 3 minutes.
4. Next, stir in the remaining ingredients and press the 'hearty soup' button.
5. Finally, transfer to the serving bowl.
Nutrition Info: Calories: 260 Fat: 4 g Total Carbs: 40 g Fiber: 5.9 g Sugar: 8 g Protein: 14 g Cholesterol: 20 mg

Roasted Butternut Squash

Servings: 4
Cooking Time: 30 Minutes
Ingredients:

- 2-pound butternut squash
- 3 tablespoon extra-virgin olive oil
- Traeger Veggie Rub, as needed

Directions:
1. Fire the Traeger Grill to 350F. Use desired wood pellets when cooking. Close the lid and preheat for 15 minutes.
2. Slice the butternut squash into ½ inch thick and remove the seeds. Season with oil and veggie rub.
3. Place the seasoned squash in a baking tray.
4. Grill for 30 minutes.

Nutrition Info: Calories per serving: 131; Protein: 1.9g; Carbs: 23.6g; Fat: 4.7g Sugar: 0g

Traeger Grilled Vegetables

Servings: 12
Cooking Time: 15 Minutes
Ingredients:
- 1 veggie tray
- 1/4 cup vegetable oil
- 1-2 tbsp Traeger veggie seasoning

Directions:
1. Preheat your Traeger to 375F.
2. Meanwhile, toss the veggies in oil placed on a sheet pan, large, then splash with the seasoning.
3. Place on the Traeger and grill for about 10-15 minutes.
4. Remove, serve, and enjoy.

Nutrition Info: Calories 44, Total fat 5g, Saturated fat 0g, Total carbs 1g, Net carbs 1g, Protein 0g, Sugars 0g, Fiber 0g, Sodium 36mg, Potassium 116mg

Wood Pellet Grill Spicy Sweet Potatoes

Servings: 6
Cooking Time: 35 Minutes
Ingredients:
- 2 lb sweet potatoes, cut into chunks
- 1 red onion, chopped
- 2 tbsp oil
- 2 tbsp orange juice
- 1 tbsp roasted cinnamon
- 1 tbsp salt
- 1/4 tbsp Chiptole chili pepper

Directions:
1. Preheat the wood pellet grill to 425°F with the lid closed.
2. Toss the sweet potatoes with onion, oil, and juice.
3. In a mixing bowl, mix cinnamon, salt, and pepper then sprinkle the mixture over the sweet potatoes.
4. Spread the potatoes on a lined baking dish in a single layer.

5. Place the baking dish in the grill and grill for 30 minutes or until the sweet potatoes ate tender.
6. Serve and enjoy.

Nutrition Info: Calories 145, Total fat 5g, Saturated fat 0g, Total Carbs 23g, Net Carbs 19g, Protein 2g, Sugar 3g, Fiber 4g, Sodium: 428mg, Potassium 230mg

Wood Pellet Smoked Mushrooms

Servings: 5
Cooking Time: 45 Minutes
Ingredients:
- 4 cup portobello, whole and cleaned
- 1 tbsp canola oil
- 1 tbsp onion powder
- 1 tbsp granulated garlic
- 1tbsp salt
- 1 tbsp pepper

Directions:
1. In a mixing bowl, add all the ingredients and mix well.
2. Set the wood pellet temperature to 180°F then place the mushrooms directly on the grill.
3. Smoke the mushrooms for 30 minutes.
4. Increase the temperature to high and cook the mushrooms for a further 15 minutes.
5. Serve and enjoy.

Nutrition Info: Calories 1680, Total fat 30g, Saturated fat 2g, Total Carbs 10g, Net Carbs 10g, Protein 4g, Sugar 0g, Fiber 0g, Sodium: 514mg, Potassium 0mg

Spinach Soup

Servings: 4
Cooking Time: 35 Minutes
Ingredients:
- 2cups Chicken Stock
- 2tbsp. Vegetable Oil
- 1Onion quartered
- 2 ½ cup Spinach
- ½ lb. Red Potatoes, sliced thinly
- 2cups Milk, whole
- 1Leek, large and sliced thinly
- Black Pepper and Sea Salt, as needed
- 1Thyme Sprigs
- 1Bay Leaf

Directions:
1. For making this healthy soup, place the oil, onion, bay leaf, and thyme in the blender pitcher.
2. Now, press the 'saute' button.
3. Once sautéed, stir in the rest of the ingredients and press the 'smooth soup' button.

4. Finally, transfer the soup to the serving bowls and serve it hot.
Nutrition Info: Calories: 403 Fat: 24 g Total Carbs: 32 g Fiber: 3 g Sugar: 5.5 g Protein: 15 g Cholesterol: 66 mg

Roasted Peach Salsa

Servings: 6
Cooking Time: 10 Minutes
Ingredients:
- 6 whole peaches, pitted and halved
- 3 tomatoes, chopped
- 2 whole onions, chopped
- ½ cup cilantro, chopped
- 2 cloves garlic, minced
- 5 teaspoons apple cider vinegar
- ½ teaspoon salt
- ¼ teaspoon black pepper
- 2 tablespoons olive oil

Directions:
1. Fire the Traeger Grill to 300F. Use desired wood pellets when cooking. Close the lid and preheat for 15 minutes.
2. Place the peaches on the grill grate and cook for 5 minutes on each side. Remove from the grill and allow to rest for 5 minutes.
3. Place the peaches, tomatoes, onion, and cilantro in a salad bowl. On a smaller bowl, stir in the garlic, apple cider vinegar, salt, pepper, and olive oil. Stir until well-combined. Pour into the salad and toss to coat.
Nutrition Info: Calories per serving: 155 ;
Protein: 3.1g; Carbs: 27.6 g; Fat: 5.1g Sugar: 20g

Mexican Street Corn With Chipotle Butter 2

Servings: 6
Cooking Time: 45 Minutes
Ingredients:
- 16 to 20 long toothpicks
- 1 pound Brussels sprouts, trimmed and wilted, leaves removed
- ½ pound bacon, cut in half
- 1 tablespoon packed brown sugar
- 1 tablespoon Cajun seasoning
- ¼ cup balsamic vinegar
- ¼ cup extra-virgin olive oil
- ¼ cup chopped fresh cilantro
- 2 teaspoons minced garlic

Directions:
1. Soak the toothpicks in water for 15 minutes.

2. Supply your smoker with wood pellets and follow the manufacturer's specific start-up procedure. Preheat, with the lid closed, to 300°F.
3. Wrap each Brussels sprout in a half slice of bacon and secure with a toothpick.
4. In a small bowl, combine the brown sugar and Cajun seasoning. Dip each wrapped Brussels sprout in this sweet rub and roll around to coat.
5. Place the sprouts on a Frogmat or parchment paper–lined baking sheet on the grill grate, close the lid, and smoke for 45 minutes to 1 hour, turning as needed, until cooked evenly and the bacon is crisp.
6. In a small bowl, whisk together the balsamic vinegar, olive oil, cilantro, and garlic.
7. Remove the toothpicks from the Brussels sprouts, transfer to a plate and serve drizzled with the cilantro-balsamic sauce.

Smoked Mushrooms

Servings: 6
Cooking Time: 10 Minutes
Ingredients:
- 4 cups baby portobello, whole and cleaned
- 1 tablespoon canola oil
- 1 teaspoon onion powder
- 1 teaspoon garlic powder
- Salt and pepper to taste

Directions:
1. Place all ingredients in a bowl and toss to coat the mushrooms with the seasoning.
2. Fire the Traeger Grill to 350F. Use desired wood pellets when cooking. Close the lid and preheat for 15 minutes.
3. Place mushrooms on the grill grate and smoke for 10 minutes. Make sure to flip the mushrooms halfway through the cooking time.
4. Remove from the grill and serve.
Nutrition Info: Calories per serving: 62;
Protein: 5.2g; Carbs: 6.6g; Fat: 2.9g Sugar: 0.3g

Minestrone Soup

Servings: 4
Cooking Time: 35 Minutes
Ingredients:
- 1/4 tsp. Black Pepper
- 2tbsp. Olive Oil
- 15 oz. Cannellini Beans
- 1Onion quartered
- 1/2 tsp. Salt
- 2Garlic cloves, minced
- 1/3 cup Parmesan Cheese, grated
- 2Rosemary sprigs, minced

- 1cup Kale leaves, chopped
- 4cups Vegetable Stock
- Juice and Zest of 1 Lemon

Directions:
1. Begin by keeping oil, onion, and garlic in the pitcher of the blender.
2. Next, select the 'saute' button.
3. Once sautéed, stir in celery, rosemary, vegetable stock, lemon zest, lemon juice, kale, parmesan, salt, and pepper.
4. Then, press the 'hearty soup' button.
5. When it takes only 5 to 6 minutes to finish, add the beans and continue cooking.

Nutrition Info: Calories: 34 Fat: 1 g Total Carbs: 4.7 g Fiber: 0.4 g Sugar: 0 g Protein: 1.8 g Cholesterol: 1 mg

Grilled Carrots And Asparagus

Servings: 6
Cooking Time: 30 Minutes
Ingredients:
- 1 pound whole carrots, with tops
- 1 bunch of asparagus, ends trimmed
- Sea salt as needed
- 1 teaspoon lemon zest
- 2 tablespoons honey
- 2 tablespoons olive oil

Directions:
1. Switch on the Traeger grill, fill the grill hopper with flavored wood pellets, power the grill on by using the control panel, select 'smoke' on the temperature dial, or set the temperature to 450 degrees F and let it preheat for a minimum of 15 minutes.
2. Meanwhile, take a medium dish, place asparagus in it, season with sea salt, drizzle with oil and toss until mixed.
3. Take a medium bowl, place carrots in it, drizzle with honey, sprinkle with sea salt and toss until combined.
4. When the grill has preheated, open the lid, place asparagus and carrots on the grill grate, shut the grill and smoke for 30 minutes.
5. When done, transfer vegetables to a dish, sprinkle with lemon zest, and then serve.

Nutrition Info: Calories: 79.8 Cal ;Fat: 4.8 g ;Carbs: 8.6 g ;Protein: 2.6 g ;Fiber: 3.5 g

Baked Cheesy Corn Pudding

Servings: 6
Cooking Time: 30 Minutes
Ingredients:
- 3 cloves of garlic, chopped

- 3 tablespoons butter
- 3 cups whole corn kernels
- 8 ounces cream cheese
- 1 cup cheddar cheese
- 1 cup parmesan cheese
- 1 tablespoon salt
- ½ tablespoon black pepper
- ½ cup dry breadcrumbs
- 1 cup mozzarella cheese, grated
- 1 tablespoon thyme, minced

Directions:
1. Fire the Traeger Grill to 350F. Use desired wood pellets when cooking. Close the lid and preheat for 15 minutes.
2. In a large saucepan, sauté the garlic and butter for 2 minutes until fragrant. Add the corn, cheddar cheese, parmesan cheese, salt, and pepper. Heat until the corn is melted then pour into a baking dish.
3. In a small bowl, combine the breadcrumbs, mozzarella cheese, and thyme.
4. Spread the cheese and bread crumb mixture on top of the corn mixture.
5. Place the baking dish on the grill grate and cook for 25 minutes.
6. Allow to rest before removing from the mold.

Nutrition Info: Calories per serving: 523; Protein: 29.4g; Carbs: 34g; Fat: 31.2g Sugar: 10.8g

Blt Pasta Salad

Servings: 6
Cooking Time: 35 To 45 Minutes
Ingredients:
- 1 pound thick-cut bacon
- 16 ounces bowtie pasta, cooked according to package directions and drained
- 2 tomatoes, chopped
- ½ cup chopped scallions
- ½ cup Italian dressing
- ½ cup ranch dressing
- 1 tablespoon chopped fresh basil
- 1 teaspoon salt
- 1 teaspoon freshly ground black pepper
- 1 teaspoon garlic powder
- 1 head lettuce, cored and torn

Directions:
1. Supply your smoker with wood pellets and follow the manufacturer's specific start-up procedure. Preheat, with the lid closed, to 225°F.
2. Arrange the bacon slices on the grill grate, close the lid, and cook for 30 to 45 minutes, flipping after 20 minutes, until crisp.
3. Remove the bacon from the grill and chop.
4. In a large bowl, combine the chopped bacon with the cooked pasta, tomatoes, scallions, Italian

dressing, ranch dressing, basil, salt, pepper, and garlic powder. Refrigerate until ready to serve.
5. Toss in the lettuce just before serving to keep it from wilting.

Smoked Baked Beans

Servings: 12
Cooking Time: 3 Hours
Ingredients:
- 1 medium yellow onion diced
- 3 jalapenos
- 56 oz pork and beans
- 3/4 cup barbeque sauce
- 1/2 cup dark brown sugar
- 1/4 cup apple cider vinegar
- 2 tbsp Dijon mustard
- 2 tbsp molasses

Directions:
1. Preheat the smoker to 250°F. Pour the beans along with all the liquid in a pan. Add brown sugar, barbeque sauce, Dijon mustard, apple cider vinegar, and molasses. Stir. Place the pan on one of the racks. Smoke for 3 hours until thickened. Remove after 3 hours. Serve
Nutrition Info: Calories: 214 Cal Fat: 2 g Carbohydrates: 42 g Protein: 7 g Fiber: 7 g

Split Pea Soup With Mushrooms

Servings: 4
Cooking Time: 35 Minutes
Ingredients:
- 2tbsp. Olive Oil
- 3Garlic cloves, minced
- 3tbsp. Parsley, fresh and chopped
- 2Carrots chopped
- 1.2/3 cup Green Peas
- 9cups Water
- 2tsp. Salt
- 1/4 tsp. Black Pepper
- 1lb. Portobello Mushrooms
- 1Bay Leaf
- 2Celery Ribs, chopped
- 1Onion quartered
- 1/2 tsp. Thyme, dried
- 6tbsp. Parmesan Cheese, grated

Directions:
1. First, keep oil, onion, and garlic in the blender pitcher.
2. Next, select the 'saute' button.
3. Once sautéed, stir in the rest of the ingredients, excluding parsley and cheese.
4. Then, press the 'hearty soup' button.

5. Finally, transfer the soup among the serving bowls and garnish it with parsley and cheese.
Nutrition Info: Calories: 61 Fat: 1.1 g Total Carbs: 10 g Fiber: 1.9 g Sugar: 3.2 g Protein: 3.2 g Cholesterol: 0

Grilled Asparagus With Wild Mushrooms

Servings: 4
Cooking Time: 10 Minutes
Ingredients:
- 2 bunches fresh asparagus, trimmed
- 4 cups wild mushrooms, sliced
- 1 large shallots, sliced into rings
- Extra virgin oil as needed
- 2 tablespoons butter, melted

Directions:
1. Fire the Traeger Grill to 500F. Use desired wood pellets when cooking. Close the lid and preheat for 15 minutes.
2. Place the asparagus, mushrooms, and shallots on a baking tray. Drizzle with oil and butter and season with salt and pepper to taste.
3. Place on a baking tray and cook for 10 minutes. Make sure to give the asparagus a good stir halfway through the cooking time for even browning.
Nutrition Info: Calories per serving: 218; Protein: 15.2g; Carbs: 26.6 g; Fat: 10g Sugar: 12.9g

Sweet Jalapeño Cornbread

Servings: 12
Cooking Time: 50 Minutes
Ingredients:
- 2/3 cup margarine, softened
- 2/3 cup white sugar
- 2cups cornmeal
- 1.1/3 cups all-purpose flour
- 4tsp baking powder
- 1tsp kosher salt
- 3eggs
- 1.2/3 cups milk
- 1cup jalapeños, deseeded and chopped
- Butter, to line baking dish

Directions:
1. Preheat pellet grill to 400°F.
2. Beat margarine and sugar together in a medium-sized bowl until smooth.
3. In another bowl, combine cornmeal, flour, baking powder, and salt.
4. In a third bowl, combine and whisk eggs and milk.
5. Pour 1/3 of the milk mixture and 1/3 of the flour mixture into the margarine mixture at a time, whisking just until mixed after each pour.

6. Once thoroughly combined, stir in chopped jalapeño.

7. Lightly butter the bottom of the baking dish. Pour cornbread mixture evenly into the baking dish.

8. Place dish on grill grates and close the lid. Cook for about 23-25 minutes, or until thoroughly cooked. The way to test is by inserting a toothpick into the center of the cornbread - it should come out clean once removed.

9. Remove dish from the grill and allow to rest for 10 minutes before slicing and serving.

Nutrition Info: Calories: 160 Fat: 6 g Cholesterol: 15 mg Carbohydrate: 25 g Fiber: 10 g Sugar: 0.5 g Protein: 3 g

Roasted Green Beans With Bacon

Servings: 6
Cooking Time: 20 Minutes
Ingredients:
- 1-pound green beans
- 4 strips bacon, cut into small pieces
- 4 tablespoons extra virgin olive oil
- 2 cloves garlic, minced
- 1 teaspoon salt

Directions:
1. Fire the Traeger Grill to 400F. Use desired wood pellets when cooking. Close the lid and preheat for 15 minutes.
2. Toss all ingredients on a sheet tray and spread out evenly.
3. Place the tray on the grill grate and roast for 20 minutes.

Nutrition Info: Calories per serving: 65 ; Protein: 1.3g; Carbs: 3.8g; Fat: 5.3g Sugar: 0.6g

Grilled Scallions

Servings: 6
Cooking Time: 20 Minutes
Ingredients:
- 10 whole scallions, chopped
- ¼ cup olive oil
- Salt and pepper to taste
- 2 tablespoons rice vinegar
- 1 whole jalapeno, sliced into rings

Directions:
1. Fire the Traeger Grill to 500F. Use desired wood pellets when cooking. Close the lid and preheat for 15 minutes.
2. Place on a bowl all ingredients and toss to coat. Transfer to a parchment-lined baking tray.
3. Place on the grill grate and cook for 20 minutes or until the scallions char.

Nutrition Info: Calories per serving: 135; Protein: 2.2 g; Carbs: 9.7 g; Fat: 10.1g Sugar: 4.6g

Shiitake Smoked Mushrooms

Servings: 4-6
Cooking Time: 45 Minutes
Ingredients:
- 4 Cup Shiitake Mushrooms
- 1 tbsp canola oil
- 1 tsp onion powder
- 1 tsp granulated garlic
- 1 tsp salt
- 1 tsp pepper

Directions:
1. Combine all the ingredients together
2. Apply the mix over the mushrooms generously.
3. Preheat the smoker at 180°F. Add wood chips and half a bowl of water in the side tray.
4. Place it in the smoker and smoke for 45 minutes.
5. Serve warm and enjoy.

Nutrition Info: Calories: 301 Cal Fat: 9 g Carbohydrates: 47.8 g Protein: 7.1 g Fiber: 4.8 g

Grilled Sweet Potato Planks

Servings: 8
Cooking Time: 30 Minutes
Ingredients:
- 5 sweet potatoes, sliced into planks
- 1 tablespoon olive oil
- 1 teaspoon onion powder
- Salt and pepper to taste

Directions:
1. Set the Traeger wood pellet grill to high.
2. Preheat it for 15 minutes while the lid is closed.
3. Coat the sweet potatoes with oil.
4. Sprinkle with onion powder, salt and pepper.
5. Grill the sweet potatoes for 15 minutes.
6. Tips: Grill for a few more minutes if you want your sweet potatoes crispier.

Wood Pellet Smoked Acorn Squash

Servings: 6
Cooking Time: 2 Hours
Ingredients:
- 3 tbsp olive oil
- 3 acorn squash, halved and seeded
- 1/4 cup unsalted butter
- 1/4 cup brown sugar
- 1 tbsp cinnamon, ground

- 1 tbsp chili powder
- 1 tbsp nutmeg, ground

Directions:
1. Brush olive oil on the acorn squash cut sides then cover the halves with foil. Poke holes on the foil to allow steam and smoke through.
2. Fire up the wood pellet to 225°F and smoke the squash for 1-1/2-2 hours.
3. Remove the squash from the smoker and allow it to sit.
4. Meanwhile, melt butter, sugar and spices in a saucepan. Stir well to combine.
5. Remove the foil from the squash and spoon the butter mixture in each squash half. Enjoy.

Nutrition Info: Calories 149, Total fat 10g, Saturated fat 5g, Total Carbs 14g, Net Carbs 12g, Protein 2g, Sugar 0g, Fiber 2g, Sodium: 19mg, Potassium 0mg

Roasted Parmesan Cheese Broccoli

Servings: 3 To 4
Cooking Time: 45 Minutes
Ingredients:
- 3cups broccoli, stems trimmed
- 1tbsp lemon juice
- 1tbsp olive oil
- 2garlic cloves, minced
- 1/2 tsp kosher salt
- 1/2 tsp ground black pepper
- 1tsp lemon zest
- 1/8 cup parmesan cheese, grated

Directions:
1. Preheat pellet grill to 375°F.
2. Place broccoli in a resealable bag. Add lemon juice, olive oil, garlic cloves, salt, and pepper. Seal the bag and toss to combine. Let the mixture marinate for 30 minutes.
3. Pour broccoli into a grill basket. Place basket on grill grates to roast. Grill broccoli for 14-18 minutes, flipping broccoli halfway through. Grill until tender yet a little crispy on the outside.
4. Remove broccoli from grill and place on a serving dish—zest with lemon and top with grated parmesan cheese. Serve immediately and enjoy!

Nutrition Info: Calories: 82.6 Fat: 4.6 g Cholesterol: 1.8 mg Carbohydrate: 8.1 g Fiber: 4.6 g Sugar: 0 Protein: 5.5

Potluck Salad With Smoked Cornbread

Servings: 6
Cooking Time: 35 To 45 Minutes
Ingredients:
- 1 cup all-purpose flour
- 1 cup yellow cornmeal

- 1 tablespoon sugar
- 2 teaspoons baking powder
- 1 teaspoon salt
- 1 cup milk
- 1 egg, beaten, at room temperature
- 4 tablespoons (½ stick) unsalted butter, melted and cooled
- Nonstick cooking spray or butter, for greasing
- ½ cup milk
- ½ cup sour cream
- 2 tablespoons dry ranch dressing mix
- 1 pound bacon, cooked and crumbled
- 3 tomatoes, chopped
- 1 bell pepper, chopped
- 1 cucumber, seeded and chopped
- 2 stalks celery, chopped (about 1 cup)
- ½ cup chopped scallions

Directions:
1. For the cornbread:
2. In a medium bowl, combine the flour, cornmeal, sugar, baking powder, and salt.
3. In a small bowl, whisk together the milk and egg. Pour in the butter, then slowly fold this mixture into the dry ingredients.
4. Supply your smoker with wood pellets and follow the manufacturer's specific start-up procedure. Preheat, with the lid closed, to 375°F.
5. Coat a cast iron skillet with cooking spray or butter.
6. Pour the batter into the skillet, place on the grill grate, close the lid, and smoke for 35 to 45 minutes, or until the cornbread is browned and pulls away from the side of the skillet.
7. Remove the cornbread from the grill and let cool, then coarsely crumble.
8. For the salad:
9. In a small bowl, whisk together the milk, sour cream, and ranch dressing mix.
10. In a medium bowl, combine the crumbled bacon, tomatoes, bell pepper, cucumber, celery, and scallions.
11. In a large serving bowl, layer half of the crumbled cornbread, half of the bacon-veggie mixture, and half of the dressing. Toss lightly.
12. Repeat the layering with the remaining cornbread, bacon-veggie mixture, and dressing. Toss again.
13. Refrigerate the salad for at least 1 hour. Serve cold.

Wood Pellet Cold Smoked Cheese

Servings: 10
Cooking Time: 2 Minutes
Ingredients:

- Ice
- 1 aluminum pan, full-size and disposable
- 1 aluminum pan, half-size and disposable
- Toothpicks
- A block of cheese

Directions:
1. Preheat the wood pellet to 165°F wit the lid closed for 15 minutes.
2. Place the small pan in the large pan. Fill the surrounding of the small pan with ice.
3. Place the cheese in the small pan on top of toothpicks then place the pan on the grill and close the lid.
4. Smoke cheese for 1 hour, flip the cheese, and smoke for 1 more hour with the lid closed.
5. Remove the cheese from the grill and wrap it in parchment paper. Store in the fridge for 2 3 days for the smoke flavor to mellow.
6. Remove from the fridge and serve. Enjoy.

Nutrition Info: Calories 1910, Total fat 7g, Saturated fat 6g, Total Carbs 2g, Net Carbs 2g, Protein 6g, Sugar 1g, Fiber 0g, Sodium: 340mg, Potassium 0mg

Smoked Baked Kale Chips

Servings: 4
Cooking Time: 30 Minutes
Ingredients:
- 2 bunches kale, stems removed
- Olive oil as needed
- Salt and pepper to taste

Directions:
1. Fire the Traeger Grill to 350F. Use desired wood pellets when cooking. Close the lid and preheat for 15 minutes.
2. Place all ingredients in a bowl and toss to coat the kale with oil.
3. Place on a baking tray and spread the leaves evenly on all surface.
4. Place in the grill and cook for 30 minutes or until the kale leaves become crispy.

Nutrition Info: Calories per serving: 206 ;
Protein: 9.9g; Carbs: 21g; Fat: 12g Sugar: 0g

Grilled Broccoli

Servings: 1-2
Cooking Time: 3 Minutes
Ingredients:
- 2cups of broccoli, fresh
- 1tablespoon of canola oil
- 1teaspoon of lemon pepper

Directions:
1. Place the grill; grate inside the unit and close the hood.

2. Preheat the grill by turning at high for 10 minutes.
3. Meanwhile, mix broccoli with lemon pepper and canola oil.
4. Toss well to coat the Ingredients: thoroughly.
5. Place it on a grill grade once add food appears.
6. Lock the unit and cook for 3 minutes at medium.
7. Take out and serve.

Nutrition Info: Calories: 96 Total Fat: 7.3g Saturated Fat: 0.5g Cholesterol: 0mg Sodium: 30mg Total Carbohydrate: 6.7g Dietary Fiber 2.7g Total Sugars: 1.6g Protein: 2.7g

Wood Pellet Smoked Asparagus

Servings: 4
Cooking Time: 1 Hour
Ingredients:
- 1 bunch fresh asparagus, ends cut
- 2 tbsp olive oil
- Salt and pepper to taste

Directions:
1. Fire up your wood pellet smoker to 230°F
2. Place the asparagus in a mixing bowl and drizzle with olive oil. Season with salt and pepper.
3. Place the asparagus in a tinfoil sheet and fold the sides such that you create a basket.
4. Smoke the asparagus for 1 hour or until soft turning after half an hour.
5. Remove from the grill and serve. Enjoy.

Nutrition Info: Calories 43, Total fat 2g, Saturated fat 0g, Total Carbs 4g, Net Carbs 2g, Protein 3g, Sugar 2g, Fiber 2g, Sodium: 148mg

Wood Pellet Grilled Stuffed Zucchini

Servings: 8
Cooking Time: 11 Minutes
Ingredients:
- 4 zucchini
- 5 tbsp olive oil
- 2 tbsp red onion, chopped
- 1/4 tbsp garlic, minced
- 1/2 cup bread crumbs
- 1/2 cup mozzarella cheese, shredded
- 1 tbsp fresh mint
- 1/2 tbsp salt
- 3 tbsp parmesan cheese

Directions:
1. Cut the zucchini lengthwise and scoop out the pulp then brush the shells with oil.
2. In a non-stick skillet sauté pulp, onion, and remaining oil. Add garlic and cook for a minute.

3. Add bread crumbs and cook until golden brown. Remove from heat and stir in mozzarella cheese, fresh mint, and salt.
4. Spoon the mixture into the shells and sprinkle parmesan cheese.
5. Place in a grill and grill for 10 minutes or until the zucchini are tender.
Nutrition Info: Calories 186, Total fat 10g, Saturated fat 5g, Total Carbs 17g, Net Carbs 14g, Protein 9g, Sugar 4g, Fiber 3g, Sodium: 553mg

Easy Smoked Vegetables

Servings: 6
Cooking Time: 1 ½ Hour
Ingredients:
- 1 cup of pecan wood chips
- 1 ear fresh corn, silk strands removed, and husks, cut corn into 1-inch pieces
- 1 medium yellow squash, 1/2-inch slices
- 1 small red onion, thin wedges
- 1 small green bell pepper, 1-inch strips
- 1 small red bell pepper, 1-inch strips
- 1 small yellow bell pepper, 1-inch strips
- 1 cup mushrooms, halved
- 2 tbsp vegetable oil
- Vegetable seasonings

Directions:
1. Take a large bowl and toss all the vegetables together in it. Sprinkle it with seasoning and coat all the vegetables well with it.
2. Place the wood chips and a bowl of water in the smoker.
3. Preheat the smoker at 100°F or ten minutes.
4. Put the vegetables in a pan and add to the middle rack of the electric smoker.
5. Smoke for thirty minutes until the vegetable becomes tender.
6. When done, serve, and enjoy.
Nutrition Info: Calories: 97 Cal Fat: 5 g Carbohydrates: 11 g   Protein: 2 g Fiber: 3 g

Grilled Corn With Honey & Butter

Servings: 4
Cooking Time: 10 Minutes
Ingredients:
- 6 pieces corn
- 2 tablespoons olive oil
- 1/2 cup butter
- 1/2 cup honey
- 1 tablespoon smoked salt
- Pepper to taste

Directions:
1. Preheat the wood pellet grill to high for 15 minutes while the lid is closed.
2. Brush the corn with oil and butter.
3. Grill the corn for 10 minutes, turning from time to time.
4. Mix honey and butter.
5. Brush corn with this mixture and sprinkle with smoked salt and pepper.
6. Tips: Slice off the kernels and serve as side dish to a main course.

POULTRY RECIPES

Wood Pellet Grilled Buffalo Chicken

Servings: 6
Cooking Time: 20 Minutes
Ingredients:
- 5 chicken breasts, boneless and skinless
- 2 tbsp homemade bbq rub
- 1 cup homemade Cholula buffalo sauce

Directions:
1. Preheat the wood pellet grill to 400°F.
2. Slice the chicken into long strips and season with bbq rub.
3. Place the chicken on the grill and paint both sides with buffalo sauce.
4. Cook for 4 minutes with the grill closed. Cook while flipping and painting with buffalo sauce every 5 minutes until the internal temperature reaches 165°F.
5. Remove from the grill and serve when warm. Enjoy.

Nutrition Info: Calories 176, Total fat 4g, Saturated fat 1g, Total carbs 1g, Net carbs 1g, Protein 32g, Sugar 1g, Fiber 0g, Sodium: 631mg

Special Occasion's Dinner Cornish Hen

Servings: 4
Cooking Time: 1 Hour
Ingredients:
- 4 Cornish game hens
- 4 fresh rosemary sprigs
- 4 tbsp. butter, melted
- 4 tsp. chicken rub

Directions:
1. Set the temperature of Traeger Grill to 375 degrees F and preheat with closed lid for 15 minutes.
2. With paper towels, pat dry the hens.
3. Tuck the wings behind the backs and with kitchen strings, tie the legs together.
4. Coat the outside of each hen with melted butter and sprinkle with rub evenly.
5. Stuff the cavity of each hen with a rosemary sprig.
6. Place the hens onto the grill and cook for about 50-60 minutes.
7. Remove the hens from grill and place onto a platter for about 10 minutes.
8. Cut each hen into desired-sized pieces and serve.

Nutrition Info: Calories per serving: 430; Carbohydrates: 2.1g; Protein: 25.4g; Fat: 33g; Sugar: 0g; Sodium: 331mg; Fiber: 0.7g

Cajun Chicken

Servings: 4
Cooking Time: 30 Minutes
Ingredients:
- 2 lb. chicken wings
- Poultry dry rub
- Cajun seasoning

Directions:
1. Season the chicken wings with the dry rub and Cajun seasoning.
2. Preheat the Traeger to 350 degrees F for 15 minutes while the lid is closed.
3. Grill for 30 minutes, flipping twice.
4. Tips: You can also smoke the chicken before grilling.

Traeger Sheet Pan Chicken Fajitas

Servings: 10
Cooking Time: 10 Minutes
Ingredients:
- 2 lb chicken breast
- 1 onion, sliced
- 1 red bell pepper, seeded and sliced
- 1 orange-red bell pepper, seeded and sliced
- 1 tbsp salt
- 1/2 tbsp onion powder
- 1/2 tbsp granulated garlic
- 2 tbsp Spiceologist Chile Margarita Seasoning
- 2 tbsp oil

Directions:
1. Preheat the Traeger to 450F and line a baking sheet with parchment paper.
2. In a mixing bowl, combine seasonings and oil then toss with the peppers and chicken.
3. Place the baking sheet in the Traeger and let heat for 10 minutes with the lid closed.
4. Open the lid and place the veggies and the chicken in a single layer. Close the lid and cook for 10 minutes or until the chicken is no longer pink.
5. Serve with warm tortillas and top with your favorite toppings.

Nutrition Info: Calories 211, Total fat 6g, Saturated fat 1g, Total carbs 5g, Net carbs 4g Protein 29g, Sugars 4g, Fiber 1g, Sodium 360mg

Spicy Bbq Chicken

Servings: 6
Cooking Time: 3 Hours
Ingredients:
- 1 whole chicken, cleaned

- For the Marinade:
- 1 medium white onion, peeled
- 6 Thai chilies
- 5 cloves of garlic, peeled
- 1 scotch bonnet
- 3 tablespoons salt
- 2 tablespoons sugar
- 2 tablespoons sweet paprika
- 4 cups grapeseed oil

Directions:

1. Prepare the marinade, and for this, place all of its ingredients in a food processor and pulse for 2 minutes until smooth.
2. Smoother whole chicken with the prepared marinade and let it marinate in the refrigerator for a minimum of 8 hours.
3. When ready to cook, switch on the Traeger grill, fill the grill hopper with apple-flavored wood pellets, power the grill on by using the control panel, select 'smoke' on the temperature dial, or set the temperature to 300 degrees F and let it preheat for a minimum of 15 minutes.
4. When the grill has preheated, open the lid, place chicken on the grill grate breast-side up, shut the grill and smoke for 3 hours until the internal temperature of chicken reaches 165 degrees F.
5. When done, transfer chicken to a cutting board, let it rest for 15 minutes, then cut into slices and serve.

Nutrition Info: Calories: 100 Cal ;Fat: 2.8 g ;Carbs: 13 g ;Protein: 3.5 g ;Fiber: 2 g

Chile-lime Rubbed Chicken

Servings: 6
Cooking Time: 40 Minutes
Ingredients:
- 3 tablespoons chili powder
- 2 tablespoons extra virgin olive oil
- 2 teaspoons lime zest
- 3 tablespoons lime juice
- 1 tablespoon garlic, minced
- 1 teaspoon ground coriander
- 1 teaspoon ground cumin
- 1 teaspoon dried oregano
- 1 ½ teaspoons salt
- 1 teaspoon ground black pepper
- A pinch of cinnamon
- 1 chicken, spatchcocked

Directions:

1. In a bowl, place the chili powder, olive oil, lime zest, juice, garlic, coriander, cumin, oregano, salt, pepper, cinnamon, and cinnamon in a bowl. Mix to form a paste.

2. Place the chicken cut-side down on a chopping board and flatten using the heel of your hand. Carefully, break the breastbone to flatten the chicken.
3. Generously rub the spices all over the chicken and make sure to massage the chicken with the spice rub. Place in a baking dish and refrigerate for 24 hours in the fridge.
4. When ready to cook, fire the Traeger Grill to 400F. Use maple wood pellets. Close the grill lid and preheat for 15 minutes.
5. Place the chicken breastbone-side down on the grill grate and cook for 40 minutes or until a thermometer inserted in the thickest part reads at 165F.
6. Make sure to flip the chicken halfway through the cooking time.
7. Once cooked, transfer to a plate and allow to rest before carving the chicken.

Nutrition Info: Calories per serving: 213; Protein: 33.1g; Carbs: 3.8g; Fat: 7g Sugar: 0.5g

Wood Pellet Smoked Spatchcock Turkey

Servings: 6
Cooking Time: 1 Hour 45 Minutes
Ingredients:
- 1 whole turkey
- 1/2 cup oil
- 1/4 cup chicken rub
- 1 tbsp onion powder
- 1 tbsp garlic powder
- 1 tbsp rubbed sage

Directions:

1. Preheat your wood pellet grill to high.
2. Meanwhile, place the turkey on a platter with the breast side down then cut on either side of the backbone to remove the spine.
3. Flip the turkey and season on both sides then place it on the preheated grill or on a pan if you want to catch the drippings.
4. Grill on high for 30 minutes, reduce the temperature to 325°F, and grill for 45 more minutes or until the internal temperature reaches 165°F
5. Remove from the grill and let rest for 20 minutes before slicing and serving. Enjoy.

Nutrition Info: Calories 156, Total fat 16g, Saturated fat 2g, Total Carbs 1g, Net Carbs 1g, Protein 2g, Sugar 0g, Fiber 0g, Sodium: 19mg

Turkey Breast

Servings: 6
Cooking Time: 8 Hours
Ingredients:
- For the Brine:

- 2 pounds turkey breast, deboned
- 2 tablespoons ground black pepper
- 1/4 cup salt
- 1 cup brown sugar
- 4 cups cold water
- For the BBQ Rub:
- 2 tablespoons dried onions
- 2 tablespoons garlic powder
- 1/4 cup paprika
- 2 tablespoons ground black pepper
- 1 tablespoon salt
- 2 tablespoons brown sugar
- 2 tablespoons red chili powder
- 1 tablespoon cayenne pepper
- 2 tablespoons sugar
- 2 tablespoons ground cumin

Directions:
1. Prepare the brine and for this, take a large bowl, add salt, black pepper, and sugar in it, pour in water, and stir until sugar has dissolved.
2. Place turkey breast in it, submerge it completely and let it soak for a minimum of 12 hours in the refrigerator.
3. Meanwhile, prepare the BBQ rub and for this, take a small bowl, place all of its ingredients in it and then stir until combined, set aside until required.
4. Then remove turkey breast from the brine and season well with the prepared BBQ rub.
5. When ready to cook, switch on the Traeger grill, fill the grill hopper with apple-flavored wood pellets, power the grill on by using the control panel, select 'smoke' on the temperature dial, or set the temperature to 180 degrees F and let it preheat for a minimum of 15 minutes.
6. When the grill has preheated, open the lid, place turkey breast on the grill grate, shut the grill, change the smoking temperature to 225 degrees F, and smoke for 8 hours until the internal temperature reaches 160 degrees F.
7. When done, transfer turkey to a cutting board, let it rest for 10 minutes, then cut it into slices and serve.

Nutrition Info: Calories: 250 Cal ;Fat: 5 g ;Carbs: 31 g ;Protein: 18 g ;Fiber: 5 g

Jamaican Jerk Chicken Quarters

Servings: 4
Cooking Time: 1 To 2 Hours
Ingredients:
- 4 chicken leg quarters, scored
- ¼ cup canola oil
- ½ cup Jamaican Jerk Paste
- 1 tablespoon whole allspice (pimento) berries

Directions:

1. Supply your smoker with wood pellets and follow the manufacturer's specific start-up procedure. Preheat, with the lid closed, to 275°F.
2. Brush the chicken with canola oil, then brush 6 tablespoons of the Jerk paste on and under the skin. Reserve the remaining 2 tablespoons of paste for basting.
3. Throw the whole allspice berries in with the wood pellets for added smoke flavor.
4. Arrange the chicken on the grill, close the lid, and smoke for 1 hour to 1 hour 30 minutes, or until a meat thermometer inserted in the thickest part of the thigh reads 165°F.
5. Let the meat rest for 5 minutes and baste with the reserved jerk paste prior to serving.

Bacon-wrapped Chicken Tenders

Servings: 6
Cooking Time: 30 Minutes
Ingredients:
- 1-pound chicken tenders
- 10 strips bacon
- 1/2 tbsp Italian seasoning
- 1/2 tbsp black pepper
- 1/2 tbsp salt
- 1 tbsp paprika
- 1 tbsp onion powder
- 1 tbsp garlic powder
- 1/3 cup light brown sugar
- 1 tbsp chili powder

Directions:
1. Preheat your wood pellet smoker to 350°F.
2. Mix seasonings
3. Sprinkle the mixture on all sides of chicken tenders
4. Wrap each chicken tender with a strip of bacon
5. Mix sugar and chili then sprinkle the mixture on the bacon-wrapped chicken.
6. Place them on the smoker and smoker for 30 minutes with the lid closed or until the chicken is cooked.
7. Serve and enjoy.

Nutrition Info: Calories: 206 Cal Fat: 7.9 g Carbohydrates: 1.5 g Protein: 30.3 g Fiber: 0 g

Smoked Lemon Chicken Breasts

Servings: 6
Cooking Time: 30 Minutes
Ingredients:
- 2 lemons, zested and juiced
- 1 clove of garlic, minced
- 2 teaspoons honey

- 2 teaspoons salt
- 1 teaspoon ground black pepper
- 2 sprigs fresh thyme
- ½ cup olive oil
- 6 boneless chicken breasts

Directions:
1. Place all ingredients in a bowl. Massage the chicken breasts so that it is coated with the marinade.
2. Place in the fridge to marinate for at least 4 hours.
3. Fire the Traeger Grill to 350F. Use apple wood pellets. Close the grill lid and preheat for 15 minutes.
4. Place the chicken breasts on the grill grate and cook for 15 minutes on both sides.
5. Serve immediately or drizzle with lemon juice.

Nutrition Info: Calories per serving: 671 ; Protein: 60.6 g; Carbs: 3.5 g; Fat: 44.9g Sugar: 2.3g

Peppered Bbq Chicken Thighs

Servings: 6
Cooking Time: 35 Minutes
Ingredients:
- 6 bone-in chicken thighs
- Salt and pepper to taste
- Traeger Big Game Rub to taste, optional

Directions:
1. Place all ingredients in a bowl and allow to marinate in the fridge for at least 4 hours.
2. When ready to cook, fire the Traeger Grill to 350F. Use apple wood pellet. Close the lid and preheat for 15 minutes.
3. Place the chicken directly on the grill grate and cook for 35 minutes. To check if the chicken is cooked thoroughly, insert a meat thermometer, and make sure that the internal temperature reads at 165F.
4. Serve the chicken immediately.

Nutrition Info: Calories per serving: 430; Protein: 32g; Carbs: 1.2g; Fat: 32.1g; Sugar: 0.4g

Hickory Smoked Chicken

Servings: 4
Cooking Time: 30 Minutes
Ingredients:
- 4 chicken breasts
- ¼ cup olive oil
- 1 teaspoon pressed garlic
- 1 tablespoon Worcestershire sauce
- Kirkland Sweet Mesquite Seasoning as needed
- 1 button Traeger Honey Bourbon Sauce

Directions:

1. Place all ingredients in a bowl except for the Bourbon sauce. Massage the chicken until all parts are coated with the seasoning.
2. Allow to marinate in the fridge for 4 hours.
3. Once ready to cook, fire the Traeger Grill to 350F. Use Hickory wood pellets and close the lid. Preheat for 15 minutes.
4. Place the chicken directly into the grill grate and cook for 30 minutes. Flip the chicken halfway through the cooking time.
5. Five minutes before the cooking time ends, brush all surfaces of the chicken with the Honey Bourbon Sauce.
6. Serve immediately.

Nutrition Info: Calories per serving: 622; Protein: 60.5g; Carbs: 1.1g; Fat: 40.3g Sugar: 0.4g

Bourbon Bbq Smoked Chicken Wings

Servings: 8
Cooking Time: 24 Minutes
Ingredients:
- 4 pounds chicken wings, patted dry
- 2 tablespoons olive oil
- Salt and pepper to taste
- ½ medium yellow onions, minced
- 5 cloves garlic, mince
- ½ cup bourbon
- 2 cups ketchup
- 1/3 cup apple cider vinegar
- 2 tablespoons liquid smoke
- ½ teaspoon kosher salt
- ½ teaspoon black pepper
- A dash of hot sauce

Directions:
1. Place the chicken in a bowl and drizzle with olive oil. Season with salt and pepper to taste. In another bowl, combine the rest of the ingredients and set aside.
2. Fire the Traeger Grill to 400F. Use hickory wood pellets. Close the lid and allow to preheat for 15 minutes.
3. Place the chicken on the grill grate and cook for 12 minutes on each side.
4. Using a brush, brush the chicken wings with bourbon sauce on all sides.
5. Flip the chicken and cook for another 12 minutes with the lid closed.

Nutrition Info: Calories per serving: 384 ; Protein: 50.7g; Carbs: 17.8 g; Fat: 11.5g Sugar: 13.1g

Cinco De Mayo Chicken Enchiladas

Servings: 6
Cooking Time: 45 Minutes

Ingredients:
- 6 cups diced cooked chicken
- 3 cups grated Monterey Jack cheese, divided
- 1 cup sour cream
- 1 (4-ounce) can chopped green chiles
- 2 (10-ounce) cans red or green enchilada sauce, divided
- 12 (8-inch) flour tortillas
- ½ cup chopped scallions
- ¼ cup chopped fresh cilantro

Directions:
1. Supply your smoker with wood pellets and follow the manufacturer's specific start-up procedure. Preheat, with the lid closed, to 350°F.
2. In a large bowl, combine the cooked chicken, 2 cups of cheese, the sour cream, and green chiles to make the filling.
3. Pour one can of enchilada sauce in the bottom of a 9-by-13-inch baking dish or aluminum pan.
4. Spoon ⅓ cup of the filling on each tortilla and roll up securely.
5. Transfer the tortillas seam-side down to the baking dish, then pour the remaining can of enchilada sauce over them, coating all exposed surfaces of the tortillas.
6. Sprinkle the remaining 1 cup of cheese over the enchiladas and cover tightly with aluminum foil.
7. Bake on the grill, with the lid closed, for 30 minutes, then remove the foil.
8. Continue baking with the lid closed for 15 minutes, or until bubbly.
9. Garnish the enchiladas with the chopped scallions and cilantro and serve immediately.

Teriyaki Wings

Servings: 8
Cooking Time: 50 Minutes
Ingredients:
- 2 ½ pounds large chicken wings
- 1 tablespoon toasted sesame seeds
- For the Marinade:
- 2 scallions, sliced
- 2 tablespoons grated ginger
- ½ teaspoon minced garlic
- 1/4 cup brown sugar
- 1/2 cup soy sauce
- 2 tablespoon rice wine vinegar
- 2 teaspoons sesame oil
- 1/4 cup water

Directions:
1. Prepare the chicken wings and for this, remove tips from the wings, cut each chicken wing through the joint into three pieces, and then place in a large plastic bag.

2. Prepare the sauce and for this, take a small saucepan, place it over medium-high heat, add all of its ingredients in it, stir until mixed, and bring it to a boil.
3. Then switch heat to medium level, simmer the sauce for 10 minutes, and when done, cool the sauce completely.
4. Pour the sauce over chicken wings, seal the bag, turn it upside down to coat chicken wings with the sauce and let it marinate for a minimum of 8 hours in the refrigerator.
5. When ready to cook, switch on the Traeger grill, fill the grill hopper with maple-flavored wood pellets, power the grill on by using the control panel, select 'smoke' on the temperature dial, or set the temperature to 350 degrees F and let it preheat for a minimum of 15 minutes.
6. Meanwhile,
7. When the grill has preheated, open the lid, place chicken wings on the grill grate, shut the grill and smoke for 50 minutes until crispy and meat is no longer pink, turning halfway.
8. When done, transfer chicken wings to a dish, sprinkle with sesame seeds and then serve.
Nutrition Info: Calories: 150 Cal ;Fat: 7.5 g ;Carbs: 6 g ;Protein: 12 g ;Fiber: 1 g

Turkey Meatballs

Servings: 8
Cooking Time: 40 Minutes
Ingredients:
- 1 1/4 lb. ground turkey
- 1/2 cup breadcrumbs
- 1 egg, beaten
- 1/4 cup milk
- 1 teaspoon onion powder
- 1/4 cup Worcestershire sauce
- Pinch garlic salt
- Salt and pepper to taste
- 1 cup cranberry jam
- 1/2 cup orange marmalade
- 1/2 cup chicken broth

Directions:
1. In a large bowl, mix the ground turkey, breadcrumbs, egg, milk, onion powder, Worcestershire sauce, garlic salt, salt and pepper.
2. Form meatballs from the mixture.
3. Preheat the Traeger wood pellet grill to 350 degrees F for 15 minutes while the lid is closed.
4. Add the turkey meatballs to a baking pan.
5. Place the baking pan on the grill.
6. Cook for 20 minutes.
7. In a pan over medium heat, simmer the rest of the ingredients for 10 minutes.
8. Add the grilled meatballs to the pan.

9. Coat with the mixture.
10. Cook for 10 minutes.
11. Tips: You can add chili powder to the meatball mixture if you want spicy flavor.

Ultimate Tasty Chicken

Servings: 5
Cooking Time: 3 Hours
Ingredients:
- For Brine:
- 1 C. brown sugar
- ½ C. kosher salt
- 16 C. water
- For Chicken:
- 1 (3-lb.) whole chicken
- 1 tbsp. garlic, crushed
- 1 tsp. onion powder
- Salt and freshly ground black pepper, to taste
- 1 medium yellow onion, quartered
- 3 whole garlic cloves, peeled
- 1 lemon, quartered
- 4-5 fresh thyme sprigs

Directions:
1. For brine: in a bucket, dissolve brown sugar and kosher salt in water.
2. Place the chicken in brine and refrigerate overnight.
3. Set the temperature of Traeger Grill to 225 degrees F and preheat with closed lid for 15 minutes.
4. Remove the chicken from brine and with paper towels, pat it dry.
5. In a small bowl, mix together crushed garlic, onion powder, salt and black pepper.
6. Rub the chicken with garlic mixture evenly.
7. Stuff the cavity of chicken with onion, garlic cloves, lemon and thyme.
8. With kitchen strings, tie the legs together.
9. Place the chicken onto grill and cook, covered for about 2½-3 hours.
10. Remove chicken from pallet grill and transfer onto a cutting board for about 10 minutes before carving.
11. With a sharp knife, cut the chicken in desired sized pieces and serve.
Nutrition Info: Calories per serving: 641; Carbohydrates: 31.7g; Protein: 79.2g; Fat: 20.2g; Sugar: 29.3g; Sodium: 11500mg; Fiber: 0.6g

Succulent Duck Breast

Servings: 4
Cooking Time: 10 Minutes
Ingredients:
- 4 (6-oz.) boneless duck breasts
- 2 tbsp. chicken rub

Directions:
1. Set the temperature of Traeger Grill to 275 degrees F and preheat with closed lid for 15 minutes.
2. With a sharp knife, score the skin of the duck into ¼-inch diamond pattern.
3. Season the duck breast with rub evenly.
4. Place the duck breasts onto the grill, meat side down and cook for about 10 minutes.
5. Now, set the temperature of Traeger Grill to 400 degrees F.
6. Now, arrange the breasts, skin side down and cook for about 10 minutes, flipping once halfway through.
7. Remove from the grill and serve.
Nutrition Info: Calories per serving: 231; Carbohydrates: 1.5g; Protein: 37.4g; Fat: 6.8g; Sugar: 0g; Sodium: 233mg; Fiber: 0g

Wood Pellet Sheet Pan Chicken Fajitas

Servings: 10
Cooking Time: 10 Minutes
Ingredients:
- 2 tbsp oil
- 2 tbsp chile margarita seasoning
- 1 tbsp salt
- 1/2 tbsp onion powder
- 1/2 tbsp garlic, granulated
- 2-pound chicken breast, thinly sliced
- 1 red bell pepper, seeded and sliced
- 1 orange bell pepper
- 1 onion, sliced

Directions:
1. Preheat the wood pellet to 450°F. Meanwhile, mix oil and seasoning then toss the chicken and the peppers. Line a sheet pan with foil then place it in the preheated grill. Let it heat for 10 minutes with the grill's lid closed. Open the grill and place the chicken with the veggies on the pan in a single layer. Cook for 10 minutes or until the chicken is cooked and no longer pink. Remove from grill and serve with tortilla or your favorite fixings.
Nutrition Info: Calories: 211 Cal Fat: 6 g Carbohydrates: 5 g   Protein: 29 g Fiber: 1 g

Chicken Fajitas On A Wood Pellet Grill

Servings: 10
Cooking Time: 20 Minutes
Ingredients:
- Chicken breast - 2 lbs, thin sliced
- Red bell pepper - 1 large

- Onion - 1 large
- Orange bell pepper - 1 large
- Seasoning mix
- Oil - 2 tbsp
- Onion powder - ½ tbsp
- Granulated garlic - ½ tbsp
- Salt - 1 tbsp

Directions:
1. Preheat the grill to 450 degrees.
2. Mix the seasonings and oil.
3. Add the chicken slices to the mix.
4. Line a large pan with a non-stick baking sheet.
5. Let the pan heat for 10 minutes.
6. Place the chicken, peppers, and other vegetables in the grill.
7. Grill for 10 minutes or until the chicken is cooked.
8. Remove it from the grill and serve with warm tortillas and vegetables.

Nutrition Info: Carbohydrates: 5 g Protein: 29 g Fat: 6 g Sodium: 360 mg Cholesterol: 77 mg

Wood Pellet Grilled Chicken

Servings: 6
Cooking Time: 1 Hour And 10 Minutes
Ingredients:
- 5 pounds whole chicken
- 1/2 cup oil
- Chicken rub

Directions:
1. Preheat your wood pellet on smoke with the lid open for 5 minutes. Close the lid, increase the temperature to 450°F and preheat for 15 more minutes.
2. Tie the chicken legs together with the baker's twine then rub the chicken with oil and coat with chicken rub.
3. Place the chicken on the grill with the breast side up.
4. Grill the chicken for 70 minutes without opening it or until the internal temperature reaches 165°F.
5. Once the chicken is out of the grill let it cool down for 15 minutes
6. Enjoy.

Nutrition Info: Calories: 935 Cal Fat: 53 g Carbohydrates: 0 g Protein: 107 g Fiber: 0 g

Skinny Smoked Chicken Breasts

Servings: 4 To 6
Cooking Time: 1 Hour 25 Minutes
Ingredients:
- 2½ pounds boneless, skinless chicken breasts
- Salt

- Freshly ground black pepper

Directions:
1. Supply your smoker with wood pellets and follow the manufacturer's specific start-up procedure. Preheat the grill, with the lid closed, to 180°F.
2. Season the chicken breasts all over with salt and pepper.
3. Place the breasts directly on the grill grate and smoke for 1 hour.
4. Increase the grill's temperature to 325°F and continue to cook until the chicken's internal temperature reaches 170°F. Remove the breasts from the grill and serve immediately.

Traeger Smoked Chicken And Potatoes

Servings: 4
Cooking Time: 1 Hour And 30 Minutes
Ingredients:
- 1 2.5-pounds rotisserie chicken
- 2 tablespoon coconut sugar
- 1 tablespoons onion powder
- 2 tablespoon garlic powder
- 1 teaspoon cayenne pepper powder
- 2 teaspoon kosher salt
- 4 tablespoons olive oil
- 2 pounds creamer potatoes, scrubbed and halved
- A dash of black pepper powder

Directions:
1. Place the chicken in a bowl. In a smaller bowl, combine the coconut sugar, onion powder, garlic powder, cayenne pepper powder, and salt. Add in the olive oil. Rub the mixture into the chicken and allow to marinate for 4 hours in the fridge.
2. Fire the Traeger Grill to 400F and close the lid. Preheat to 15 minutes.
3. Place the seasoned chicken in a heat-proof dish and place the potatoes around the chicken. Season the potatoes with salt.
4. Place in the grill and cook for 30 minutes. Lower the heat to 250F and cook for another hour.
5. Insert a meat thermometer in the thickest part of the chicken and make sure that the temperature reads at 165F. Flip the chicken halfway through the cooking time for even browning.

Nutrition Info: Calories per serving: 991; Protein: 79.7g; Carbs: 49.8g; Fat: 73.6g Sugar: 6.5g

Spatchcocked Turkey

Servings: 10 To 14
Cooking Time: 2 Hours
Ingredients:
- 1 whole turkey

- 2 tablespoons olive oil
- 1 batch Chicken Rub

Directions:

1. Supply your smoker with wood pellets and follow the manufacturer's specific start-up procedure. Preheat the grill, with the lid closed, to 350°F.
2. To remove the turkey's backbone, place the turkey on a work surface, on its breast. Using kitchen shears, cut along one side of the turkey's backbone and then the other. Pull out the bone.
3. Once the backbone is removed, turn the turkey breast-side up and flatten it.
4. Coat the turkey with olive oil and season it on both sides with the rub. Using your hands, work the rub into the meat and skin.
5. Place the turkey directly on the grill grate, breast-side up, and cook until its internal temperature reaches 170°F.
6. Remove the turkey from the grill and let it rest for 10 minutes, before carving and serving.

Garlic Parmesan Chicken Wings

Servings: 6
Cooking Time: 20 Minutes

Ingredients:

- 5 pounds of chicken wings
- 1/2 cup chicken rub
- 3 tablespoons chopped parsley
- 1 cup shredded parmesan cheese
- For the Sauce:
- 5 teaspoons minced garlic
- 2 tablespoons chicken rub
- 1 cup butter, unsalted

Directions:

1. Switch on the Traeger grill, fill the grill hopper with cherry flavored wood pellets, power the grill on by using the control panel, select 'smoke' on the temperature dial, or set the temperature to 450 degrees F and let it preheat for a minimum of 15 minutes.
2. Meanwhile, take a large bowl, place chicken wings in it, sprinkle with chicken rub and toss until well coated.
3. When the grill has preheated, open the lid, place chicken wings on the grill grate, shut the grill, and smoke for 10 minutes per side until the internal temperature reaches 165 degrees F.
4. Meanwhile, prepare the sauce and for this, take a medium saucepan, place it over medium heat, add all the ingredients for the sauce in it and cook for 10 minutes until smooth, set aside until required.
5. When done, transfer chicken wings to a dish, top with prepared sauce, toss until mixed, garnish with cheese and parsley and then serve.

Nutrition Info: Calories: 180 Cal ;Fat: 1 g ;Carbs: 8 g ;Protein: 0 g ;Fiber: 0 g

Wood Pellet Smoked Cornish Hens

Servings: 6
Cooking Time: 1 Hour

Ingredients:

- 6 Cornish hens
- 3 tbsp avocado oil
- 6 tbsp rub of choice

Directions:

1. Fire up the wood pellet and preheat it to 275°F.
2. Rub the hens with oil then coat generously with rub. Place the hens on the grill with the chest breast side down.
3. Smoke for 30 minutes. Flip the hens and increase the grill temperature to 400°F. Cook until the internal temperature reaches 165°F.
4. Remove from the grill and let rest for 10 minutes before serving. Enjoy.

Nutrition Info: Calories: 696 Cal Fat: 50 g Carbohydrates: 1 g Protein: 57 g Fiber: 0 g

Game Day Chicken Drumsticks

Servings: 8
Cooking Time: 1 Hour

Ingredients:

- For Brine:
- ½ C. brown sugar
- ½ C. kosher salt
- 5 C. water
- 2 (12-oz.) bottles beer
- 8 chicken drumsticks
- For Coating:
- ¼ C. olive oil
- ½ C. BBQ rub
- 1 tbsp. fresh parsley, minced
- 1 tbsp. fresh chives, minced
- ¾ C. BBQ sauce
- ¼ C. beer

Directions:

1. For brine: in a bucket, dissolve brown sugar and kosher salt in water and beer.
2. Place the chicken drumsticks in brine and refrigerate, covered for about 3 hours.
3. Set the temperature of Traeger Grill to 275 degrees F and preheat with closed lid for 15 minutes.
4. Remove chicken drumsticks from brine and rinse under cold running water.
5. With paper towels, pat dry chicken drumsticks.
6. Coat drumsticks with olive oil and rub with BBQ rub evenly.

7. Sprinkle the drumsticks with parsley and chives.
8. Arrange the chicken drumsticks onto the grill and cook for about 45 minutes.
9. Meanwhile, in a bowl, mix together BBQ sauce and beer.
10. Remove from grill and coat the drumsticks with BBQ sauce evenly.
11. Cook for about 15 minutes more.
12. Serve immediately.

Nutrition Info: Calories per serving: 448; Carbohydrates: 20.5g; Protein: 47.2g; Fat: 16.1g; Sugar: 14.9g; Sodium: 9700mg; Fiber: 0.2g

Herb Roasted Turkey

Servings: 12
Cooking Time: 3 Hours And 30 Minutes
Ingredients:
- 14 pounds turkey, cleaned
- 2 tablespoons chopped mixed herbs
- Pork and poultry rub as needed
- 1/4 teaspoon ground black pepper
- 3 tablespoons butter, unsalted, melted
- 8 tablespoons butter, unsalted, softened
- 2 cups chicken broth

Directions:
1. Clean the turkey by removing the giblets, wash it inside out, pat dry with paper towels, then place it on a roasting pan and tuck the turkey wings by tiring with butcher's string.
2. Switch on the Traeger grill, fill the grill hopper with hickory flavored wood pellets, power the grill on by using the control panel, select 'smoke' on the temperature dial, or set the temperature to 325 degrees F and let it preheat for a minimum of 15 minutes.
3. Meanwhile, prepared herb butter and for this, take a small bowl, place the softened butter in it, add black pepper and mixed herbs and beat until fluffy.
4. Place some of the prepared herb butter underneath the skin of turkey by using a handle of a wooden spoon, and massage the skin to distribute butter evenly.
5. Then rub the exterior of the turkey with melted butter, season with pork and poultry rub, and pour the broth in the roasting pan.
6. When the grill has preheated, open the lid, place roasting pan containing turkey on the grill grate, shut the grill and smoke for 3 hours and 30 minutes until the internal temperature reaches 165 degrees F and the top has turned golden brown.
7. When done, transfer turkey to a cutting board, let it rest for 30 minutes, then carve it into slices and serve.

Nutrition Info: Calories: 154.6 Cal ;Fat: 3.1 g ;Carbs: 8.4 g ;Protein: 28.8 g ;Fiber: 0.4 g

Mini Turducken Roulade

Servings: 6
Cooking Time: 2 Hours
Ingredients:
- 1 (16-ounce) boneless turkey breast
- 1 (8-to 10-ounce) boneless duck breast
- 1 (8-ounce) boneless, skinless chicken breast
- Salt
- Freshly ground black pepper
- 2 cups Italian dressing
- 2 tablespoons Cajun seasoning
- 1 cup prepared seasoned stuffing mix
- 8 slices bacon
- Butcher's string

Directions:
1. Butterfly the turkey, duck, and chicken breasts, cover with plastic wrap and, using a mallet, flatten each ½ inch thick.
2. Season all the meat on both sides with a little salt and pepper.
3. In a medium bowl, combine the Italian dressing and Cajun seasoning. Spread one-fourth of the mixture on top of the flattened turkey breast.
4. Place the duck breast on top of the turkey, spread it with one-fourth of the dressing mixture, and top with the stuffing mix.
5. Place the chicken breast on top of the duck and spread with one-fourth of the dressing mixture.
6. Supply your smoker with wood pellets and follow the manufacturer's specific start-up procedure. Preheat, with the lid closed, to 275°F.
7. Tightly roll up the stack, tie with butcher's string, and slather the whole thing with the remaining dressing mixture.
8. Wrap the bacon slices around the turducken and secure with toothpicks, or try making a bacon weave (see the technique for this in the Jalapeño-Bacon Pork Tenderloin recipe).
9. Place the turducken roulade in a roasting pan. Transfer to the grill, close the lid, and roast for 2 hours, or until a meat thermometer inserted in the turducken reads 165°F. Tent with aluminum foil in the last 30 minutes, if necessary, to keep from overbrowning.
10. Let the turducken rest for 15 to 20 minutes before carving. Serve warm.

Smoked Turkey Breast

Servings: 2 To 4
Cooking Time: 1 To 2 Hours
Ingredients:
- 1 (3-pound) turkey breast

- Salt
- Freshly ground black pepper
- 1 teaspoon garlic powder

Directions:
1. Supply your smoker with wood pellets and follow the manufacturer's specific start-up procedure. Preheat the grill, with the lid closed, to 180°F.
2. Season the turkey breast all over with salt, pepper, and garlic powder.
3. Place the breast directly on the grill grate and smoke for 1 hour.
4. Increase the grill's temperature to 350°F and continue to cook until the turkey's internal temperature reaches 170°F. Remove the breast from the grill and serve immediately.

Turkey With Apricot Barbecue Glaze

Servings: 4
Cooking Time: 30 Minutes
Ingredients:
- 4 turkey breast fillets
- 4 tablespoons chicken rub
- 1 cup apricot barbecue sauce

Directions:
1. Preheat the Traeger wood pellet grill to 365 degrees F for 15 minutes while the lid is closed.
2. Season the turkey fillets with the chicken run.
3. Grill the turkey fillets for 5 minutes per side.
4. Brush both sides with the barbecue sauce and grill for another 5 minutes per side.
5. Tips: You can sprinkle turkey with chili powder if you want your dish spicy.

Wood Pellet Chicken Wings With Spicy Miso

Servings: 6
Cooking Time: 25 Minutes
Ingredients:
- 2-pound chicken wings
- 3/4 cup soy
- 1/2 cup pineapple juice
- 1 tbsp sriracha
- 1/8 cup miso
- 1/8 cup gochujang
- 1/2 cup water
- 1/2 cup oil
- Togarashi

Directions:
1. Mix all ingredients then toss the chicken wings until well coated. Refrigerate for 12 minutes.
2. Preheat your wood pellet grill to 375°F. Place the chicken wings on the grill grates and close the lid.

Cook until the internal temperature reaches 165°F. Remove the wings from the grill and sprinkle with togarashi. Serve when hot and enjoy.
Nutrition Info: Calories: 704 Cal Fat: 56 g Carbohydrates: 24 g   Protein: 27 g Fiber: 1 g

Smoked Whole Chicken

Servings: 6 To 8
Cooking Time: 4 Hours
Ingredients:
- 1 whole chicken
- 2 cups Tea Injectable (using Not-Just-for-Pork Rub)
- 2 tablespoons olive oil
- 1 batch Chicken Rub
- 2 tablespoons butter, melted

Directions:
1. Supply your smoker with wood pellets and follow the manufacturer's specific start-up procedure. Preheat the grill, with the lid closed, to 180°F.
2. Inject the chicken throughout with the tea injectable.
3. Coat the chicken all over with olive oil and season it with the rub. Using your hands, work the rub into the meat.
4. Place the chicken directly on the grill grate and smoke for 3 hours.
5. Baste the chicken with the butter and increase the grill's temperature to 375°F. Continue to cook the chicken until its internal temperature reaches 170°F.
6. Remove the chicken from the grill and let it rest for 10 minutes, before carving and serving.

Smoked Chicken Thighs

Servings: 6
Cooking Time: 24 Minutes.
Ingredients:
- 6 chicken thighs
- ½ cup commercial BBQ sauce of your choice
- 1 ½ tablespoon poultry spice
- 4 tablespoons butter

Directions:
1. Place all ingredients in a bowl except for the butter. Massage the chicken to make sure that the chicken is coated with the marinade.
2. Place in the fridge to marinate for 4 hours.
3. Fire the Traeger Grill to 350F. Use hickory wood pellets. Close the lid and preheat for 15 minutes.
4. When ready to cook, place the chicken on the grill grate and cook for 12 minutes on each side.
5. Before serving the chicken, brush with butter on top.

Nutrition Info: Calories per serving: 504; Protein: 32.4g; Carbs: 2.7g; Fat: 39.9g Sugar: 0.9g

Wood Pellet Grilled Buffalo Chicken

Servings: 6
Cooking Time: 20 Minutes
Ingredients:
- 5 chicken breasts, boneless and skinless
- 2 tbsp homemade barbeque rub
- 1 cup homemade Cholula buffalo sauce

Directions:
1. Preheat the wood pellet grill to 400°F.
2. Slice the chicken into long strips and season with barbeque rub.
3. Place the chicken on the grill and paint both sides with buffalo sauce.
4. Cook for 4 minutes with the grill closed. Cook while flipping and painting with buffalo sauce every 5 minutes until the internal temperature reaches 165°F.
5. Remove from the grill and serve when warm. Enjoy.

Nutrition Info: Calories: 176 Cal Fat: 4 g Carbohydrates: 1 g Protein: 32 g Fiber: 0 g

Honey Garlic Chicken Wings

Servings: 4
Cooking Time: 1 Hour And 15 Minutes
Ingredients:
- 2 1/2 lb. chicken wings
- Poultry dry rub
- 4 tablespoons butter
- 3 cloves garlic, minced
- 1/2 cup hot sauce
- 1/4 cup honey

Directions:
1. Sprinkle chicken wings with dry rub.
2. Place on a baking pan.
3. Set the Traeger wood pellet grill to 350 degrees F.
4. Preheat for 15 minutes while the lid is closed.
5. Place the baking pan on the grill.
6. Cook for 50 minutes.
7. Add butter to a pan over medium heat.
8. Sauté garlic for 3 minutes.
9. Stir in hot sauce and honey.
10. Cook for 5 minutes while stirring.
11. Coat the chicken wings with the mixture.
12. Grill for 10 more minutes.
13. Tips: You can make the sauce in advance to reduce preparation time.

Smoked Airline Chicken

Servings: 4
Cooking Time: 1 To 2 Hours
Ingredients:
- 2 boneless chicken breasts with drumettes attached
- ½ cup soy sauce
- ½ cup teriyaki sauce
- ¼ cup canola oil
- ¼ cup white vinegar
- 1 tablespoon minced garlic
- ¼ cup chopped scallions
- 2 teaspoons freshly ground black pepper
- 1 teaspoon ground mustard

Directions:
1. Place the chicken in a baking dish.
2. In a bowl, whisk together the soy sauce, teriyaki sauce, canola oil, vinegar, garlic, scallions, pepper and ground mustard, then pour this marinade over the chicken, coating both sides.
3. Refrigerate the chicken in marinade for 4 hours, turning over every hour.
4. When ready to smoke the chicken, supply your smoker with wood pellets and follow the manufacturer's specific start-up procedure. Preheat, with the lid closed, to 250°F.
5. Remove the chicken from the marinade but do not rinse. Discard the marinade.
6. Arrange the chicken directly on the grill, close the lid, and smoke for 1 hour 30 minutes to 2 hours, or until a meat thermometer inserted in the thickest part of the meat reads 165°F.
7. Let the meat rest for 3 minutes before serving.

Paprika Chicken

Servings: 7
Cooking Time: 2 – 4 Hours
Ingredients:
- 4-6 chicken breast
- 4 tablespoons olive oil
- 2tablespoons smoked paprika
- ½ tablespoon salt
- ¼ teaspoon pepper
- 2teaspoons garlic powder
- 2teaspoons garlic salt
- 2teaspoons pepper
- 1teaspoon cayenne pepper
- 1teaspoon rosemary

Directions:
1. Preheat your smoker to 220 degrees Fahrenheit using your favorite wood Pellets
2. Prepare your chicken breast according to your desired shapes and transfer to a greased baking dish
3. Take a medium bowl and add spices, stir well

4. Press the spice mix over chicken and transfer the chicken to smoker
5. Smoke for 1-1 and a ½ hours
6. Turn-over and cook for 30 minutes more
7. Once the internal temperature reaches 165 degrees Fahrenheit
8. Remove from the smoker and cover with foil
9. Allow it to rest for 15 minutes
10. Enjoy!
Nutrition Info: Calories: 237 Fats: 6.1g Carbs: 14g Fiber: 3g

Turkey Legs

Servings: 4
Cooking Time: 5 Hours
Ingredients:
- 4 turkey legs
- For the Brine:
- 1/2 cup curing salt
- 1 tablespoon whole black peppercorns
- 1 cup BBQ rub
- 1/2 cup brown sugar
- 2 bay leaves
- 2 teaspoons liquid smoke
- 16 cups of warm water
- 4 cups ice
- 8 cups of cold water

Directions:
1. Prepare the brine and for this, take a large stockpot, place it over high heat, pour warm water in it, add peppercorn, bay leaves, and liquid smoke, stir in salt, sugar, and BBQ rub and bring it to a boil.
2. Remove pot from heat, bring it to room temperature, then pour in cold water, add ice cubes and let the brine chill in the refrigerator.
3. Then add turkey legs in it, submerge them completely, and let soak for 24 hours in the refrigerator.
4. After 24 hours, remove turkey legs from the brine, rinse well and pat dry with paper towels.
5. When ready to cook, switch on the Traeger grill, fill the grill hopper with hickory flavored wood pellets, power the grill on by using the control panel, select 'smoke' on the temperature dial, or set the temperature to 250 degrees F and let it preheat for a minimum of 15 minutes.
6. When the grill has preheated, open the lid, place turkey legs on the grill grate, shut the grill, and smoke for 5 hours until nicely browned and the internal temperature reaches 165 degrees F.
7. Serve immediately.
Nutrition Info: Calories: 416 Cal ;Fat: 13.3 g ;Carbs: 0 g ;Protein: 69.8 g ;Fiber: 0 g

Wood Pellet Grilled Chicken Kabobs

Servings: 6
Cooking Time: 12 Minutes
Ingredients:
- 1/2 cup olive oil
- 2 tbsp white vinegar
- 1 tbsp lemon juice
- 1-1/2 tbsp salt
- 1/2 tbsp pepper, coarsely ground
- 2 tbsp chives, freshly chopped
- 1-1/2 tbsp thyme, freshly chopped
- 2 tbsp Italian parsley freshly chopped
- 1tbsp garlic, minced
- Kabobs
- 1 each orange, red, and yellow pepper
- 1-1/2 pounds chicken breast, boneless and skinless
- 12 mini mushrooms

Directions:
1. In a mixing bowl, add all the marinade ingredients and mix well. Toss the chicken and mushrooms in the marinade then refrigerate for 30 minutes.
2. Meanwhile, soak the skewers in hot water. Remove the chicken from the fridge and start assembling the kabobs.
3. Preheat your wood pellet to 450°F.
4. Grill the kabobs in the wood pellet for 6 minutes, flip them and grill for 6 more minutes.
5. Remove from the grill and let rest. Heat up the naan bread on the grill for 2 minutes.
6. Serve and enjoy.
Nutrition Info: Calories: 165 Cal Fat: 13 g Carbohydrates: 1 g   Protein: 33 g Fiber: 0 g

Chicken Cordon Bleu

Servings: 6
Cooking Time: 40 Minutes
Ingredients:
- 6 boneless skinless chicken breasts
- 6 slices of ham
- 12 slices swiss cheese
- 1cup panko breadcrumbs
- ½ cup all-purpose flour
- 1tsp ground black pepper or to taste
- 1tsp salt or to taste
- 4tbsp grated parmesan cheese
- 2tbsp melted butter
- ½ tsp garlic powder
- ½ tsp thyme
- ¼ tsp parsley

Directions:

1. Butterfly the chicken breast with a pairing knife. Place the chicken breast in between 2 plastic wraps and pound with a mallet until the chicken breasts are ¼ inch thick.
2. Place a plastic wrap on a flat surface. Place one fat chicken breast on it.
3. Place one slice of swiss cheese on the chicken. Place one slice of ham over the cheese and place another cheese slice over the ham.
4. Roll the chicken breast tightly. Fold both ends of the roll tightly. Pin both ends of the rolled chicken breast with a toothpick.
5. Repeat step 3 and 4 for the remaining chicken breasts
6. In a mixing bowl, combine the all-purpose flour, ½ tsp salt, and ½ tsp pepper. Set aside.
7. In another mixing bowl, combine breadcrumbs, parmesan, butter, garlic, thyme, parsley, ½ tsp salt, and ½ tsp pepper. Set aside.
8. Break the eggs into another mixing bowl and whisk. Set aside.
9. Grease a baking sheet.
10. Bake one chicken breast roll. Dip into the flour mixture, brush with eggs and dip into breadcrumb mixture. The chicken breast should be coated.
11. Place it on the baking sheet.
12. Repeat steps 9 and 10 for the remaining breast rolls.
13. Preheat your grill to 375°F with the lid closed for 15 minutes.
14. Place the baking sheet on the grill and cook for about 40 minutes, or until the chicken is golden brown.
15. Remove the baking sheet from the grill and let the chicken rest for a few minutes.
16. Slice cordon bleu and serve.
Nutrition Info: Calories: 560 Total Fat: 27.4 g Saturated Fat: 15.9 g Cholesterol: 156mg Sodium: 1158 mg Total Carbohydrate: 23.2 g Dietary Fiber: 1.1 g Total Sugars: 1.2 g Protein: 54.3 g

Wood Pellet Chile Lime Chicken

Servings: 1
Cooking Time: 15 Minutes
Ingredients:
- 1 chicken breast
- 1 tbsp oil
- 1 tbsp chile-lime seasoning
Directions:
1. Preheat your wood pellet to 400°F.
2. Brush the chicken breast with oil on all sides.
3. Sprinkle with seasoning and salt to taste.
4. Grill for 7 minutes per side or until the internal temperature reaches 165°F.
5. Serve when hot or cold and enjoy.

Nutrition Info: Calories: 131 Cal Fat: 5 g Carbohydrates: 4 g   Protein: 19 g Fiber: 1 g

Rustic Maple Smoked Chicken Wings

Servings: 16
Cooking Time: 35 Minutes
Ingredients:
- 16 chicken wings
- 1 tablespoon olive oil
- 1 tablespoon Traeger Chicken Rub
- 1 cup Traeger 'Que BBQ Sauce or other commercial BBQ sauce of choice
Directions:
1. Place all ingredients in a bowl except for the BBQ sauce. Massage the chicken breasts so that it is coated with the marinade.
2. Place in the fridge to marinate for at least 4 hours.
3. Fire the Traeger Grill to 350F. Use maple wood pellets. Close the grill lid and preheat for 15 minutes.
4. Place the wings on the grill grate and cook for 12 minutes on each side with the lid closed.
5. Once the chicken wings are done, place in a clean bowl.
6. Pour over the BBQ sauce and toss to coat with the sauce.
Nutrition Info: Calories per serving: 230 ; Protein: 37.5g; Carbs: 2.2g; Fat: 7g Sugar: 1.3g

Budget Friendly Chicken Legs

Servings: 6
Cooking Time: 1½ Hours
Ingredients:
- For Brine:
- 1 C. kosher salt
- ¾ C. light brown sugar
- 16 C. water
- 6 chicken leg quarters
- For Glaze:
- ½ C. mayonnaise
- 2 tbsp. BBQ rub
- 2 tbsp. fresh chives, minced
- 1 tbsp. garlic, minced
Directions:
1. For brine: in a bucket, dissolve salt and brown sugar in water.
2. Place the chicken quarters in brine and refrigerate, covered for about 4 hours.
3. Set the temperature of Traeger Grill to 275 degrees F and preheat with closed lid for 15 minutes.
4. Remove chicken quarters from brine and rinse under cold running water.

5. With paper towels, pat dry chicken quarters.
6. For glaze: in a bowl, add all ingredients and mix till ell combined.
7. Coat chicken quarters with glaze evenly.
8. Place the chicken leg quarters onto grill and cook for about 1-1½ hours.
9. Serve immediately.
Nutrition Info: Calories per serving: 399; Carbohydrates: 17.2g; Protein: 29.1g; Fat: 24.7g; Sugar: 14.2g; Sodium: 15000mg; Fiber: 0g

Beer Can Chicken

Servings: 6
Cooking Time: 1 Hour And 15 Minutes
Ingredients:
- 5-pound chicken
- 1/2 cup dry chicken rub
- 1 can beer

Directions:
1. Preheat your wood pellet grill on smoke for 5 minutes with the lid open.
2. The lid must then be closed and then preheated up to 450 degrees Fahrenheit
3. Pour out half of the beer then shove the can in the chicken and use the legs like a tripod.
4. Place the chicken on the grill until the internal temperature reaches 165°F.
5. Remove from the grill and let rest for 20 minutes before serving. Enjoy.
Nutrition Info: Calories: 882 Cal Fat: 51 g Carbohydrates: 2 g Protein: 94 g Fiber: 0 g

Thanksgiving Dinner Turkey

Servings: 16
Cooking Time: 4 Hours
Ingredients:
- ½ lb. butter, softened
- 2 tbsp. fresh thyme, chopped
- 2 tbsp. fresh rosemary, chopped
- 6 garlic cloves, crushed
- 1 (20-lb.) whole turkey, neck and giblets removed
- Salt and freshly ground black pepper, to taste

Directions:
1. Set the temperature of Traeger Grill to 300 degrees F and preheat with closed lid for 15 minutes, using charcoal.
2. In a bowl, place butter, fresh herbs, garlic, salt and black pepper and mix well.
3. With your fingers, separate the turkey skin from breast to create a pocket.
4. Stuff the breast pocket with ¼-inch thick layer of butter mixture.

5. Season the turkey with salt and black pepper evenly.
6. Arrange the turkey onto the grill and cook for 3-4 hours.
7. Remove the turkey from grill and place onto a cutting board for about 15-20 minutes before carving.
8. With a sharp knife, cut the turkey into desired-sized pieces and serve.
Nutrition Info: Calories per serving: 965; Carbohydrates: 0.6g; Protein: 106.5g; Fat: 52g; Sugar: 0g; Sodium: 1916mg; Fiber: 0.2g

Wood Pellet Grilled Buffalo Chicken Leg

Servings: 6
Cooking Time: 25 Minutes
Ingredients:
- 12 chicken legs
- 1/2 tbsp salt
- 1 tbsp buffalo seasoning
- 1 cup buffalo sauce

Directions:
1. Preheat your wood pellet grill to 325°F.
2. Toss the legs in salt and buffalo seasoning then place them on the preheated grill.
3. Grill for 40 minutes ensuring you turn them twice through the cooking.
4. Brush the legs with buffalo sauce and cook for an additional 10 minutes or until the internal temperature reaches 165°F.
5. Remove the legs from the grill, brush with more sauce, and serve when hot.
Nutrition Info: Calories: 956 Cal Fat: 47 g Carbohydrates: 1 g Protein: 124 g Fiber: 0 g

Beer Can–smoked Chicken

Servings: 3 To 4
Cooking Time: 3 To 4 Hours
Ingredients:
- 8 tablespoons (1 stick) unsalted butter, melted
- ½ cup apple cider vinegar
- ½ cup Cajun seasoning, divided
- 1 teaspoon garlic powder
- 1 teaspoon onion powder
- 1 (4-pound) whole chicken, giblets removed
- Extra-virgin olive oil, for rubbing
- 1 (12-ounce) can beer
- 1 cup apple juice
- ½ cup extra-virgin olive oil

Directions:
1. In a small bowl, whisk together the butter, vinegar, ¼ cup of Cajun seasoning, garlic powder, and onion powder.

2. Use a meat-injecting syringe to inject the liquid into various spots in the chicken. Inject about half of the mixture into the breasts and the other half throughout the rest of the chicken.

3. Rub the chicken all over with olive oil and apply the remaining ¼ cup of Cajun seasoning, being sure to rub under the skin as well.

4. Drink or discard half the beer and place the opened beer can on a stable surface.

5. Place the bird's cavity on top of the can and position the chicken so it will sit up by itself. Prop the legs forward to make the bird more stable, or buy an inexpensive, specially made stand to hold the beer can and chicken in place.

6. Supply your smoker with wood pellets and follow the manufacturer's specific start-up procedure. Preheat, with the lid closed, to 250°F.

7. In a clean 12-ounce spray bottle, combine the apple juice and olive oil. Cover and shake the mop sauce well before each use.

8. Carefully put the chicken on the grill. Close the lid and smoke the chicken for 3 to 4 hours, spraying with the mop sauce every hour, until golden brown and a meat thermometer inserted in the thickest part of the thigh reads 165°F. Keep a piece of aluminum foil handy to loosely cover the chicken if the skin begins to brown too quickly.

9. Let the meat rest for 5 minutes before carving.

6. Squeeze 3 orange wedges into brine.

7. Add goose, 4 onion wedges, bay leaves, juniper berries and peppercorns in brine and refrigerate for 24 hours.

8. Set the temperature of Traeger Grill to 350 degrees F and preheat with closed lid for 15 minutes.

9. Remove the goose from brine and with paper towels, pat dry completely.

10. Season the in and outside of goose with salt and black pepper evenly.

11. Stuff the cavity with apple wedges, herbs, remaining orange and onion wedges.

12. With kitchen strings, tie the legs together loosely.

13. Place the goose onto a rack arranged in a shallow roasting pan.

14. Arrange the goose on grill and cook for about 1 hour.

15. With a basting bulb, remove some of the fat from the pan and cook for about 1 hour.

16. Again, remove excess fat from the pan and cook for about ½-1 hour more.

17. Remove goose from grill and place onto a cutting board for about 20 minutes before carving.

18. With a sharp knife, cut the goose into desired-sized pieces and serve.

Nutrition Info: Calories per serving: 907; Carbohydrates: 23.5g; Protein: 5.6g; Fat: 60.3g; Sugar: 19.9g; Sodium: 8000mg; Fiber: 1.1g

Christmas Dinner Goose

Servings: 12
Cooking Time: 3 Hours
Ingredients:
- 1½ C. kosher salt
- 1 C. brown sugar
- 20 C. water
- 1 (12-lb.) whole goose, giblets removed
- 1 naval orange, cut into 6 wedges
- 1 large onion, cut into 8 wedges
- 2 bay leaves
- ¼ C. juniper berries, crushed
- 12 black peppercorns
- Salt and freshly ground black pepper, to taste
- 1 apple, cut into 6 wedges
- 2-3 fresh parsley sprigs

Directions:
1. Trim off any loose neck skin.
2. Then, trim the first two joints off the wings.
3. Wash the goose under cold running water and with paper towels, pat dry it.
4. With the tip of a paring knife, prick the goose all over the skin.
5. In a large pitcher, dissolve kosher salt and brown sugar in water.

Chicken Tenders

Servings: 2 To 4
Cooking Time: 1 Hour, 20 Minutes
Ingredients:
- 1 pound boneless, skinless chicken breast tenders
- 1 batch Chicken Rub

Directions:
1. Supply your smoker with wood pellets and follow the manufacturer's specific start-up procedure. Preheat the grill, with the lid closed, to 180°F.
2. Season the chicken tenders with the rub. Using your hands, work the rub into the meat.
3. Place the tenders directly on the grill grate and smoke for 1 hour.
4. Increase the grill's temperature to 300°F and continue to cook until the tenders' internal temperature reaches 170°F. Remove the tenders from the grill and serve immediately.

Trager Smoked Spatchcock Turkey

Servings: 8
Cooking Time: 1 Hour 15 Minutes;
Ingredients:

- 1 turkey
- 1/2 cup melted butter
- 1/4 cup Traeger chicken rub
- 1 tbsp onion powder
- 1 tbsp garlic powder
- 1 tbsp rubbed sage

Directions:
1. Preheat your Traeger to high temperature.
2. Place the turkey on a chopping board with the breast side down and the legs pointing towards you.
3. Cut either side of the turkey backbone, to remove the spine. Flip the turkey and place it on a pan
4. Season both sides with the seasonings and place it on the grill skin side up on the grill.
5. Cook for 30 minutes, reduce temperature, and cook for 45 more minutes or until the internal temperature reaches 165F.
6. Remove from the Traeger and let rest for 15 minutes before slicing and serving.

Nutrition Info: Calories 156, Total fat 16g, Saturated fat 2g, Total carbs 1g, Net carbs 1g Protein 2g, Sugars 0g, Fiber 0g, Sodium 19mg

Wood Pellet Smoked Spatchcock Turkey

Servings: 6
Cooking Time: 1 Hour And 45 Minutes
Ingredients:
- 1 whole turkey
- 1/2 cup oil
- 1/4 cup chicken rub
- 1 tbsp onion powder
- 1 tbsp garlic powder
- 1 tbsp rubbed sage

Directions:
1. Preheat your wood pellet grill to high.
2. Meanwhile, place the turkey on a platter with the breast side down then cut on either side of the backbone to remove the spine.
3. Flip the turkey and season on both sides then place it on the preheated grill or on a pan if you want to catch the drippings. Grill on high for 30 minutes, reduce the temperature to 325°F, and grill for 45 more minutes or until the internal temperature reaches 165°F Remove from the grill and let rest for 20 minutes before slicing and serving. Enjoy.

Nutrition Info: Calories: 156 Cal Fat: 16 g Carbohydrates: 1 g Protein: 2 g Fiber: 0 g

Smoked Chicken With Apricot Bbq Glaze

Servings: 6
Cooking Time: 30 Minutes
Ingredients:

- 2 whole chicken, halved
- 4 tablespoon Traeger Chicken Rub
- 1 cup Trager Apricot BBQ Sauce

Directions:
1. Massage the chicken with the chicken rub. Allow to marinate for 2 hours in the fridge.
2. When ready to cook, fire the Traeger Grill to 350F. Use preferred wood pellets. Close the grill lid and preheat for 15 minutes.
3. Place the chicken on the grill grate and grill for 15 minutes on each side. Baste the chicken with Apricot BBQ glaze.
4. Once cooked, allow to rest for 10 minutes before slicing.

Nutrition Info: Calories per serving: 304; Protein: 49g; Carbs: 10.2g; Fat: 6.5g Sugar: 8.7g

Bbq Sauce Smothered Chicken Breasts

Servings: 4
Cooking Time: 30 Minutes
Ingredients:
- 1 tsp. garlic, crushed
- ¼ C. olive oil
- 1 tbsp. Worcestershire sauce
- 1 tbsp. sweet mesquite seasoning
- 4 chicken breasts
- 2 tbsp. regular BBQ sauce
- 2 tbsp. spicy BBQ sauce
- 2 tbsp. honey bourbon BBQ sauce

Directions:
1. Set the temperature of Traeger Grill to 450 degrees F and preheat with closed lid for 15 minutes.
2. In a large bowl, mix together garlic, oil, Worcestershire sauce and mesquite seasoning.
3. Coat chicken breasts with seasoning mixture evenly.
4. Place the chicken breasts onto the grill and cook for about 20-30 minutes.
5. Meanwhile, in a bowl, mix together all 3 BBQ sauces.
6. In the last 4-5 minutes of cooking, coat breast with BBQ sauce mixture.
7. Serve hot.

Nutrition Info: Calories per serving: 421; Carbohydrates: 10.1g; Protein: 41,2g; Fat: 23.3g; Sugar: 6.9g; Sodium: 763mg; Fiber: 0.2g

Lemon Chicken

Servings: 6
Cooking Time: 10 Minutes
Ingredients:
- 2 teaspoons honey
- 1 tablespoon lemon juice

- 1 teaspoon lemon zest
- 1 clove garlic, coarsely chopped
- 2 sprigs thyme
- Salt and pepper to taste
- ½ cup olive oil
- 6 chicken breast fillets

Directions:
1. Mix the honey, lemon juice, lemon zest, garlic, thyme, salt and pepper in a bowl.
2. Gradually add olive oil to the mixture.
3. Soak the chicken fillets in the mixture.
4. Cover and refrigerate for 4 hours.
5. Preheat the Traeger wood pellet grill to 400 degrees F for 15 minutes while the lid is closed.
6. Grill the chicken for 5 minutes per side.
7. Tips: You can also make additional marinade to be used for basting during grill time.

Easy Smoked Chicken Breasts

Servings: 4
Cooking Time: 30 Minutes
Ingredients:
- 4 large chicken breasts, bones and skin removed
- 1 tablespoon olive oil
- 2 tablespoons brown sugar
- 2 tablespoons maple syrup
- 1 teaspoon celery seeds
- 2 tablespoons paprika
- 2 tablespoons salt
- 1 teaspoon black pepper
- 2 tablespoons garlic powder
- 2 tablespoons onion powder

Directions:
1. Place all ingredients in a bowl and massage the chicken with your hands. Place in the fridge to marinate for at least 4 hours.
2. Fire the Traeger Grill to 350F and use maple wood pellets. Close the lid and allow to preheat to 15 minutes.
3. Place the chicken on the grill a and cook for 15 minutes with the lid closed.
4. Turn the chicken over and cook for another 10 minutes.
5. Insert a thermometer into the thickest part of the chicken and make sure that the temperature reads to 165F.
6. Remove the chicken from the grill and allow to rest for 5 minutes before slicing.
Nutrition Info: Calories per serving: 327 ; Protein: 40 g; Carbs: 23g; Fat: 9g Sugar: 13g

Maple Turkey Breast

Servings: 4
Cooking Time: 2 Hours
Ingredients:
- 3 tablespoons olive oil
- 3 tablespoons dark brown sugar
- 3 tablespoons garlic, minced
- 2 tablespoons Cajun seasoning
- 2 tablespoons Worcestershire sauce
- 6 lb. turkey breast fillets

Directions:
1. Combine olive oil, sugar, garlic, Cajun seasoning and Worcestershire sauce in a bowl.
2. Soak the turkey breast fillets in the marinade.
3. Cover and marinate for 4 hours.
4. Grill the turkey at 180 degrees F for 2 hours.
5. Tips: You can also sprinkle dry rub on the turkey before grilling.

Sweet Sriracha Bbq Chicken

Servings: 5
Cooking Time: 1 And ½-2 Hours
Ingredients:
- 1cup sriracha
- ½ cup butter
- ½ cup molasses
- ½ cup ketchup
- ¼ cup firmly packed brown sugar
- 1teaspoon salt
- 1teaspoon fresh ground black pepper
- 1whole chicken, cut into pieces
- ½ teaspoon fresh parsley leaves, chopped

Directions:
1. Preheat your smoker to 250 degrees Fahrenheit using cherry wood
2. Take a medium saucepan and place it over low heat, stir in butter, sriracha, ketchup, molasses, brown sugar, mustard, pepper and salt and keep stirring until the sugar and salt dissolves
3. Divide the sauce into two portions
4. Brush the chicken half with the sauce and reserve the remaining for serving
5. Make sure to keep the sauce for serving on the side, and keep the other portion for basting
6. Transfer chicken to your smoker rack and smoke for about 1 and a ½ to 2 hours until the internal temperature reaches 165 degrees Fahrenheit
7. Sprinkle chicken with parsley and serve with reserved BBQ sauce
8. Enjoy!
Nutrition Info: Calories: 148 Fats: 0.6g Carbs: 10g Fiber: 1g

Barbecue Chicken Wings

Servings: 4
Cooking Time: 15 Minutes
Ingredients:
- Fresh chicken wings
- Salt to taste
- Pepper to taste
- Garlic powder
- Onion powder
- Cayenne
- Paprika
- Seasoning salt
- Bbq sauce to taste

Directions:
1. Preheat the wood pellet grill to low.
2. In a mixing bowl, mix all the seasoning ingredients then toss the chicken wings until well coated.
3. Place the wings on the grill and cook for 20 minutes or until the wings are fully cooked.
4. Let rest to cool for 5 minutes then toss with bbq sauce.
5. Serve with orzo and salad. Enjoy.

Nutrition Info: Calories 311, Total fat 22g, Saturated fat 4g, Total carbs 22g, Net carbs 19g, Protein 22g, Sugar 12g, Fiber 3g, Sodium: 1400mg

Smoked Turkey Wings

Servings: 2
Cooking Time: 1 Hour
Ingredients:
- 4 turkey wings
- 1 batch Sweet and Spicy Cinnamon Rub

Directions:
1. Supply your smoker with wood pellets and follow the manufacturer's specific start-up procedure. Preheat the grill, with the lid closed, to 180°F.
2. Using your hands, work the rub into the turkey wings, coating them completely.
3. Place the wings directly on the grill grate and cook for 30 minutes.
4. Increase the grill's temperature to 325°F and continue to cook until the turkey's internal temperature reaches 170°F. Remove the wings from the grill and serve immediately.

South-east-asian Chicken Drumsticks

Servings: 6
Cooking Time: 2 Hours
Ingredients:
- 1 C. fresh orange juice
- ¼ C. honey
- 2 tbsp. sweet chili sauce
- 2 tbsp. hoisin sauce
- 2 tbsp. fresh ginger, grated finely
- 2 tbsp. garlic, minced
- 1 tsp. Sriracha
- ½ tsp. sesame oil
- 6 chicken drumsticks

Directions:
1. Set the temperature of Traeger Grill to 225 degrees F and preheat with closed lid for 15 minutes, using charcoal.
2. In a bowl, place all ingredients except for chicken drumsticks and mix until well combined.
3. Reserve half of honey mixture in a small bowl.
4. In the bowl of remaining sauce, add drumsticks and mix well.
5. Arrange the chicken drumsticks onto the grill and cook for about 2 hours, basting with remaining sauce occasionally.
6. Serve hot.

Nutrition Info: Calories per serving: 385; Carbohydrates: 22.7g; Protein: 47.6g; Fat: 10.5g; Sugar: 18.6g; Sodium: 270mg; Fiber: 0.6g

Rosemary Orange Chicken

Servings: 6
Cooking Time: 45 Minutes
Ingredients:
- 4 pounds chicken, backbone removed
- For the Marinade:
- 2 teaspoons salt
- 3 tablespoons chopped rosemary leaves
- 2 teaspoons Dijon mustard
- 1 orange, zested
- 1/4 cup olive oil
- ¼ cup of orange juice

Directions:
1. Prepare the chicken and for this, rinse the chicken, pat dry with paper towels and then place in a large baking dish.
2. Prepare the marinade and for this, take a medium bowl, place all of its ingredients in it and whisk until combined.
3. Cover chicken with the prepared marinade, cover with a plastic wrap, and then marinate for a minimum of 2 hours in the refrigerator, turning halfway.
4. When ready to cook, switch on the Traeger grill, fill the grill hopper with flavored wood pellets, power the grill on by using the control panel, select 'smoke' on the temperature dial, or set the temperature to 350 degrees F and let it preheat for a minimum of 5 minutes.

5. When the grill has preheated, open the lid, place chicken on the grill grate skin-side down, shut the grill and smoke for 45 minutes until well browned, and the internal temperature reaches 165 degrees F.
6. When done, transfer chicken to a cutting board, let it rest for 10 minutes, cut it into slices, and then serve.
Nutrition Info: Calories: 258 Cal ;Fat: 17.4 g ;Carbs: 5.2 g ;Protein: 19.3 g ;Fiber: 0.3 g

Buttered Thanksgiving Turkey

Servings: 12 To 14
Cooking Time: 5 To 6 Hours
Ingredients:
- 1 whole turkey (make sure the turkey is not pre-brined)
- 2 batches Garlic Butter Injectable
- 3 tablespoons olive oil
- 1 batch Chicken Rub
- 2 tablespoons butter

Directions:
1. Supply your smoker with wood pellets and follow the manufacturer's specific start-up procedure. Preheat the grill, with the lid closed, to 180°F.
2. Inject the turkey throughout with the garlic butter injectable. Coat the turkey with olive oil and season it with the rub. Using your hands, work the rub into the meat and skin.
3. Place the turkey directly on the grill grate and smoke for 3 or 4 hours (for an 8- to 12-pound turkey, cook for 3 hours; for a turkey over 12 pounds, cook for 4 hours), basting it with butter every hour.
4. Increase the grill's temperature to 375°F and continue to cook until the turkey's internal temperature reaches 170°F.
5. Remove the turkey from the grill and let it rest for 10 minutes, before carving and serving.

Traeger Smoked Cornish Hens

Servings: 6
Cooking Time: 1 Hour
Ingredients:
- 6 Cornish hens
- 3 tbsp canola oil
- 6 tbsp rub

Directions:
1. Preheat your Traeger to 275F.
2. Meanwhile, rub the hens with canola oil then with your favorite rub.
3. Place the hens on the grill with the breast side down. Smoke for 30 minutes.

4. Flip the hens and increase the Traeger temperature to 400F. Cook until the internal temperature reaches 165F.
5. Remove the hens from the grill and let rest for 10 minutes before serving.
Nutrition Info: Calories 696, Total fat 50g, Saturated fat 13g, Total carbs 1g, Net carbs 1g Protein 57g, Sugars 0g, Fiber 0g, Sodium 165mg

Buffalo Wings

Servings: 2 To 3
Cooking Time: 35 Minutes
Ingredients:
- 1 pound chicken wings
- 1 batch Chicken Rub
- 1 cup Frank's Red-Hot Sauce, Buffalo wing sauce, or similar

Directions:
1. Supply your smoker with wood pellets and follow the manufacturer's specific start-up procedure. Preheat the grill, with the lid closed, to 300°F.
2. Season the chicken wings with the rub. Using your hands, work the rub into the meat.
3. Place the wings directly on the grill grate and smoke until their internal temperature reaches 160°F.
4. Baste the wings with the sauce and continue to smoke until the wings' internal temperature reaches 170°F.

Lemon Rosemary And Beer Marinated Chicken

Servings: 6
Cooking Time: 55 Minutes
Ingredients:
- 1 whole chicken
- 1 lemon, zested and juiced
- 1 teaspoon salt
- 1 teaspoon ground black pepper
- 1 teaspoon rosemary, chopped
- 12-ounce beer, apple-flavored

Directions:
1. Place all ingredients in a bowl and allow the chicken to marinate for at least 12 hours in the fridge.
2. When ready to cook, fire the Traeger Grill to 350F. Use preferred wood pellets. Close the grill lid and preheat for 15 minutes.
3. Place the chicken on the grill grate and cook for 55 minutes.
4. Cook until the internal temperature reads at 165F.
5. Take the chicken out and allow to rest before carving.

Nutrition Info: Calories per serving: 288; Protein: 36.1g; Carbs: 4.4g; Fat: 13.1g Sugar: 0.7g

Traeger Chile Lime Chicken

Servings: 1
Cooking Time: 15 Minutes
Ingredients:
- 1 chicken breast
- 1 tbsp oil
- 1 tbsp spiceology Chile Lime Seasoning

Directions:
1. Preheat your Traeger to 400F.
2. Brush the chicken breast with oil then sprinkle the chile-lime seasoning and salt.
3. Place the chicken breast on the grill and cook for 7 minutes on each side or until the internal temperature reaches 165F.
4. Serve when hot and enjoy.

Nutrition Info: Calories 131, Total fat 5g, Saturated fat 1g, Total carbs 4g, Net carbs 3g Protein 19g, Sugars 1g, Fiber 1g, Sodium 235mg

Traeger Asian Miso Chicken Wings

Servings: 6
Cooking Time: 25 Minutes
Ingredients:
- 2 lb chicken wings
- 3/4 cup soy
- 1/2 cup pineapple juice
- 1 tbsp sriracha
- 1/8 cup miso
- 1/8 cup gochujang
- 1/2 cup water
- 1/2 cup oil
- Togarashi

Directions:
1. Preheat the Traeger to 375F.
2. Combine all the ingredients except togarashi in a zip lock bag. Toss until the chicken wings are well coated. Refrigerate for 12 hours
3. Pace the wings on the grill grates and close the lid. Cook for 25 minutes or until the internal temperature reaches 165F
4. Remove the wings from the Traeger and sprinkle Togarashi.
5. Serve when hot and enjoy.

Nutrition Info: Calories 703, Total fat 56g, Saturated fat 14g, Total carbs 24g, Net carbs 23g Protein 27g, Sugars 6g, Fiber 1g, Sodium 1156mg

Lemon Chicken Breast

Servings: 4
Cooking Time: 30 Minutes
Ingredients:
- 6 chicken breasts, skinless and boneless
- ½ cup oil
- 1-3 fresh thyme sprigs
- 1teaspoon ground black pepper
- 2teaspoon salt
- 2teaspoons honey
- 1garlic clove, chopped
- 1lemon, juiced and zested
- Lemon wedges

Directions:
1. Take a bowl and prepare the marinade by mixing thyme, pepper, salt, honey, garlic, lemon zest, and juice. Mix well until dissolved
2. Add oil and whisk
3. Clean breasts and pat them dry, place in a bag alongside marinade and let them sit in the fridge for 4 hours
4. Preheat your smoker to 400 degrees F
5. Drain chicken and smoke until the internal temperature reaches 165 degrees, for about 15 minutes
6. Serve and enjoy!

Nutrition Info: Calories: 230 Fats: 7g Carbs: 1g Fiber: 2g

Roasted Chicken With Pimenton Potatoes

Servings: 16
Cooking Time: 1 Hour
Ingredients:
- 2 whole chicken
- 6 clove garlic, minced
- 2 tablespoons salt
- 3 tablespoons pimento (smoked paprika)
- 3 tablespoons extra virgin olive oil
- 2 bunch fresh thyme
- 3 pounds Yukon gold potatoes

Directions:
1. Season the whole chicken with garlic, salt, paprika, olive oil, and thyme. Massage the chicken to coat all surface of the chicken with the spices. Tie the legs together with a string. Place in a baking dish and place the potatoes on the side. Season the potatoes with salt and olive oil.
2. Allow the chicken to rest in the fridge for 4 hours.
3. When ready to cook, fire the Traeger Grill to 300F. Use preferred wood pellets. Close the grill lid and preheat for 15 minutes.

4. Place the chicken and potatoes in the grill and cook for 1 hour until a thermometer inserted in the thickest part of the chicken comes out clean.

5. Remove from the grill and allow to rest before carving.

Nutrition Info: Calories per serving: 210; Protein: 26.1g; Carbs: 15.3g; Fat: 4.4g Sugar: 0.7g

Korean Chicken Wings

Servings: 6
Cooking Time: 1 Hour
Ingredients:
- 3 pounds of chicken wings
- 2 tablespoons olive oil
- For the Brine:
- 1 head garlic, halved
- 1 lemon, halved
- 1/2 cup sugar
- 1 cup of sea salt
- 4 sprigs of thyme
- 10 peppercorns
- 16 cups of water
- For the Sauce:
- 2 teaspoons minced garlic
- 1/2 cup gochujang hot pepper paste
- 1 tablespoon grated ginger
- 2 tablespoons of rice wine vinegar
- 1/3 cup honey
- 1/4 cup soy sauce
- 2 tablespoons lime juice
- 2 tablespoons toasted sesame oil
- 1/4 cup melted butter

Directions:
1. Prepare the brine and for this, take a large stockpot, place it over high heat, pour in water, stir in salt and sugar until dissolved, and bring to a boil.
2. Then remove the pot from heat, add remaining ingredients for the brine, and bring the brine to room temperature.
3. Add chicken wings, submerge them completely, cover the pot and let wings soak for a minimum of 4 hours in the refrigerator.
4. When ready to cook, switch on the Traeger grill, fill the grill hopper with flavored wood pellets, power the grill on by using the control panel, select 'smoke' on the temperature dial, or set the temperature to 375 degrees F and let it preheat for a minimum of 15 minutes.
5. Meanwhile, remove chicken wings from the brine, pat dry with paper towels, place them in a large bowl, drizzle with oil and toss until well coated.
6. When the grill has preheated, open the lid, place chicken wings on the grill grate, shut the grill, and smoke for 1 hour until the internal temperature reaches 165 degrees F.
7. Meanwhile, prepare the sauce and for this, take a medium bowl, place all of the sauce ingredients in it and whisk until smooth.
8. When done, transfer chicken wings to a dish, top with prepared sauce, toss until coated, and then serve.

Nutrition Info: Calories: 137 Cal ;Fat: 9 g ;Carbs: 4 g ;Protein: 8 g ;Fiber: 1 g

Smoked Chicken Drumsticks

Servings: 5
Cooking Time: 2 Hours 30 Minutes
Ingredients:
- 10 chicken drumsticks
- 2tsp garlic powder
- 1tsp salt
- 1tsp onion powder
- 1/2 tsp ground black pepper
- ½ tsp cayenne pepper
- 1tsp brown sugar
- 1/3 cup hot sauce
- 1tsp paprika
- ½ tsp thyme

Directions:
1. In a large mixing bowl, combine the garlic powder, sugar, hot sauce, paprika, thyme, cayenne, salt, and ground pepper. Add the drumsticks and toss to combine.
2. Cover the bowl and refrigerate for 1 hour.
3. Remove the drumsticks from the marinade and let them sit for about 1 hour until they are at room temperature.
4. Arrange the drumsticks into a rack.
5. Start your pellet grill on smoke, leaving the lid open for 5 minutes for the fire to start.
6. Close the lid and preheat grill to 250°F, using hickory or apple hardwood pellets.
7. Place the rack on the grill and smoke drumsticks for 2 hours, 30 minutes, or until the drumsticks' internal temperature reaches 180°F.
8. Remove drumsticks from heat and let them rest for a few minutes.
9. Serve.

Nutrition Info: Calories: 167 Total Fat: 5.4 g Saturated Fat: 1.4 g Cholesterol: 81 mg Sodium: 946 mg Total Carbohydrate: 2.6 g Dietary Fiber: 0.5 g Total Sugars: 1.3 g Protein: 25.7 g

Chicken Tikka Masala

Servings: 4
Cooking Time: 1 Hour

Ingredients:
- 1 tablespoon garam masala
- 1 tablespoon smoked paprika
- 1 tablespoon ground coriander
- 1 tablespoon ground cumin
- 1 teaspoon ground cayenne pepper
- 1 teaspoon turmeric
- 1 onion, sliced
- 6 cloves garlic, minced
- 1/4 cup olive oil
- 1 tablespoon ginger, chopped
- 1 tablespoon lemon juice
- 1 1/2 cups Greek yogurt
- 1 tablespoon lime juice
- 1 tablespoon curry powder
- Salt to taste
- 1 tablespoon lime juice
- 12 chicken drumsticks
- Chopped cilantro

Directions:
1. Make the marinade by mixing all the spices, onion, garlic, olive oil, ginger, lemon juice, yogurt, lime juice, curry powder and salt.
2. Transfer to a food processor.
3. Pulse until smooth.
4. Divide the mixture into two.
5. Marinade the chicken in the first bowl.
6. Cover the bowl and refrigerate for 12 hours.
7. Set the Traeger wood pellet grill to high.
8. Preheat it for 15 minutes while the lid is closed.
9. Grill the chicken for 50 minutes.
10. Garnish with the chopped cilantro.
11. Tips: You can also smoke the chicken before grilling.

Traeger Grilled Buffalo Chicken
Servings: 6
Cooking Time: 20 Minutes
Ingredients:
- 5 chicken breasts, boneless and skinless
- 2 tbsp homemade BBQ rub
- 1 cup homemade Cholula Buffalo sauce

Directions:
1. Preheat the Traeger to 400F.
2. Slice the chicken breast lengthwise into strips. Season the slices with BBQ rub.
3. Place the chicken slices on the grill and paint both sides with buffalo sauce.
4. Cook for 4 minutes with the lid closed. Flip the breasts, paint again with sauce and cook until the internal temperature reaches 165F.
5. Remove the chicken from the Traeger and serve when warm.

Nutrition Info: Calories 176, Total fat 4g, Saturated fat 1g, Total carbs 1g, Net carbs 1g Protein 32g, Sugars 1g, Fiber 0g, Sodium 631mg

Chicken Wings
Servings: 4
Cooking Time: 15 Minutes
Ingredients:
- Fresh chicken wings
- Salt to taste
- Pepper to taste
- Garlic powder
- Onion powder
- Cayenne
- Paprika
- Seasoning salt
- Barbeque sauce to taste

Directions:
1. Preheat the wood pellet grill to low. Mix seasoning and coat on chicken. Put the wings on the grill and cook. Place the wings on the grill and cook for 20 minutes or until the wings are fully cooked. Let rest to cool for 5 minutes then toss with barbeque sauce. Serve with orzo and salad. Enjoy.

Nutrition Info: Calories: 311 Cal Fat: 22 g Carbohydrates: 22 g   Protein: 22 g Fiber: 3 g

Traeger Grilled Chicken
Servings: 6
Cooking Time: 1 Hour 10 Minutes;
Ingredients:
- 5 lb. whole chicken
- 1/2 cup oil
- Traeger chicken rub

Directions:
1. Preheat the Traeger on the smoke setting with the lid open for 5 minutes. Close the lid and let it heat for 15 minutes or until it reaches 450..
2. Use bakers twine to tie the chicken legs together then rub it with oil. Coat the chicken with the rub and place it on the grill.
3. Grill for 70 minutes with the lid closed or until it reaches an internal temperature of 165F.
4. Remove the chicken from the Traeger and let rest for 15 minutes. Cut and serve.

Nutrition Info: Calories 935, Total fat 53g, Saturated fat 15g, Total carbs 0g, Net carbs 0g Protein 107g, Sugars 0g, Fiber 0g, Sodium 320mg

Cornish Game Hen
Servings: 4

Cooking Time: 2 To 3 Hours

Ingredients:
- 4 Cornish game hens
- Extra-virgin olive oil, for rubbing
- 2 teaspoons salt
- 1 teaspoon freshly ground black pepper
- 1 teaspoon celery seeds

Directions:
1. Supply your smoker with wood pellets and follow the manufacturer's specific start-up procedure. Preheat, with the lid closed, to 275°F.
2. Rub the game hens over and under the skin with olive oil and season all over with the salt, pepper, and celery seeds.
3. Place the birds directly on the grill grate, close the lid, and smoke for 2 to 3 hours, or until a meat thermometer inserted in each bird reads 170°F.
4. Serve the Cornish game hens hot.

4. Sprinkle prepared rub on the chicken wings and then toss until well coated.
5. Meanwhile,
6. When the grill has preheated, open the lid, place chicken wings on the grill grate, shut the grill and smoke for 40 minutes until golden brown and skin have turned crisp, turning halfway.
7. Meanwhile, prepare the sauce and for this, take a small saucepan, place it over medium-low heat, add butter in it and when it melts, add jalapeno and cook for 4 minutes.
8. Then stir in hot sauce and cilantro until mixed and remove the pan from heat.
9. When done, transfer chicken wings to a dish, top with prepared sauce, toss until coated, and then serve.

Nutrition Info: Calories: 250 Cal ;Fat: 15 g ;Carbs: 11 g ;Protein: 19 g ;Fiber: 1 g

Hellfire Chicken Wings

Servings: 6
Cooking Time: 40 Minutes
Ingredients:
- 3 pounds chicken wings, tips removed
- 2 tablespoons olive oil
- For the Rub:
- 1 teaspoon onion powder
- 1 teaspoon salt
- 1 teaspoon garlic powder
- 1 tablespoon paprika
- 1 teaspoon ground black pepper
- 1 teaspoon celery seed
- 1 teaspoon cayenne pepper
- 2 teaspoons brown sugar
- For the Sauce:
- 4 jalapeno peppers, sliced crosswise
- 8 tablespoons butter, unsalted
- 1/2 cup hot sauce
- 1/2 cup cilantro leaves

Directions:
1. Switch on the Traeger grill, fill the grill hopper with hickory flavored wood pellets, power the grill on by using the control panel, select 'smoke' on the temperature dial, or set the temperature to 350 degrees F and let it preheat for a minimum of 15 minutes.
2. Prepare the chicken wings and for this, remove tips from the wings, cut each chicken wing through the joint into two pieces, and then place in a large bowl.
3. Prepare the rub and for this, take a small bowl, place all of its ingredients in it and then stir until combined.

Wild West Wings

Servings: 4
Cooking Time: 1 Hour
Ingredients:
- 2 pounds chicken wings
- 2 tablespoons extra-virgin olive oil
- 2 packages ranch dressing mix (such as Hidden Valley brand)
- ¼ cup prepared ranch dressing (optional)

Directions:
1. Supply your smoker with wood pellets and follow the manufacturer's specific start-up procedure. Preheat, with the lid closed, to 350°F.
2. Place the chicken wings in a large bowl and toss with the olive oil and ranch dressing mix.
3. Arrange the wings directly on the grill, or line the grill with aluminum foil for easy cleanup, close the lid, and smoke for 25 minutes.
4. Flip and smoke for 20 to 35 minutes more, or until a meat thermometer inserted in the thickest part of the wings reads 165°F and the wings are crispy. (Note: The wings will likely be done after 45 minutes, but an extra 10 to 15 minutes makes them crispy without drying the meat.)
5. Serve warm with ranch dressing (if using).

Bbq Half Chickens

Servings: 4
Cooking Time: 75 Minutes
Ingredients:
- 3.5-pound whole chicken, cleaned, halved
- Summer rub as needed
- Apricot BBQ sauce as needed

Directions:

1. Switch on the Traeger grill, fill the grill hopper with apple-flavored wood pellets, power the grill on by using the control panel, select 'smoke' on the temperature dial, or set the temperature to 375 degrees F and let it preheat for a minimum of 15 minutes.
2. Meanwhile, cut chicken in half along with backbone and then season with summer rub.
3. When the grill has preheated, open the lid, place chicken halves on the grill grate skin-side up, shut the grill, change the smoking temperature to 225 degrees F, and smoke for 1 hour and 30 minutes until the internal temperature reaches 160 degrees F.
4. Then brush chicken generously with apricot sauce and continue grilling for 10 minutes until glazed.
5. When done, transfer chicken to cutting to a dish, let it rest for 5 minutes, and then serve.
Nutrition Info: Calories: 435 Cal ;Fat: 20 g ;Carbs: 20 g ;Protein: 42 g ;Fiber: 1 g

Authentic Holiday Turkey Breast

Servings: 6
Cooking Time: 4 Hours
Ingredients:
- ½ C. honey
- ¼ C. dry sherry
- 1 tbsp. butter
- 2 tbsp. fresh lemon juice
- Salt, to taste
- 1 (3-3½-pound) skinless, boneless turkey breast

Directions:
1. In a small pan, place honey, sherry and butter over low heat and cook until the mixture becomes smooth, stirring continuously.
2. Remove from heat and stir in lemon juice and salt. Set aside to cool.
3. Transfer the honey mixture and turkey breast in a sealable bag.
4. Seal the bag and shake to coat well.
5. Refrigerate for about 6-10 hours.
6. Set the temperature of Traeger Grill to 225-250 degrees F and preheat with closed lid for 15 minutes.
7. Place the turkey breast onto the grill and cook for about 2½-4 hours or until desired doneness.
8. Remove turkey breast from grill and place onto a cutting board for about 15-20 minutes before slicing.
9. With a sharp knife, cut the turkey breast into desired-sized slices and serve.
Nutrition Info: Calories per serving: 443; Carbohydrates: 23.7g; Protein: 59.2g; Fat: 11.4g; Sugar: 23.4g; Sodium: 138mg; Fiber: 0.1g

Traeger Chicken Breast

Servings: 6
Cooking Time: 15 Minutes
Ingredients:
- 3 chicken breasts
- 1 tbsp avocado oil
- 1/4 tbsp garlic powder
- 1/4 tbsp onion powder
- 3/4 tbsp salt
- 1/4 tbsp pepper

Directions:
1. Preheat your Traeger to 375F
2. Cut the chicken breast into halves lengthwise then coat with avocado oil.
3. Season with garlic powder, onion powder, salt, and pepper.
4. Place the chicken on the grill and cook for 7 minutes on each side or until the internal temperature reaches 165F
Nutrition Info: Calories 120, Total fat 4g, Saturated fat 1g, Total carbs 0g, Net carbs 0g Protein 19g, Sugars 0g, Fiber 0g, Sodium 309mg

Applewood-smoked Whole Turkey

Servings: 6 To 8
Cooking Time: 5 To 6 Hours
Ingredients:
- 1 (10- to 12-pound) turkey, giblets removed
- Extra-virgin olive oil, for rubbing
- ¼ cup poultry seasoning
- 8 tablespoons (1 stick) unsalted butter, melted
- ½ cup apple juice
- 2 teaspoons dried sage
- 2 teaspoons dried thyme

Directions:
1. Supply your smoker with wood pellets and follow the manufacturer's specific start-up procedure. Preheat, with the lid closed, to 250°F.
2. Rub the turkey with oil and season with the poultry seasoning inside and out, getting under the skin.
3. In a bowl, combine the melted butter, apple juice, sage, and thyme to use for basting.
4. Put the turkey in a roasting pan, place on the grill, close the lid, and grill for 5 to 6 hours, basting every hour, until the skin is brown and crispy, or until a meat thermometer inserted in the thickest part of the thigh reads 165°F.
5. Let the bird rest for 15 to 20 minutes before carving.

Serrano Chicken Wings

Servings: 4
Cooking Time: 40 Minutes
Ingredients:
- 4 lb. chicken wings
- 2 cups beer
- 2 teaspoons crushed red pepper
- Cajun seasoning powder
- 1 lb. Serrano chili peppers
- 1 teaspoon fresh basil
- 1 teaspoon dried oregano
- 4 cloves garlic
- 1 cup vinegar
- Salt and pepper to taste

Directions:
1. Soak the chicken wings in beer.
2. Sprinkle with crushed red pepper.
3. Cover and refrigerate for 12 hours.
4. Remove chicken from brine.
5. Season with Cajun seasoning.
6. Preheat your Traeger wood pellet grill to 325 degrees F for 15 minutes while the lid is closed.
7. Add the chicken wings and Serrano chili peppers on the grill.
8. Grill for 5 minutes per side.
9. Remove chili peppers and place in a food processor.
10. Grill the chicken for another 20 minutes.
11. Add the rest of the ingredients to the food processor.
12. Pulse until smooth.
13. Dip the chicken wings in the sauce.
14. Grill for 5 minutes and serve.
15. Tips: You can also use prepared pepper sauce to save time.

Maple And Bacon Chicken

Servings: 7
Cooking Time: 1 And ½ Hours
Ingredients:
- 4 boneless and skinless chicken breast
- Salt as needed
- Fresh pepper
- 12 slices bacon, uncooked
- 1cup maple syrup
- ½ cup melted butter
- 1teaspoon liquid smoke

Directions:
1. Preheat your smoker to 250 degrees Fahrenheit
2. Season the chicken with pepper and salt
3. Wrap the breast with 3 bacon slices and cover the entire surface
4. Secure the bacon with toothpicks

5. Take a medium-sized bowl and stir in maple syrup, butter, liquid smoke, and mix well
6. Reserve 1/3rd of this mixture for later use
7. Submerge the chicken breast into the butter mix and coat them well
8. Place a pan in your smoker and transfer the chicken to your smoker
9. Smoker for 1 to 1 and a ½ hours
10. Brush the chicken with reserved butter and smoke for 30 minutes more until the internal temperature reaches 165 degrees Fahrenheit
11. Enjoy!
Nutrition Info: Calories: 458 Fats: 20g Carbs: 65g Fiber: 1g

Peach And Basil Grilled Chicken

Servings: 4
Cooking Time: 35 Minutes
Ingredients:
- 4 boneless chicken breasts
- ½ cup peach preserves, unsweetened
- ½ cup olive oil
- ¼ cup apple cider vinegar
- 3 tablespoons lemon juice
- 2 tablespoons Dijon mustard
- 1 garlic clove, crushed
- ½ teaspoon red hot sauce
- ½ cup fresh basil leaves, chopped
- Salt to taste
- 4 peaches, halved, pit removed

Directions:
1. Place chicken in a bowl and stir in the peach preserves, olive oil, vinegar, lemon juice, Dijon mustard, garlic, red hot sauce, and basil leaves.
2. Massage the chicken until all surfaces are coated with the marinade. Marinate in the fridge for 4 hours.
3. Once ready to cook, fire the Traeger Grill to 400F. Use apple wood pellets. Close the lid and preheat for 15 minutes.
4. Place the chicken directly on the grill grate and cook for 35 minutes.
5. Flip the chicken halfway through the cooking time.
6. Ten minutes before the cooking time ends, place the peach halves and grill.
7. Serve with the chicken.
Nutrition Info: Calories per serving: 777; Protein: 61g; Carbs: 9.8g; Fat: 54.2g Sugar: 8g

Smoked Cornish Chicken In Wood Pellets

Servings: 6
Cooking Time: 1 Hour 10 Minutes
Ingredients:

- Cornish hens - 6
- Canola or avocado oil - 2-3 tbsp
- Spice mix - 6 tbsp

Directions:
1. Preheat your wood pellet grill to 275 degrees.
2. Rub the whole hen with oil and the spice mix. Use both of these ingredients liberally.
3. Place the breast area of the hen on the grill and smoke for 30 minutes.
4. Flip the hen, so the breast side is facing up. Increase the temperature to 400 degrees.
5. Cook until the temperature goes down to 165 degrees.
6. Pull it out and leave it for 10 minutes.
7. Serve warm with a side dish of your choice.

Nutrition Info: Carbohydrates: 1 g Protein: 57 g Fat: 50 g Sodium: 165 mg Cholesterol: 337 mg

Perfectly Smoked Turkey Legs

Servings: 6
Cooking Time: 4 Hours
Ingredients:
- For Turkey:
- 3 tbsp. Worcestershire sauce
- 1 tbsp. canola oil
- 6 turkey legs
- For Rub:
- ¼ C. chipotle seasoning
- 1 tbsp. brown sugar
- 1 tbsp. paprika
- For Sauce:
- 1 C. white vinegar
- 1 tbsp. canola oil
- 1 tbsp. chipotle BBQ sauce

Directions:
1. For turkey in a bowl, add the Worcestershire sauce and canola oil and mix well.
2. With your fingers, loosen the skin of legs.
3. With your fingers coat the legs under the skin with oil mixture.
4. In another bowl, mix together rub ingredients.
5. Rub the spice mixture under and outer surface of turkey legs generously.
6. Transfer the legs into a large sealable bag and refrigerate for about 2-4 hours.
7. Remove the turkey legs from refrigerator and set aside at room temperature for at least 30 minutes before cooking.
8. Set the temperature of Traeger Grill to 200-220 degrees F and preheat with closed lid for 15 minutes.
9. In a small pan, mix together all sauce ingredients on low heat and cook until warmed completely, stirring continuously.

10. Place the turkey legs onto the grill cook for about 3½-4 hours, coating with sauce after every 45 minutes.
11. Serve hot.

Nutrition Info: Calories per serving: 430; Carbohydrates: 4.9g; Protein: 51.2g; Fat: 19.5g; Sugar: 3.9g; Sodium: 1474mg; Fiber: 0.5g

Smoked Whole Duck

Servings: 6
Cooking Time: 2 Hours 30 Minutes
Ingredients:
- 5 pounds whole duck (trimmed of any excess fat)
- 1small onion (quartered)
- 1apple (wedged)
- 1orange (quartered)
- 1tbsp freshly chopped parsley
- 1tbsp freshly chopped sage
- ½ tsp onion powder
- 2tsp smoked paprika
- 1tsp dried Italian seasoning
- 1tbsp dried Greek seasoning
- 1tsp pepper or to taste
- 1tsp sea salt or to taste

Directions:
1. Remove giblets and rinse duck, inside and pour, under cold running water.
2. Pat dry with paper towels.
3. Use the tip of a sharp knife to cut the duck skin all over. Be careful not to cut through the meat. Tie the duck legs together with butcher's string.
4. To make a rub, combine the onion powder, pepper, salt, Italian seasoning, Greek seasoning, and paprika in a mixing bowl.
5. Insert the orange, onion, and apple to the duck cavity. Stuff the duck with freshly chopped parsley and sage.
6. Season all sides of the duck generously with rub mixture.
7. Start your pellet grill on smoke mode, leaving the lip open or until the fire starts.
8. Close the lid and preheat the grill to 325°F for 10 minutes.
9. Place the duck on the grill grate.
10. Roast for 2 to 21/2 hours, or until the duck skin is brown and the internal temperature of the thigh reaches 160°F.
11. Remove the duck from heat and let it rest for a few minutes.
12. Cut into sizes and serve.

Nutrition Info: Calories: 809 Total Fat: 42.9 g Saturated Fat: 15.8 g Cholesterol: 337 mg Sodium: 638 mg Total Carbohydrate: 11.7 g Dietary Fiber: 2.4 g Total Sugars: 7.5 g Protein: 89.6 g

Traeger Grilled Buffalo Chicken Legs

Servings: 8
Cooking Time: 1 Hour 15 Minutes;
Ingredients:
- 12 chicken legs
- 1/2 tbsp salt
- 1 tbsp buffalo seasoning
- 1 cup Buffalo sauce

Directions:
1. Preheat your Traeger to 325F.
2. Toss the chicken legs in salt and seasoning then place them on the preheated grill.
3. Grill for 40 minutes turning twice through the cooking.
4. Increase the heat and cook for 10 more minutes. Brush the chicken legs and brush with buffalo sauce. Cook for an additional 10 minutes or until the internal temperature reaches 165F.
5. Remove from the Traeger and brush with more buffalo sauce.
6. Serve with blue cheese, celery, and hot ranch.

Nutrition Info: Calories 956, Total fat 47g, Saturated fat 13g, Total carbs 1g, Net carbs 1g Protein 124g, Sugars 0g, Fiber 0g, Sodium 1750mg

Grilled Sweet And Sour Chicken

Servings: 6
Cooking Time: 35 Minutes
Ingredients:
- 6 cups water
- 1/3 cup salt
- ¼ cup brown sugar
- ¼ cup soy sauce
- 6 chicken breasts, boneless
- 1 cup granulated white sugar
- ½ cup ketchup
- 1 cup apple cider vinegar
- 2 tablespoons soy sauce
- 1 teaspoon garlic powder

Directions:
1. Place the water, salt, brown sugar, and soy sauce in a large bowl. Stir until well combined. Add in the chicken breasts into the brine and allow to soak for 24 hours in the refrigerator.
2. Fire the Traeger Grill to 350F. Use maple wood pellets. Close the grill lid and preheat for 15 minutes.
3. Place the breasts on the grill grate and cook for 35 minutes on each side with the lid closed. Flip the chicken halfway through the cooking time.
4. Meanwhile, place the remaining ingredients in a bowl and stir until combined.

5. Ten minutes before the chicken breasts are cooked, brush with the sauce.
6. Serve immediately.
Nutrition Info: Calories per serving: 675 ;
Protein: 61.9g; Carbs: 35.8g; Fat: 29.7g Sugar: 32.7g

Wild Turkey Egg Rolls

Servings: 4-6
Cooking Time: 40 Minutes
Ingredients:
- Corn - ½ cup
- Leftover wild turkey meat - 2 cups
- Black beans - ½ cup
- Taco seasoning - 3 tbsp
- Water ½ cup
- Rotel chilies and tomatoes - 1 can
- Egg roll wrappers- 12
- Cloves of minced garlic- 4
- 1 chopped Poblano pepper or 2 jalapeno peppers
- Chopped white onion - ½ cup

Directions:
1. Add some olive oil to a fairly large skillet. Heat it over medium heat on a stove.
2. Add peppers and onions. Sauté the mixture for 2-3 minutes until it turns soft.
3. Add some garlic and sauté for another 30 seconds. Add the Rotel chilies and beans to the mixture. Keeping mixing the content gently. Reduce the heat and then simmer.
4. After about 4-5 minutes, pour in the taco seasoning and ⅓ cup of water over the meat. Mix everything and coat the meat thoroughly. If you feel that it is a bit dry, you can add 2 tbsp of water. Keep cooking until everything is heated all the way through.
5. Remove the content from the heat and box it to store in a refrigerator. Before you stuff the mixture into the egg wrappers, it should be completely cool to avoid breaking the rolls.
6. Place a spoonful of the cooked mixture in each wrapper and then wrap it securely and tightly. Do the same with all the wrappers.
7. Preheat the pellet grill and brush it with some oil. Cook the egg rolls for 15 minutes on both sides until the exterior is nice and crispy.
8. Remove them from the grill and enjoy with your favorite salsa!

Nutrition Info: Carbohydrates: 26.1 g Protein: 9.2 g Fat: 4.2 g Sodium: 373.4 mg Cholesterol: 19.8 mg

Hickory Smoked Chicken Leg And Thigh Quarters

Servings: 6
Cooking Time: 2 Hours
Ingredients:
- 6 chicken legs (with thigh and drumsticks)
- 2 tablespoons olive oil
- Traeger Poultry Rub to taste

Directions:
1. Place all ingredients in a bowl and mix until the chicken pieces are coated in oil and rub. Allow to marinate for at least 2 hours.
2. Fire the Traeger Grill to 180F. Close the lid and allow to preheat for 10 minutes. Use hickory wood pellets to smoke your chicken.
3. Arrange the chicken on the grill grate and smoke for one hour. Increase the temperature to 350F and continue cooking for another hour until the chicken is golden and the juices run clean.
4. To check if the meat is cooked, insert a meat thermometer, and make sure that the temperature on the thickest part of the chicken registers at 165F.
5. Remove the chicken and serve.
Nutrition Info: Calories per serving: 358 ; Protein: 50.8g; Carbs: 0g; Fat: 15.7g Sugar:0 g

Buffalo Chicken Wraps

Servings: 4
Cooking Time: 20 Minutes
Ingredients:
- 2 teaspoons poultry seasoning
- 1 teaspoon freshly ground black pepper
- 1 teaspoon garlic powder
- 1 to 1½ pounds chicken tenders
- 4 tablespoons (½ stick) unsalted butter, melted
- ½ cup hot sauce (such as Frank's RedHot)
- 4 (10-inch) flour tortillas
- 1 cup shredded lettuce
- ½ cup diced tomato
- ½ cup diced celery
- ½ cup diced red onion
- ½ cup shredded Cheddar cheese
- ¼ cup blue cheese crumbles
- ¼ cup prepared ranch dressing
- 2 tablespoons sliced pickled jalapeño peppers (optional)

Directions:
1. Supply your smoker with wood pellets and follow the manufacturer's specific start-up procedure. Preheat, with the lid closed, to 350°F.
2. In a small bowl, stir together the poultry seasoning, pepper, and garlic powder to create an all-purpose rub, and season the chicken tenders with it.
3. Arrange the tenders directly on the grill, close the lid, and smoke for 20 minutes, or until a meat thermometer inserted in the thickest part of the meat reads 170°F.
4. In another bowl, stir together the melted butter and hot sauce and coat the smoked chicken with it.
5. To serve, heat the tortillas on the grill for less than a minute on each side and place on a plate.
6. Top each tortilla with some of the lettuce, tomato, celery, red onion, Cheddar cheese, blue cheese crumbles, ranch dressing, and jalapeños (if using).
7. Divide the chicken among the tortillas, close up securely, and serve.

Smoked And Fried Chicken Wings

Servings: 6
Cooking Time: 2 Hours
Ingredients:
- 3 pounds chicken wings
- 1 tbsp Goya adobo all-purpose seasoning
- Sauce of your choice

Directions:
1. Fire up your wood pellet grill and set it to smoke.
2. Meanwhile, coat the chicken wings with adobo all-purpose seasoning. Place the chicken on the grill and smoke for 2 hours.
3. Remove the wings from the grill.
4. Preheat oil to 375°F in a frying pan. Drop the wings in batches and let fry for 5 minutes or until the skin is crispy.
5. Drain the oil and proceed with drizzling preferred sauce
6. Drain oil and drizzle preferred sauce
7. Enjoy.
Nutrition Info: Calories: 755 Cal Fat: 55 g Carbohydrates: 24 g   Protein: 39 g Fiber: 1 g

Whole Smoked Chicken

Servings: 6
Cooking Time: 3 Hours
Ingredients:
- ½ cup salt
- 1 cup brown sugar
- 1 whole chicken (3 ½ pounds)
- 1 teaspoon minced garlic
- 1 lemon, halved
- 1 medium onion, quartered
- 3 whole cloves
- 5 sprigs of thyme

Directions:

1. Dissolve the salt and sugar in 4 liters of water. Once dissolved, place the chicken in the brine and allow to marinate for 24 hours.
2. When ready to cook, fire the Traeger Grill up to 250F and allow to preheat for 15 minutes with the lid closed. Use any wood pellet desired but we recommend using the maple wood pellet.
3. While the grill is preheating, remove the chicken from the brine and pat dry using paper towel. Rub the minced garlic all over the chicken. Stuff the cavity of the chicken with the remaining ingredients.
4. Tie the legs together with a natural string.
5. Place the stuffed chicken directly on the grill grate and smoke for 3 hours until the internal temperature of the chicken is 160F particularly in the breast part.
6. Take the chicken out and grill.
Nutrition Info: Calories per serving: 251; Protein: 32.6g; Carbs: 19g; Fat: 4.3g Sugar: 17.3g

Smoked Fried Chicken

Servings: 6
Cooking Time: 3 Hours
Ingredients:
- 3.5 lb. chicken
- Vegetable oil
- Salt and pepper to taste
- 2 tablespoons hot sauce
- 1 quart buttermilk
- 2 tablespoons brown sugar
- 1 tablespoon poultry dry rub
- 2 tablespoons onion powder
- 2 tablespoons garlic powder
- 2 1/2 cups all-purpose flour
- Peanut oil

Directions:
1. Set the Traeger wood pellet grill to 200 degrees F.
2. Preheat it for 15 minutes while the lid is closed.
3. Drizzle chicken with vegetable oil and sprinkle with salt and pepper.
4. Smoke chicken for 2 hours and 30 minutes.
5. In a bowl, mix the hot sauce, buttermilk and sugar.
6. Soak the smoked chicken in the mixture.
7. Cover and refrigerate for 1 hour.
8. In another bowl, mix the dry rub, onion powder, garlic powder and flour.
9. Coat the chicken with the mixture.
10. Heat the peanut oil in a pan over medium heat.
11. Fry the chicken until golden and crispy.
12. Tips: Drain chicken on paper towels before serving.

Smoke-roasted Chicken Thighs

Servings: 12 To 15
Cooking Time: 1 To 2 Hours
Ingredients:
- 3 pounds chicken thighs
- 2 teaspoons salt
- 2 teaspoons freshly ground black pepper
- 2 teaspoons garlic powder
- 2 teaspoons onion powder
- 2 cups prepared Italian dressing

Directions:
1. Place the chicken thighs in a shallow dish and sprinkle with the salt, pepper, garlic powder, and onion powder, being sure to get under the skin.
2. Cover with the Italian dressing, coating all sides, and refrigerate for 1 hour.
3. Supply your smoker with wood pellets and follow the manufacturer's specific start-up procedure. Preheat, with the lid closed, to 250°F.
4. Remove the chicken thighs from the marinade and place directly on the grill, skin-side down. Discard the marinade.
5. Close the lid and roast the chicken for 1 hour 30 minutes to 2 hours, or until a meat thermometer inserted in the thickest part of the thighs reads 165°F. Do not turn the thighs during the smoking process.

Lemon Chicken Breasts

Servings: 6
Cooking Time: 40 Minutes
Ingredients:
- 1 clove of garlic, minced
- 2 teaspoons honey
- 2 teaspoons salt
- 1 teaspoon black pepper, ground
- 2 sprigs fresh thyme leaves
- 1 lemon, zested and juiced
- ½ cup olive oil
- 6 boneless chicken breasts

Directions:
1. Make the marinade by combining the garlic, honey, salt, pepper, thyme, lemon zest, and juice in a bowl. Whisk until well-combined.
2. Place the chicken into the marinade and mix with hands to coat the meat with the marinade. Refrigerate for 4 hours.
3. When ready to grill, fire the Traeger Grill to 400F. Close the lid and preheat for 10 minutes.
4. Drain the chicken and discard the marinade.
5. Arrange the chicken breasts directly on to the grill grate and cook for 40 minutes or until the internal temperature of the thickest part of the chicken reaches to 165F.
6. Drizzle with more lemon juice before serving.

Nutrition Info: Calories per serving: 669;
Protein: 60.6g; Carbs: 3g; Fat: 44.9g Sugar: 2.1g

Smoked Drumsticks

Servings: 2 To 4
Cooking Time: 25 Minutes
Ingredients:
- 1 pound chicken drumsticks
- 2 tablespoons olive oil
- 1 batch Sweet and Spicy Cinnamon Rub

Directions:
1. Supply your smoker with wood pellets and follow the manufacturer's specific start-up procedure. Preheat the grill, with the lid closed, to 350°F.
2. Coat the drumsticks all over with olive oil and season with the rub. Using your hands, work the rub into the meat.
3. Place the drumsticks directly on the grill grate and smoke until their internal temperature reaches 170°F. Remove the drumsticks from the grill and serve immediately.

Chili Barbecue Chicken

Servings: 4
Cooking Time: 2 Hours And 10 Minutes
Ingredients:
- 1 tablespoon brown sugar
- 1 tablespoon lime zest
- 1 tablespoon chili powder
- 1/2 teaspoon ground cumin
- 1/2 tablespoon ground espresso
- Salt to taste
- 2 tablespoons olive oil
- 8 chicken legs
- 1/2 cup barbecue sauce

Directions:
1. Combine sugar, lime zest, chili powder, cumin, ground espresso and salt.
2. Drizzle the chicken legs with oil.
3. Sprinkle sugar mixture all over the chicken.
4. Cover with foil and refrigerate for 5 hours.
5. Set the Traeger wood pellet grill to 180 degrees F.
6. Preheat it for 15 minutes while the lid is closed.
7. Smoke the chicken legs for 1 hour.
8. Increase temperature to 350 degrees F.
9. Grill the chicken legs for another 1 hour, flipping once.
10. Brush the chicken with barbecue sauce and grill for another 10 minutes.
11. Tips: You can also add chili powder to the barbecue sauce.

Buffalo Chicken Flatbread

Servings: 6
Cooking Time: 30 Minutes
Ingredients:
- 6 mini pita bread
- 1-1/2 cups buffalo sauce
- 4 cups chicken breasts, cooked and cubed
- 3 cups mozzarella cheese
- Blue cheese for drizzling

Directions:
1. Preheat the wood pellet grill to 375-400°F.
2. Place the breads on a flat surface and evenly spread sauce over all of them.
3. Toss the chicken with the remaining buffalo sauce and place it on the pita breads.
4. Top with cheese then place the breads on the grill but indirectly from the heat. Close the grill lid.
5. Cook for 7 minutes or until the cheese has melted and the edges are toasty.
6. Remove from grill and drizzle with blue cheese. Serve and enjoy.

Nutrition Info: Calories: 254 Cal Fat: 13 g
Carbohydrates: 4 g   Protein: 33 g Fiber: 3 g

Wood-fired Chicken Breasts

Servings: 2 To 4
Cooking Time: 45 Minutes
Ingredients:
- 2 (1-pound) bone-in, skin-on chicken breasts
- 1 batch Chicken Rub

Directions:
1. Supply your smoker with wood pellets and follow the manufacturer's specific start-up procedure. Preheat the grill, with the lid closed, to 350°F.
2. Season the chicken breasts all over with the rub. Using your hands, work the rub into the meat.
3. Place the breasts directly on the grill grate and smoke until their internal temperature reaches 170°F. Remove the breasts from the grill and serve immediately.

Smoked Quarters

Servings: 2 To 4
Cooking Time: 2 Hours
Ingredients:
- 4 chicken quarters
- 2 tablespoons olive oil
- 1 batch Chicken Rub
- 2 tablespoons butter

Directions:

1. Supply your smoker with wood pellets and follow the manufacturer's specific start-up procedure. Preheat the grill, with the lid closed, to 180°F.
2. Coat the chicken quarters all over with olive oil and season them with the rub. Using your hands, work the rub into the meat.
3. Place the quarters directly on the grill grate and smoke for 1½ hours.
4. Baste the quarters with the butter and increase the grill's temperature to 375°F. Continue to cook until the chicken's internal temperature reaches 170°F.
5. Remove the quarters from the grill and let them rest for 10 minutes before serving.

Savory-sweet Turkey Legs

Servings: 4
Cooking Time: 4 To 5 Hours
Ingredients:
- 1 gallon hot water
- 1 cup curing salt (such as Morton Tender Quick)
- ¼ cup packed light brown sugar
- 1 teaspoon freshly ground black pepper
- 1 teaspoon ground cloves
- 1 bay leaf
- 2 teaspoons liquid smoke
- 4 turkey legs
- Mandarin Glaze, for serving

Directions:
1. In a large container with a lid, stir together the water, curing salt, brown sugar, pepper, cloves, bay leaf, and liquid smoke until the salt and sugar are dissolved; let come to room temperature.
2. Submerge the turkey legs in the seasoned brine, cover, and refrigerate overnight.
3. When ready to smoke, remove the turkey legs from the brine and rinse them; discard the brine.
4. Supply your smoker with wood pellets and follow the manufacturer's specific start-up procedure. Preheat, with the lid closed, to 225°F.
5. Arrange the turkey legs on the grill, close the lid, and smoke for 4 to 5 hours, or until dark brown and a meat thermometer inserted in the thickest part of the meat reads 165°F.
6. Serve with Mandarin Glaze on the side or drizzled over the turkey legs.

Wood Pellet Chicken Breasts

Servings: 6
Cooking Time: 15 Minutes
Ingredients:
- 3 chicken breasts
- 1 tbsp avocado oil

- 1/4 tbsp garlic powder
- 1/4 tbsp onion powder
- 3/4 tbsp salt
- 1/4 tbsp pepper

Directions:
1. Preheat your pellet to 375°F.
2. Half the chicken breasts lengthwise then coat with avocado oil.
3. With the spices, drizzle it on all sides to season
4. Drizzle spices to season the chicken. Put the chicken on top of the grill and begin to cook until its internal temperature approaches 165 degrees Fahrenheit. Put the chicken on top of the grill and begin to cook until it rises to a temperature of 165 degrees Fahrenheit
5. Serve and enjoy.
Nutrition Info: Calories: 120 Cal Fat: 4 g Carbohydrates: 0 g Protein: 19 g Fiber: 0 g

Traeger Grill Bbq Chicken Breasts

Servings: 4
Cooking Time: 30 Minutes
Ingredients:
- 4 whole chicken breasts, deboned
- ¼ cup olive oil
- 1 teaspoon pressed garlic
- 1 teaspoon Worcestershire sauce
- 1 teaspoon cayenne pepper powder
- ½ cup Traeger 'Que BBQ Sauce

Directions:
1. In a bowl, combine all ingredients except for the Traeger 'Que BBQ Sauce and make sure to rub the chicken breasts until coated with the mixture. Allow to marinate in the fridge for at least overnight.
2. Place the preferred wood pellets into the Traeger Grill and fire the grill. Allow the temperature to rise to 500F and preheat for 5 minutes. Reduce the temperature to 165F.
3. Place the chicken on the grill grate and cook for 30 minutes.
4. Five minutes before the chicken is done, glaze the chicken with Traeger's BBQ sauce.
5. Serve immediately.
Nutrition Info: Calories per serving: 631; Protein: 61g; Carbs: 2.9g; Fat: 40.5g Sugar: 1.5g

Crispy & Juicy Chicken

Servings: 6
Cooking Time: 5 Hours
Ingredients:
- ¾ C. dark brown sugar
- ½ C. ground espresso beans
- 1 tbsp. ground cumin

- 1 tbsp. ground cinnamon
- 1 tbsp. garlic powder
- 1 tbsp. cayenne pepper
- Salt and freshly ground black pepper, to taste
- 1 (4-lb.) whole chicken, neck and giblets removed

Directions:

1. Set the temperature of Traeger Grill to 200-225 degrees F and preheat with closed lid for 15 minutes.
2. In a bowl, mix together brown sugar, ground espresso, spices, salt and black pepper.
3. Rub the chicken with spice mixture generously.
4. Place the chicken onto the grill and cook for about 3-5 hours.
5. Remove chicken from grill and place onto a cutting board for about 10 minutes before carving.
6. With a sharp knife, cut the chicken into desired-sized pieces and serve.

Nutrition Info: Calories per serving: 540; Carbohydrates: 20.7g; Protein: 88.3g; Fat: 9.6g; Sugar: 18.1g; Sodium: 226mg; Fiber: 1.2g

Traditional Bbq Chicken

Servings: 8

Cooking Time: 1 To 2 Hours

Ingredients:

- 8 boneless, skinless chicken breasts
- 2 teaspoons salt
- 2 teaspoons freshly ground black pepper
- 2 teaspoons garlic powder
- 2 cups The Ultimate BBQ Sauce or your preferred barbecue sauce, divided

Directions:

1. Supply your smoker with wood pellets and follow the manufacturer's specific start-up procedure. Preheat, with the lid closed, to 250°F.
2. Place the chicken breasts in a large pan and sprinkle both sides with the salt, pepper, and garlic powder, being sure to rub under the skin.
3. Place the roasting pan on the grill, close the lid, and smoke for 1 hour 30 minutes to 2 hours, or until a meat thermometer inserted in the thickest part of each breast reads 165°F. During the last 15 minutes of cooking, cover the chicken with 1 cup of barbecue sauce.
4. Serve the chicken warm with the remaining 1 cup of barbecue sauce.

BEEF,PORK & LAMB RECIPES

Traeger Smoked Leg

Servings: 6
Cooking Time: 3 Hours
Ingredients:
- 1 leg of lamb, boneless
- 2 tbsp oil
- 4 garlic cloves, minced
- 2 tbsp oregano
- 1 tbsp thyme
- 2 tbsp salt
- 1 tbsp black pepper, freshly ground

Directions:
1. Trim excess fat from the lamb ensuring you keep the meat in an even thickness for even cooking.
2. In a mixing bowl, mix oil, garlic, and all spices. Rub the mixture all over the lamb then cover with a plastic wrap.
3. Place the lamb in a fridge and let marinate for an hour.
4. Transfer the lamb on a smoker rack and set the Traeger to smoke at 250F.
5. Smoke the meat for 4 hours or until the internal temperature reaches 145F
6. Remove from the Traeger and serve immediately.
Nutrition Info: Calories 356, Total fat 16g, Saturated fat 5g, Total carbs 3g, Net carbs 2g Protein 49g, Sugars 1g, Fiber 1g, Sodium 2474mg

Brown Sugar Lamb Chops

Servings: 4
Cooking Time: 10-15 Minutes
Ingredients:
- Pepper
- One t. garlic powder
- Salt
- Two t. tarragon
- One t. cinnamon
- ¼ c. brown sugar
- 4 lamb chops
- Two t. ginger

Directions:
1. Combine the salt, garlic powder, pepper, cinnamon, tarragon, ginger, and sugar. Coat the lamb chops in the mixture and chill for two hours.
2. Add wood pellets to your smoker and follow your cooker's startup procedure. Preheat your smoker, with your lid closed, until it reaches 450. Place the chops on the grill, cover, and smoke for 10-15 minutes per side. Serve.
Nutrition Info: Calories: 210 Cal Fat: 11 g Carbohydrates: 3 g Protein: 25 g Fiber: 1 g

Pineapple-pepper Pork Kebabs

Servings: 12 To 15
Cooking Time: 1 To 4 Hours
Ingredients:
- 1 (20-ounce) bottle hoisin sauce
- ½ cup Sriracha
- ¼ cup honey
- ¼ cup apple cider vinegar
- 2 tablespoons canola oil
- 2 teaspoons minced garlic
- 2 teaspoons onion powder
- 1 teaspoon ground ginger
- 1 teaspoon salt
- 1 teaspoon freshly ground black pepper
- 2 pounds thick-cut pork chops or pork loin, cut into 2-inch cubes
- 10 ounces fresh pineapple, cut into chunks
- 1 red onion, cut into wedges
- 1 bag mini sweet peppers, tops removed and seeded
- 12 metal or wooden skewers (soaked in water for 30 minutes if wooden)

Directions:
1. In a small bowl, stir together the hoisin, Sriracha, honey, vinegar, oil, minced garlic, onion powder, ginger, salt, and black pepper to create the marinade. Reserve ¼ cup for basting.
2. Toss the pork cubes, pineapple chunks, onion wedges, and mini peppers in the remaining marinade. Cover and refrigerate for at least 1 hour or up to 4 hours.
3. Supply your smoker with wood pellets and follow the manufacturer's specific start-up procedure. Preheat, with the lid closed, to 450°F.
4. Remove the pork, pineapple, and veggies from the marinade; do not rinse. Discard the marinade.
5. Use the double-skewer technique to assemble the kebabs (see Tip below). Thread each of 6 skewers with a piece of pork, a piece of pineapple, a piece of onion, and a sweet mini pepper, making sure that the skewer goes through the left side of the ingredients. Repeat the threading on each skewer two more times. Double-skewer the kebabs by sticking another 6 skewers through the right side of the ingredients.
6. Place the kebabs directly on the grill, close the lid, and smoke for 10 to 12 minutes, turning once. They are done when a meat thermometer inserted in the pork reads 160°F.

Citrus Pork Chops

Servings: 4
Cooking Time: 30 Minutes
Ingredients:
- 2 oranges, sliced into wedges
- 2 lemons, sliced into wedges
- 6 sprigs rosemary, chopped
- 2 sticks butter, softened
- 1 clove garlic, minced
- 4 tablespoons fresh thyme leaves, chopped
- 1 teaspoon black pepper
- 5 pork chops

Directions:
1. Set the Traeger wood pellet grill to smoke.
2. Wait for it to establish fire for 5 minutes.
3. Set temperature to high.
4. Squeeze lemons and oranges into a bowl.
5. Stir in the rest of the ingredients except the pork chops.
6. Marinate the pork chops in the mixture for 3 hours.
7. Grill for 10 minutes per side.
8. Tips: Use bone-in pork chops for this recipe.

Bacon-swiss Cheesesteak Meatloaf

Servings: 4
Cooking Time: 2 Hours
Ingredients:
- 1 tablespoon canola oil
- 2 garlic cloves, finely chopped
- 1 medium onion, finely chopped
- 1 poblano chile, stemmed, seeded, and finely chopped
- 2 pounds extra-lean ground beef
- 2 tablespoons Montreal steak seasoning
- 1 tablespoon A.Steak Sauce
- ½ pound bacon, cooked and crumbled
- 2 cups shredded Swiss cheese
- 1 egg, beaten
- 2 cups breadcrumbs
- ½ cup Tiger Sauce

Directions:
1. On your stove top, heat the canola oil in a medium sauté pan over medium-high heat. Add the garlic, onion, and poblano, and sauté for 3 to 5 minutes, or until the onion is just barely translucent
2. Supply your smoker with wood pellets and follow the manufacturer's specific start-up procedure. Preheat, with the lid closed, to 225°F.
3. In a large bowl, combine the sautéed vegetables, ground beef, steak seasoning, steak sauce, bacon, Swiss cheese, egg, and breadcrumbs. Mix with your hands until well incorporated, then shape into a loaf.

4. Put the meatloaf in a cast iron skillet and place it on the grill. Close the lid and smoke for 2 hours, or until a meat thermometer inserted in the loaf reads 165°F.
5. Top with the meatloaf with the Tiger Sauce, remove from the grill, and let rest for about 10 minutes before serving.

Grilled Lamb Sandwiches

Servings: 6
Cooking Time: 50 Minutes
Ingredients:
- 1 (4 pounds) boneless lamb.
- 1 cup of raspberry vinegar.
- 2 tablespoons of olive oil.
- 1 tablespoon of chopped fresh thyme.
- 2 pressed garlic cloves.
- 1/4 teaspoon of salt to taste.
- 1/4 teaspoon of ground pepper.
- Sliced bread.

Directions:
1. Using a large mixing bowl, add in the raspberry vinegar, oil, and thyme then mix properly to combine. Add in the lamb, toss to combine then let it sit in the refrigerator for about eight hours or overnight. Next, discard the marinade the season the lamb with salt and pepper to taste. Preheat a Wood Pellet Smoker and grill t0 400-500 degrees F, add in the seasoned lamb and grill for about thirty to forty minutes until it attains a temperature of 150 degrees F. Once cooked, let the lamb cool for a few minutes, slice as desired then serve on the bread with your favorite topping.

Nutrition Info: Calories: 407 Cal Fat: 23 g Carbohydrates: 26 g Protein: 72 g Fiber: 2.3 g

Cocoa Crusted Grilled Flank Steak

Servings: 7
Cooking Time: 6 Minutes
Ingredients:
- 1 tbsp cocoa powder
- 2 tbsp chili powder
- 1 tbsp chipotle chili powder
- 1/2 tbsp garlic powder
- 1/2 tbsp onion powder
- 1-1/2 tbsp brown sugar
- 1 tbsp cumin
- 1 tbsp smoked paprika
- 1 tbsp kosher salt
- 1/2 tbsp black pepper
- Olive oil
- 4 lb Flank steak

Directions:
1. Whisk together cocoa, chili powder, garlic powder, onion powder, sugar, cumin, paprika, salt, and pepper in a mixing bowl.
2. Drizzle the steak with oil then rub with the cocoa mixture on both sides.
3. Preheat your wood pellet grill for 15 minutes with the lid closed.
4. Cook the meat on the grill grate for 5 minutes or until the internal temperature reaches 135°F.
5. Remove the meat from the grill and let it cool for 15 minutes to allow the juices to redistribute.
6. Slice the meat against the grain and on a sharp diagonal.
7. Serve and enjoy.

Nutrition Info: Calories 420, Total fat 26g, Saturated fat 8g, Total carbs 21g, Net carbs 13g, Protein 3g, Sugar 7g, Fiber 8g, Sodium: 2410mg

Wood Pellet Pulled Pork

Servings: 12
Cooking Time: 12 Hours
Ingredients:
- 8 lb pork shoulder roast, bone-in
- BBQ rub
- 3 cups apple cider, dry hard

Directions:
1. Fire up the wood pellet grill and set it to smoke.
2. Meanwhile, rub the pork with bbq rub on all sides then place it on the grill grates. cook for 5 hours, flipping it every 1 hour.
3. Increase the heat to 225°F and continue cooking for 3 hours directly on the grate.
4. Transfer the pork to a foil pan and place the apple cider at the bottom of the pan.
5. Cook until the internal temperature reaches 200°F then remove it from the grill. Wrap the pork loosely with foil then let it rest for 1 hour.
6. Remove the fat layer and use forks to shred it.
7. Serve and enjoy.

Nutrition Info: Calories 912, Total fat 65g, Saturated fat 24g, Total Carbs 7g, Net Carbs 7g, Protein 70g, Sugar 6g, Fiber 0g, Sodium: 208mg

Smoked Baby Back Ribs

Servings: 10
Cooking Time: 2 Hours
Ingredients:
- 3 racks baby back ribs
- Salt and pepper to taste

Directions:
1. Clean the ribs by removing the extra membrane that covers it. Pat dry the ribs with a clean paper towel. Season the baby back ribs with salt and pepper to taste. Allow to rest in the fridge for at least 4 hours before cooking.
2. Once ready to cook, fire the Traeger Grill to 225F. Use hickory wood pellets when cooking the ribs. Close the lid and preheat for 15 minutes.
3. Place the ribs on the grill grate and cook for two hours. Carefully flipping the ribs halfway through the cooking time for even cooking.

Nutrition Info: Calories per serving: 1037; Protein: 92.5g; Carbs: 1.4g; Fat: 73.7g Sugar: 0.2g

Smoked Beef Ribs

Servings: 4 To 8
Cooking Time: 4 To 6 Hours
Ingredients:
- 2 (2- or 3-pound) racks beef ribs
- 2 tablespoons yellow mustard
- 1 batch Sweet and Spicy Cinnamon Rub

Directions:
1. Supply your Traeger with wood pellets and follow the start-up procedure. Preheat the grill, with the lid closed, to 225°F.
2. Remove the membrane from the backside of the ribs. This can be done by cutting just through the membrane in an X pattern and working a paper towel between the membrane and the ribs to pull it off.
3. Coat the ribs all over with mustard and season them with the rub. Using your hands, work the rub into the meat.
4. Place the ribs directly on the grill grate and smoke until their internal temperature reaches between 190°F and 200°F.
5. Remove the racks from the grill and cut them into individual ribs. Serve immediately.

Sweet Heat Burnt Ends

Servings: 8 To 10
Cooking Time: 6 Hours
Ingredients:
- 1 (6-pound) brisket point
- 2 tablespoons yellow mustard
- 1 batch Sweet Brown Sugar Rub
- 2 tablespoons honey
- 1 cup barbecue sauce
- 2 tablespoons light brown sugar

Directions:
1. Supply your Traeger with wood pellets and follow the start-up procedure. Preheat the grill, with the lid closed, to 225°F.

2. Using a boning knife, carefully remove all but about ½ inch of the large layer of fat covering one side of your brisket point.
3. Coat the point all over with mustard and season it with the rub. Using your hands, work the rub into the meat.
4. Place the point directly on the grill grate and smoke until its internal temperature reaches 165°F.
5. Pull the brisket from the grill and wrap it completely in aluminum foil or butcher paper.
6. Increase the grill's temperature to 350°F and return the wrapped brisket to it. Continue to cook until its internal temperature reaches 185°F.
7. Remove the point from the grill, unwrap it, and cut the meat into 1-inch cubes. Place the cubes in an aluminum pan and stir in the honey, barbecue sauce, and brown sugar.
8. Place the pan in the grill and smoke the beef cubes for 1 hour more, uncovered. Remove the burnt ends from the grill and serve immediately.

Traeger Grilled Leg Of Lamb Steak

Servings: 4
Cooking Time: 10 Minutes
Ingredients:
- 4 eaches lamb steaks, bone-in
- 1/4 cup olive oil
- 4 garlic cloves, minced
- 1 tbsp rosemary, freshly chopped
- Salt and pepper to taste

Directions:
1. Arrange the steak in a dish in a single layer. Cover the meat with oil, garlic, fresh rosemary, salt, and pepper.
2. Flip the meat to coat on all sides and let it marinate. For 30 minutes.
3. Preheat your Traeger and lightly oil the grates cook the meat on the grill until well browned on both sides and the internal temperature reaches 140F.
4. Serve and enjoy.
Nutrition Info: Calories 327.3, Total fat 21.9g, Saturated fat 5.3g, Total carbs 1.7g, Net carbs 1.5g Protein 29.6g, Sugars 0.1g, Fiber 0.2g, Sodium 112.1mg, Potassium 409.8mg

Traeger Bacon

Servings: 6
Cooking Time: 25 Minutes
Ingredients:
- 1lb bacon

Directions:
1. Preheat your Traeger to 375F.

2. Line a baking sheet with parchment paper then arrange the thick-cut bacon on it in a single layer.
3. Bake the bacon in the Traeger for 20 minutes. Flip the bacon pieces and cook for 20 more minutes or until the bacon is no longer floppy.
4. Serve and enjoy.
Nutrition Info: Calories 315, Total fat 10g, Saturated fat 0g, Total carbs 0g, Net carbs 0g Protein 9g, Sugars 0g, Fiber 0g, Sodium 500mg

Smoked Porchetta With Italian Salsa Verde

Servings: 8 To 12
Cooking Time: 3 Hours
Ingredients:
- 3 Tablespoon dried fennel seed
- 2 Tablespoon red pepper flakes
- 2 Tablespoon sage, minced
- 1 Tablespoon rosemary, minced
- 3 Clove garlic, minced
- As Needed lemon zest
- As Needed orange zest
- To Taste salt and pepper
- 6 Pound Pork Belly, skin on
- As Needed salt and pepper
- 1 Whole shallot, thinly sliced
- 6 Tablespoon parsley, minced
- 2 Tablespoon freshly minced chives
- 1 Tablespoon Oregano, fresh
- 3 Tablespoon white wine vinegar
- 1/2 Teaspoon kosher salt
- 3/4 Cup olive oil
- 1/2 Teaspoon Dijon mustard
- As Needed fresh lemon juice

Directions:
1. Prepare herb mixture: In a medium bowl, mix together fennel seeds, red pepper flakes, sage, rosemary, garlic, citrus zest, salt and pepper.
2. Place pork belly skin side up on a clean work surface and score in a crosshatch pattern. Flip the pork belly over and season flesh side with salt, pepper and half of the herb mixture.
3. Place trimmed pork loin in the center of the belly and rub with remaining herb mixture. Season with salt and pepper.
4. Roll the pork belly around the loin to form a cylindrical shape and tie tightly with kitchen twine at 1" intervals.
5. Season the outside with salt and pepper and transfer to refrigerator, uncovered and let air dry overnight.
6. When ready to cook, start the Traeger grill and set to Smoke.

7. Fit a rimmed baking sheet with a rack and place the pork on the rack seam side down.
8. Place the pan directly on the grill grate and smoke for 1 hour.
9. Increase the grill temperature to 325 degrees F and roast until the internal temperature of the meat reaches 135 degrees, about 2 1/2 hours. If the exterior begins to burn before the desired internal temperature is reached, tent with foil.
10. Remove from grill and let stand 30 minutes before slicing.
11. 1To make the Italian salsa verde: Combine shallot, parsley, chives, vinegar, oregano and salt in a medium bowl. Whisk in olive oil then stir in mustard and lemon juice.

Tender Flank Steak

Servings: 6
Cooking Time: 10 Minutes
Ingredients:
- ½ C. olive oil
- 1/3 C. fresh lemon juice
- 1/3 C. soy sauce
- ¼ C. brown sugar
- 2 tbsp. Worcestershire sauce
- 5 garlic cloves, minced
- 1 tsp. red chili powder
- 1 tsp. red pepper flakes, crushed
- 2 lb. flank steak

Directions:
1. In a resealable plastic bag, add all ingredients except for steak and mix well.
2. Place the steak and seal the bag.
3. Shake the bag vigorously to coat well.
4. Refrigerate to marinate overnight.
5. Set the temperature of Traeger Grill to 450 degrees F and preheat with closed lid for 15 minutes.
6. Place the steak onto the grill and cook for about 5 minutes per side.
7. Remove the steak from grill and place onto a cutting board for about 10 minutes before slicing.
8. With a sharp knife, cut the steak into slices across the grain.
Nutrition Info: Calories per serving: 482; Carbohydrates: 9.5g; Protein: 43.3g; Fat: 29.6g; Sugar: 7.5g; Sodium: 948mg; Fiber: 0.4g

Sweet & Spicy Pork Roast

Servings: 4
Cooking Time: 1 Hour And 30 Minutes
Ingredients:
- 3 lb. pork loin
- 1/2 teaspoon Chinese 5 spice

- 1 can coconut milk
- 1 habanero pepper
- 1 teaspoon curry powder
- 1 tablespoon paprika
- 1 teaspoon ginger, grated
- 1 tablespoon garlic, minced
- 1 tablespoon lime juice

Directions:
1. Place pork in a bowl.
2. In another bowl, combine the remaining ingredients.
3. Pour the mixture over the pork and marinate overnight covered in the refrigerator.
4. Set the Traeger wood pellet grill to 300 degrees F.
5. Preheat for 15 minutes while the lid is closed.
6. Add the pork to the grill.
7. Cook for 1 hour.
8. Flip and cook for another 30 minutes.
9. Tips: You can also marinate for at least 4 hours.

Traeger Tri-tip Roast

Servings: 6
Cooking Time: 3 Hours And 45 Minutes
Ingredients:
- 1 tri-tip roast
- Traeger 'Que BBQ Sauce, as needed
- Traeger Prime Rib Rub, as needed
- ½ cup beef broth

Directions:
1. Marinate the tri-trip roast in the Traeger Que BBQ Sauce overnight inside the fridge.
2. Once ready to cook, remove the beef from the marinade and season with the Prime Rib Rub.
3. Fire the Traeger Grill to 180F. Use desired wood pellets when cooking. Close the lid and preheat for 15 minutes.
4. Place the beef on the grill grate and cook for 3 hours.
5. Remove from the grill and place the beef on an aluminum foil sheet. Crimp the edges of the aluminum foil to create a sleeve.
6. Place the roast in the aluminum sleeve on the grill grate and pour over the beef broth.
7. Pour over the broth and increase the heat to 300F. Cook for 45 minutes.
Nutrition Info: Calories per serving: 357; Protein: 48g; Carbs: 1.7g; Fat: 16g Sugar: 0g

Apricot Pork Tenderloin

Servings: 4
Cooking Time: 1 ½ Hours
Ingredients:

- 2 pounds pork tenderloin
- 3 ounces Traeger Big Game Rub
- 1 cup Traeger Apricot BBQ Sauce

Directions:
1. Place the pork tenderloin in a bowl and massage with the Big Game Rub. Allow to rest in the fridge for 2 hours.
2. When ready to cook, fire the Traeger Grill to 355F. Use desired wood pellets when cooking. Close the lid and preheat for 15 minutes.
3. Place the seasoned pork tenderloin on the grill grate and close the lid. Cook for 1 ½ hours. Make sure to flip the pork tenderloin halfway through the cooking time.
4. 10 minutes before the cooking time ends, baste the meat with the apricot BBQ sauce.
5. Allow to rest for 10 minutes before slicing.

Nutrition Info: Calories per serving: 426; Protein: 65.3g; Carbs: 20.4g; Fat: 8.4g Sugar: 17.8g

Supper Beef Roast

Servings: 7
Cooking Time: 3 Hours
Ingredients:
- 3-1/2 beef top round
- 3 tbsp vegetable oil
- Prime rib rub
- 2 cups beef broth
- 1 russet potato, peeled and sliced
- 2 carrots, peeled and sliced
- 2 celery stalks, chopped
- 1 onion, sliced
- 2 thyme sprigs

Directions:
1. Rub the roast with vegetable oil and place it on the roasting fat side up. Season with prime rib rub then pour the beef broth.
2. Set the temperature to 500°F and preheat the wood pellet grill for 15 minutes with the lid closed.
3. Cook for 30 minutes or until the roast is well seared.
4. Reduce temperature to 225°F. Add the veggies and thyme and cover with foil. Cook for 3 more hours o until the internal temperature reaches 135°F.
5. Remove from the grill and let rest for 10 minutes. Slice against the grain and serve with vegetables and the pan dippings.
6. Enjoy.

Nutrition Info: Calories 697, Total fat 10g, Saturated fat 4.7g, Total Carbs 127g, Net Carbs 3106g, Protein 34g, Sugar 14g, Fiber 22g, Sodium: 3466mg, Potassium 2329mg

Bbq Brown Sugar Bacon

Servings: 3
Cooking Time: 30 Minutes
Ingredients:
- ½ cup brown sugar
- 1 tablespoon fennel, ground
- 2 teaspoons salt
- 1 teaspoon black pepper
- 1-pound pork belly, sliced thinly into bacon

Directions:
1. Place all ingredients in a bowl and mix until well combined. Allow seasoned pork to rest in the fridge for at least 3 hours.
2. When ready to cook, fire the Traeger Grill to 255F. Use maple wood pellets when cooking. Close the lid and preheat for 15 minutes.
3. Place the bacon on the grill grate and close the lid. Smoke for 20 to 30 minutes.

Nutrition Info: Calories per serving: 331 ; Protein: 26.2g; Carbs: 39.7g; Fat: 8.5g Sugar: 26.7g

Buttered Tenderloin

Servings: 8
Cooking Time: 45 Minutes
Ingredients:
- 1 (4-lb.) beef tenderloin, trimmed
- Smoked salt and cracked black pepper, to taste
- 3 tbsp. butter, melted

Directions:
1. Set the temperature of Traeger Grill to 300 degrees F and preheat with closed lid for 15 minutes.
2. Season the tenderloin with salt and black pepper generously and then rub with butter.
3. Place the tenderloin onto the grill and cook for about 45 minutes.
4. Remove the tenderloin from grill and place onto a cutting board for about 10-15 minutes before serving.
5. With a sharp knife, cut the tenderloin into desired-sized slices and serve.

Nutrition Info: Calories per serving: 505; Carbohydrates: 0g; Protein: 65.7g; Fat: 25.1g; Sugar: 0g; Sodium: 184mg; Fiber: 0g

Smoked Roast Beef

Servings: 5 To 8
Cooking Time: 12 To 14 Hours
Ingredients:
- 1 (4-pound) top round roast
- 1 batch Espresso Brisket Rub
- 1 tablespoon butter

Directions:

1. Supply your Traeger with wood pellets and follow the start-up procedure. Preheat the grill, with the lid closed, to 180°F.
2. Season the top round roast with the rub. Using your hands, work the rub into the meat.
3. Place the roast directly on the grill grate and smoke until its internal temperature reaches 140°F. Remove the roast from the grill.
4. Place a cast-iron skillet on the grill grate and increase the grill's temperature to 450°F. Place the roast in the skillet, add the butter, and cook until its internal temperature reaches 145°F, flipping once after about 3 minutes.
5. Remove the roast from the grill and let it rest for 10 to 15 minutes, before slicing and serving.

Traeger Blackened Pork Chops

Servings: 6
Cooking Time: 20 Minutes
Ingredients:
- 6 pork chops
- 1/4 cup blackening seasoning
- Salt and pepper

Directions:
1. Preheat your Traeger to 375F.
2. Generously season the pork chops with the blackening seasoning, salt, and pepper.
3. Place the chops on the Traeger grill and cook for 8 minutes on one side then flip.
4. Cook until the internal temperature reaches 1420F.
5. Let the pork chops rest for 10 minutes before slicing and serving.
Nutrition Info: Calories 333, Total fat 18g, Saturated fat 6g, Total carbs 1g, Net carbs 0g Protein 40g, Sugars 0g, Fiber 1g, Sodium 3175mg

Bbq Beef Short Ribs

Servings: 8
Cooking Time: 10 Hours
Ingredients:
- 4 beef short rib racks, membrane removed, containing 4 bones
- 1/2 cup beef rub
- 1 cup apple juice

Directions:
1. Switch on the Traeger grill, fill the grill hopper with apple-flavored wood pellets, power the grill on by using the control panel, select 'smoke' on the temperature dial, or set the temperature to 225 degrees F and let it preheat for a minimum of 15 minutes.

2. Meanwhile, prepare the ribs, and for this, sprinkle beef rub on both sides until well coated.
3. When the grill has preheated, open the lid, place ribs on the grill grate bone-side down, shut the grill, and smoke for 10 hours until internal temperature reaches 205 degrees F, spritzing with apple juice every hour.
4. When done, transfer ribs to a cutting board, let rest for 10 minutes, then cut into slices and serve.
Nutrition Info: Calories: 280 Cal ;Fat: 15 g ;Carbs: 17 g ;Protein: 20 g ;Fiber: 1 g

Easy-to-prepare Lamb Chops

Servings: 6
Cooking Time: 12 Minutes
Ingredients:
- 6 (6-oz.) lamb chops
- 3 tbsp. olive oil
- Salt and freshly ground black pepper, to taste

Directions:
1. Set the temperature of Traeger Grill to 450 degrees F and preheat with closed lid for 15 minutes.
2. Coat the lamb chops with oil and then, season with salt and black pepper evenly.
3. Arrange the chops onto the grill and cook for about 4-6 minutes per side.
4. Remove the chops from grill and serve hot.
Nutrition Info: Calories per serving: 376; Carbohydrates: 0g; Protein: 47.8g; Fat: 19.5g; Sugar: 0g; Sodium: 156mg; Fiber: 0g

Texas Smoked Brisket

Servings: 12 To 15
Cooking Time: 16 To 20 Hours
Ingredients:
- 1 (12-pound) full packer brisket
- 2 tablespoons yellow mustard
- 1 batch Espresso Brisket Rub
- Worcestershire Mop and Spritz, for spritzing

Directions:
1. Supply your Traeger with wood pellets and follow the start-up procedure. Preheat the grill, with the lid closed, to 225°F.
2. Using a boning knife, carefully remove all but about ½ inch of the large layer of fat covering one side of your brisket.
3. Coat the brisket all over with mustard and season it with the rub. Using your hands, work the rub into the meat. Pour the mop into a spray bottle.
4. Place the brisket directly on the grill grate and smoke until its internal temperature reaches 195°F, spritzing it every hour with the mop.

5. Pull the brisket from the grill and wrap it completely in aluminum foil or butcher paper. Place the wrapped brisket in a cooler, cover the cooler, and let it rest for 1 or 2 hours.
6. Remove the brisket from the cooler and unwrap it.
7. Separate the brisket point from the flat by cutting along the fat layer and slice the flat. The point can be saved for burnt ends (see Sweet Heat Burnt Ends), or sliced and served as well.

Smoked Midnight Brisket

Servings: 6
Cooking Time: 12 Hours
Ingredients:
- 1 tbsp Worcestershire sauce
- 1 tbsp Traeger beef Rub
- 1 tbsp Traeger Chicken rub
- 1 tbsp Traeger Blackened Saskatchewan rub
- 5 lb flat cut brisket
- 1 cup beef broth

Directions:
1. Rub the sauce and rubs in a mixing bowl then rub the mixture on the meat.
2. Preheat your grill to 180°F with the lid closed for 15 minutes. You can use super smoke if you desire.
3. Place the meat on the grill and grill for 6 hours or until the internal temperature reaches 160°F.
4. Remove the meat from the grill and double wrap it with foil.
5. Add beef broth and return to grill with the temperature increased to 225°F. Cook for 4 hours or until the internal temperature reaches 204°F.
6. Remove from grill and let rest for 30 minutes. Serve and enjoy with your favorite BBQ sauce.
Nutrition Info: Calories 200, Total fat 14g, Saturated fat 6g, Total carbs 3g, Net carbs 3g, Protein 14g, Sugar 0g, Fiber 0g, Sodium: 680mg

Simply Delicious Tri Tip Roast

Servings: 8
Cooking Time: 35 Minutes
Ingredients:
- 1 tbsp. granulated onion
- 1 tbsp. granulated garlic
- Salt and freshly ground black pepper, to taste
- 1 (3-lb.) tri tip roast, trimmed

Directions:
1. In a bowl, add all ingredients except for roast and mix well.
2. Coat the roast with spice mixture generously.
3. Set aside at room temperature until grill heats.

4. Set the temperature of Traeger Grill to 250 degrees F and preheat with closed lid for 15 minutes.
5. Place the roast onto the grill and cook for about 25 minutes.
6. Now, set the grill to 350-400 degrees F and preheat with closed lid for 15 minutes. and sear roast for about 3-5 minutes per side.
7. Remove the roast from grill and place onto a cutting board for about 15-20 minutes before slicing.
8. With a sharp knife, cut the roast into slices across the grain and serve.
Nutrition Info: Calories per serving: 313; Carbohydrates: 0.8g; Protein: 45.7g; Fat: 14.2g; Sugar: 0.3g; Sodium: 115mg; Fiber: 0.1g

Wood Pellet Smoked Beef Jerky

Servings: 10
Cooking Time: 5 Hours
Ingredients:
- 3 lb sirloin steaks, sliced into 1/4 inch thickness
- 2 cups soy sauce
- 1/2 cup brown sugar
- 1 cup pineapple juice
- 2 tbsp sriracha
- 2 tbsp red pepper flake
- 2 tbsp hoisin
- 2 tbsp onion powder
- 2 tbsp rice wine vinegar
- 2 tbsp garlic, minced

Directions:
1. Mix all the ingredients in a ziplock bag. Seal the bag and mix until the beef is well coated. Ensure you get as much air as possible from the ziplock bag.
2. Put the bag in the fridge overnight to let marinate. Remove the bag from the fridge 1 hour prior to cooking.
3. Startup your wood pallet grill and set it to smoke setting. Layout the meat on the grill with half-inch space between them.
4. Let them cook for 5 hours while turning after every 2-1/2 hours.
5. Transfer from the grill and let cool for 30 minutes before serving.
6. enjoy.
Nutrition Info: Calories 80, Total fat 1g, Saturated fat 0g, Total carbs 5g, Net carbs 5g, Protein 14g, Sugar 5g, Fiber 0g, Sodium: 650mg

Corned Beef And Cabbage

Servings: 6-8
Cooking Time: 4-5 Hours
Ingredients:
- 1-gallon water

- 1 (3- to 4-pound) point cut corned beef brisket with pickling spice packet
- 1 tablespoon freshly ground black pepper
- 1 tablespoon garlic powder
- ½ cup molasses
- 1 teaspoon ground mustard
- 1 head green cabbage
- 4 tablespoons (½ stick) butter
- 2 tablespoons rendered bacon fat
- 1 chicken bouillon cube, crushed

Directions:
1. Refrigerate overnight, changing the water as often as you remember to do so—ideally, every 3 hours while you're awake—to soak out some of the curing salt initially added.
2. Supply your smoker with wood pellets and follow the manufacturer's specific start-up procedure. Preheat, with the lid closed, to 275°F.
3. Remove the meat from the brining liquid, pat it dry, and generously rub with the black pepper and garlic powder.
4. Put the seasoned corned beef directly on the grill, fat-side up, close the lid, and grill for 2 hours. Remove from the grill when done.
5. In a small bowl, combine the molasses and ground mustard and pour half of this mixture into the bottom of a disposable aluminum pan.
6. Transfer the meat to the pan, fat-side up, and pour the remaining molasses mixture on top, spreading it evenly over the meat. Cover tightly with aluminum foil.
7. Transfer the pan to the grill, close the lid, and continue smoking the corned beef for 2 to 3 hours, or until a meat thermometer inserted in the thickest part reads 185°F.
8. Rest meat
9. Serve.

Nutrition Info: Calories: 295 Cal Fat: 17 g Carbohydrates: 19 g   Protein: 18 g Fiber: 6 g

Simple Traeger Grilled Lamb Chops

Servings: 6
Cooking Time: 20 Minutes
Ingredients:
- 1/4 cup white vinegar, distilled
- 2 tbsp olive oil
- 2 tbsp salt
- 1/2 tbsp black pepper
- 1 tbsp minced garlic
- 1 onion, thinly sliced
- 2 lb lamb chops

Directions:

1. In a resealable bag, mix vinegar, oil, salt, black pepper, garlic, and sliced onions until all salt has dissolved.
2. Add the lamb and toss until evenly coated. Place in a fridge to marinate for 2 hours.
3. Preheat your Traeger.
4. Remove the lamb from the resealable bag and leave any onion that is stuck on the meat. Use an aluminum foil to cover any exposed bone ends.
5. Grill until the desired doneness is achieved. Serve and enjoy when hot.

Nutrition Info: Calories 519, Total fat 44.8g, Saturated fat 18.4g, Total carbs 2.3g, Net carbs 1.9g Protein 25g, Sugars 0.8g, Fiber 0.4g, Sodium 861mg, Potassium 358.6mg

Traeger Beef Tenderloin

Servings: 6
Cooking Time: 45 Minutes
Ingredients:
- 4 lb beef tenderloin
- 3 tbsp steak rub
- 1 tbsp kosher salt

Directions:
1. Preheat the Traeger to high heat.
2. Meanwhile, trim excess fat from the beef and cut it into 3 pieces.
3. Coat the steak with rub and kosher salt. Place it on the grill.
4. Close the lid and cook for 10 minutes. Open the lid, flip the beef and cook for 10 more minutes.
5. Reduce the temperature of the grill until 225F and smoke the beef until the internal temperature reaches 130F.
6. Remove the beef from the grill and let rest for 15 minutes before slicing and serving.

Nutrition Info: Calories 999, Total fat 76g, Saturated fat 30g, Total carbs 0g, Net carbs 0g Protein 74g, Sugars 0g, Fiber 0g, Sodium 1234mmg

Simple Wood Pellet Smoked Pork Ribs

Servings: 7
Cooking Time: 5 Hours
Ingredients:
- 3 rack baby back ribs
- 3/4 cup pork and poultry rub
- 3/4 cup Que BBQ Sauce

Directions:
1. Peel the membrane from the backside of the ribs and trim any fat.
2. Season the pork generously with the rub.
3. Set the wood pellet grill to 180°F and preheat for 15 minutes with the lid closed.

4. Place the pork ribs on the grill and smoke them for 5 hours.
5. Remove the pork from the grill and wrap them in a foil with the BBQ sauce.
6. Place back the pork and increase the temperature to 350°F. Cook for 45 more minutes.
7. Remove the pork from the grill and let it rest for 20 minutes before serving. Enjoy.
Nutrition Info: Calories 762, Total fat 57g, Saturated fat 17g, Total Carbs 23g, Net Carbs 22.7g, Protein 39g, Sugar 18g, Fiber 0.5g, Sodium: 737mg, Potassium 618mg

Cocoa Crusted Pork Tenderloin

Servings: 5
Cooking Time: 25 Minutes
Ingredients:
- 1 pork tenderloin
- 1/2 tbsp fennel, ground
- 2 tbsp cocoa powder, unsweetened
- 1 tbsp smoked paprika
- 1/2 tbsp kosher salt
- 1/2 tbsp black pepper
- 1 tbsp extra virgin olive oil
- 3 green onion

Directions:
1. Remove the silver skin and the connective tissues from the pork loin.
2. Combine the rest of the ingredients in a mixing bowl, then rub the mixture on the pork. Refrigerate for 30 minutes.
3. Preheat the wood pellet grill for 15 minutes with the lid closed.
4. Sear all sides of the loin at the front of the grill then reduce the temperature to 350°F and move the pork to the centre grill.
5. Cook for 15 more minutes or until the internal temperature is 145°F.
6. Remove from grill and let rest for 10 minutes before slicing. Enjoy
Nutrition Info: Calories 264, Total fat 13.1g, Saturated fat 6g, Total Carbs 4.6g, Net Carbs 1.2g, Protein 33g, Sugar 0g, Fiber 3.4g, Sodium: 66mg

Sweet Smoked Country Ribs

Servings: 12 To 15
Cooking Time: 4 Hours
Ingredients:
- 2 pounds country-style ribs
- 1 batch Sweet Brown Sugar Rub
- 2 tablespoons light brown sugar
- 1 cup Pepsi or other cola
- ¼ cup The Ultimate BBQ Sauce

Directions:
1. Supply your smoker with wood pellets and follow the manufacturer's specific start-up procedure. Preheat the grill, with the lid closed, to 180°F.
2. Sprinkle the ribs with the rub and use your hands to work the rub into the meat.
3. Place the ribs directly on the grill grate and smoke for 3 hours.
4. Remove the ribs from the grill and place them on enough aluminum foil to wrap them completely. Dust the brown sugar over the ribs.
5. Increase the grill's temperature to 300°F.
6. Fold in three sides of the foil around the ribs and add the cola. Fold in the last side, completely enclosing the ribs and liquid. Return the ribs to the grill and cook for 45 minutes.
7. Remove the ribs from the foil and place them on the grill grate. Baste all sides of the ribs with barbecue sauce. Cook for 15 minutes more to caramelize the sauce.
8. Remove the ribs from the grill and serve immediately.

Rosemary Prime Rib

Servings: 8
Cooking Time: 1 Hour
Ingredients:
- 8 pounds whole ribeye roast
- 4 tablespoons olive oil
- 4 tablespoons peppercorns
- 3 whole rosemary sprigs
- ½ cup garlic, minced
- ½ cup smoked salt

Directions:
1. Fire the Traeger Grill to 500F. Use desired wood pellets when cooking. Close the lid and preheat for 15 minutes.
2. Cut the rib loin in half and sear the halves in oil over high heat until golden brown. Set aside.
3. Place the peppercorns in a bag and crush with a rolling pin. Next, strip the rosemary leaves from the stem and mix with garlic and salt.
4. Season the seared steak with the spice mixture.
5. Place in the grill and roast for 30 minutes and reduce the heat to 300F. Cook for another 30 minutes.
6. Once cooked, remove from the grill, and allow to rest for 20 minutes before slicing.
Nutrition Info: Calories per serving: 954; Protein: 128.5g; Carbs: 4.1g; Fat: 47.7g Sugar: 0.3g

Kalbi Beef Ribs

Servings: 6
Cooking Time: 23 Minutes

Ingredients:
- Thinly sliced beef ribs - 2 ½ lbs
- Soy sauce - ½ cup
- Brown sugar - ½ cup
- Rice wine or mirin - ⅛ cup
- Minced garlic - 2 tbsp
- Sesame oil - 1 tbsp
- Grated onion - ⅛ cup

Directions:
1. In a medium-sized bowl, mix the mirin, soy sauce, sesame oil, brown sugar, garlic, and grated onion.
2. Add the ribs to the bowl to marinate and cover it properly with cling wrap. Put it in the refrigerator for up to 6 hours.
3. Once you remove the marinated ribs from the refrigerator, immediately put them on the grill. Close the grill quickly, so no heat is lost. Also, make sure the grill is preheated well before you place the ribs on it.
4. Cook on one side for 4 minutes and then flip it. Cook the other side for 4 minutes.
5. Pull it out once it looks fully cooked. Serve it with rice or any other side dish

Nutrition Info: Carbohydrates: 22 g Protein: 28 g Fat: 6 g Sodium: 1213 mg Cholesterol: 81 mg

Grilled Butter Basted Porterhouse Steak

Servings: 4
Cooking Time: 8 Minutes
Ingredients:
- 4 tablespoons melted butter
- 2 tablespoons Worcestershire sauce
- 2 tablespoons Dijon mustard
- Traeger Prime Rib Rub, as needed
- 2 porterhouse steaks, 1 ½ inch thick

Directions:
1. Fire the Traeger Grill to 255F. Use desired wood pellets when cooking. Close the lid and preheat for 15 minutes.
2. In a bowl, mix the butter, Worcestershire sauce, mustard, and Prime Rib Rub.
3. Massage all over the steak on all sides. Allow steak to rest for an hour before cooking.
4. When ready to cook, fire the Traeger Grill to 500F. Use desired wood pellets when cooking. Close the lid and preheat for 15 minutes.
5. Place the steaks on the grill grates and cook for 4 minutes on each side or until the internal temperature reads at 130F for medium rare steaks.
6. Remove from the grill and allow to rest for 10 minutes before slicing.

Nutrition Info: Calories per serving: 515 ; Protein: 65.3g; Carbs: 2.1g; Fat: 27.7g Sugar: 0.9g

2-ingredients Filet Mignon

Servings: 2
Cooking Time: 10 Minutes
Ingredients:
- 2 filet mignons
- Salt and freshly ground black pepper, to taste

Directions:
1. Set the temperature of Traeger Grill to 450 degrees F and preheat with closed lid for 15 minutes.
2. Season the steaks with salt and black pepper generously.
3. Place the filet mignons onto the grill and grill and cook for about 5 minutes per side.
4. Remove from grill and serve immediately.

Nutrition Info: Calories per serving: 254; Carbohydrates: 0g; Protein: 39.8g; Fat: 9.3g; Sugar: 0g; Sodium: 161mg; Fiber: 0g

Traeger Smoked Pork Ribs

Servings: 4
Cooking Time: 10 Hours
Ingredients:
- 2 racks back ribs
- 1 cup homemade bbq rub
- 2 12-oz hard apple cider
- 1 cup dark brown sugar
- 2 batches homemade BBQ sauce

Directions:
1. Turn the Traeger to smoke setting and remove any membrane from the meat.
2. Place the pork in the Traeger and smoke for 5 hours or until it reaches an internal temperature of 175.
3. Increase the grill temperature to 225F. Transfer the meat to a pan sprayed with cooking spray.
4. Pour one bottle of hard apple cider to the pan and rub the brown sugar on top of the ribs.
5. Cover the pan with tin foil and place it back to the Traeger. Cook for 4 hours.
6. Remove the tin foil, increase the temperature to 300F, and place the ribs on the grill grates.
7. Cook for 1 hour brushing the ribs with BBQ sauce 3 times.
8. The ribs should now be falling off the bone. Let rest for 5 minutes before serving.

Nutrition Info: Calories 1073, Total fat 42g, Saturated fat 15g, Total carbs 111g, Net carbs 109g Protein 61g, Sugars 99g, Fiber 3g, Sodium 1663mg

Pulled Beef

Servings: 5 To 8
Cooking Time: 12 To 14 Hours
Ingredients:
- 1 (4-pound) top round roast
- 2 tablespoons yellow mustard
- 1 batch Espresso Brisket Rub
- ½ cup beef broth

Directions:
1.   Supply your Traeger with wood pellets and follow the start-up procedure. Preheat the grill, with the lid closed, to 225°F.
2.   Coat the top round roast all over with mustard and season it with the rub. Using your hands, work the rub into the meat.
3.   Place the roast directly on the grill grate and smoke until its internal temperature reaches 160°F and a dark bark has formed.
4.   Pull the roast from the grill and place it on enough aluminum foil to wrap it completely.
5.   Increase the grill's temperature to 350°F.
6.   Fold in three sides of the foil around the roast and add the beef broth. Fold in the last side, completely enclosing the roast and liquid. Return the wrapped roast to the grill and cook until its internal temperature reaches 195°F.
7.   Pull the roast from the grill and place it in a cooler. Cover the cooler and let the roast rest for 1 or 2 hours.
8.   Remove the roast from the cooler and unwrap it. Pull apart the beef using just your fingers. Serve immediately.

Traeger Grilled Pork Chops

Servings: 6
Cooking Time: 20 Minutes
Ingredients:
- 6 thick-cut pork chops
- BBQ rub

Directions:
1.   Preheat your Traeger to 450F.
2.   Season the pork chops with the BBQ rub.
3.   Place the chops on the Traeger and cook for 6 minutes on each side or until the internal temperature reaches 145F.
4.   Remove the chops from the Traeger and let cool for 5 minutes before serving.
Nutrition Info: Calories 398, Total fat 19g, Saturated fat 6g, Total carbs 8g, Net carbs 7g Protein 46g, Sugars 6g, Fiber 1g, Sodium 363mg

Stunning Prime Rib Roast

Servings: 10
Cooking Time: 3 Hours 50 Minutes
Ingredients:
- 1 (5-lb.) prime rib roast
- Salt, to taste
- 5 tbsp. olive oil
- 4 tsp. dried rosemary, crushed
- 2 tsp. garlic powder
- 1 tsp. onion powder
- 1 tsp. paprika
- ½ tsp. cayenne pepper
- Freshly ground black pepper, to taste

Directions:
1.   Season the roast with salt generously.
2.   With a plastic wrap, cover the roast and refrigerate for about 24 hours.
3.   In a bowl, mix together remaining ingredients and set aside for about 1 hour.
4.   Rub the roast with oil mixture from both sides evenly.
5.   Arrange the roast in a large baking sheet and refrigerate for about 6-12 hours.
6.   Set the temperature of Traeger Grill to 225-230 degrees F and preheat with closed lid for 15 minutes. , using pecan wood chips.
7.   Place the roast onto the grill and cook for about 3-3½ hours.
8.   Meanwhile, preheat the oven to 500 degrees F.
9.   Remove the roast from grill and place onto a large baking sheet.
10.   Place the baking sheet in oven and roast for about 15-20 minutes.
11.   Remove the roast from oven and place onto a cutting board for about 10-15 minutes before serving.
12.   With a sharp knife, cut the roast into desired-sized slices and serve.
Nutrition Info: Calories per serving: 605; Carbohydrates: 3.8g; Protein: 38g; Fat: 47.6g; Sugar: 0.3g; Sodium: 1285mg; Fiber: 0.3g Stunning Prime Rib Roast

Thai Beef Salad

Servings: 4
Cooking Time: 10 Minutes
Ingredients:
- 1 ½ pound skirt steak
- 1 ½ teaspoon salt
- 1 teaspoon ground white pepper
- For the Dressing:
- 4 jalapeño peppers, minced
- ½ teaspoon minced garlic
- 4 tablespoons Thai fish sauce
- 4 tablespoons lime juice

- 1 tablespoon brown sugar
- For the Salad:
- 1 small red onion, peeled, thinly sliced
- 6 cherry tomatoes, halved
- 2 green onions, ¼-inch diced
- 1 cucumber, deseeded, thinly sliced
- 1 heart of romaine lettuce, chopped
- ½ cup chopped mint
- 2 tablespoons cilantro
- ½ teaspoon red pepper flakes
- 1 tablespoon lime juice
- 2 tablespoons fish sauce

Directions:
1. Switch on the Traeger grill, fill the grill hopper with cherry flavored wood pellets, power the grill on by using the control panel, select 'smoke' on the temperature dial, or set the temperature to 450 degrees F and let it preheat for a minimum of 15 minutes.
2. Meanwhile, prepare the steak, and for this, season it with salt and black pepper until well coated.
3. When the grill has preheated, open the lid, place steak on the grill grate, shut the grill and smoke for 10 minutes until internal temperature reaches 130 degrees F.
4. Meanwhile, prepare the dressing and for this, take a medium bowl, place all of its ingredients in it and then stir until combined.
5. Take a large salad, place all the ingredients for the salad in it, drizzle with dressing and toss until well coated and mixed.
6. When done, transfer steak to a cutting board, let it rest for 10 minutes and then cut it into slices.
7. Add steak slices into the salad, toss until mixed, and then serve.

Nutrition Info: Calories: 128 Cal ;Fat: 6 g ;Carbs: 6 g ;Protein: 12 g ;Fiber: 1 g

Beautiful Christmas Ham

Servings: 16
Cooking Time: 1 Hour 20 Minutes
Ingredients:
- 1 C. honey
- ¼ C. dark corn syrup
- 1 (7-lb.) ready-to-eat ham
- ¼ C. whole cloves
- ½ C. butter, softened

Directions:
1. Set the temperature of Traeger Grill to 325 degrees F and preheat with closed lid for 15 minutes, using charcoal.
2. In a small pan, add honey and corn syrup and cook until heated slightly, stirring continuously.
3. Remove the pan of glaze from heat and set aside.

4. With a sharp knife, score the ham in a cross pattern.
5. Insert whole cloves at the crossings.
6. Coat the ham with butter evenly.
7. Arrange ham in foil-lined roasting pan and top with ¾ of glaze evenly.
8. Place the pan onto the grill and cook for about 1¼ hours, coating with remain glaze after every 10-15 minutes.
9. Remove the ham from grill and place onto a cutting board for about 20-25 minutes before serving.
10. With a sharp knife, cut the ham into desired-sized slices and serve.

Nutrition Info: Calories per serving: 457; Carbohydrates: 29.7g; Protein: 33.2g; Fat: 23.1g; Sugar: 18.7g; Sodium: 2633mg; Fiber: 3.2g

Reverse-seared Tri-tip

Servings: 4
Cooking Time: 2 To 3 Hours
Ingredients:
- 1½ pounds tri-tip roast
- 1 batch Espresso Brisket Rub

Directions:
1. Supply your Traeger with wood pellets and follow the start-up procedure. Preheat the grill, with the lid closed, to 180°F.
2. Season the tri-tip roast with the rub. Using your hands, work the rub into the meat.
3. Place the roast directly on the grill grate and smoke until its internal temperature reaches 140°F.
4. Increase the grill's temperature to 450°F and continue to cook until the roast's internal temperature reaches 145°F. This same technique can be done over an open flame or in a cast-iron skillet with some butter.
5. Remove the tri-tip roast from the grill and let it rest 10 to 15 minutes, before slicing and serving.

Thai Beef Skewers

Servings: 6
Cooking Time: 8 Minutes
Ingredients:
- ½ of medium red bell pepper, destemmed, cored, cut into a ¼-inch piece
- ½ of beef sirloin, fat trimmed
- ½ cup salted peanuts, roasted, chopped
- For the Marinade:
- 1 teaspoon minced garlic
- 1 tablespoon grated ginger
- 1 lime, juiced
- 1 teaspoon ground black pepper
- 1 tablespoon sugar

- 1/4 cup soy sauce
- 1/4 cup olive oil

Directions:
1. Prepare the marinade and for this, take a small bowl, place all of its ingredients in it, whisk until combined, and then pour it into a large plastic bag.
2. Cut into beef sirloin 1-1/4-inch dice, add to the plastic bag containing marinade, seal the bag, turn it upside down to coat beef pieces with the marinade and let it marinate for a minimum of 2 hours in the refrigerator.
3. When ready to cook, switch on the Traeger grill, fill the grill hopper with cherry flavored wood pellets, power the grill on by using the control panel, select 'smoke' on the temperature dial, or set the temperature to 425 degrees F and let it preheat for a minimum of 5 minutes.
4. Meanwhile, remove beef pieces from the marinade and then thread onto skewers.
5. When the grill has preheated, open the lid, place prepared skewers on the grill grate, shut the grill, and smoke for 4 minutes per side until done.
6. When done, transfer skewers to a dish, sprinkle with peanuts and red pepper, and then serve.

Nutrition Info: Calories: 124 Cal ;Fat: 5.5 g ;Carbs: 1.7 g ;Protein: 15.6 g ;Fiber: 0 g

Grilled Lamb Burgers

Servings: 5
Cooking Time: 15 Minutes
Ingredients:
- 1 1/4 pounds of ground lamb.
- 1 egg.
- 1 teaspoon of dried oregano.
- 1 teaspoon of dry sherry.
- 1 teaspoon of white wine vinegar.
- 4 minced cloves of garlic.
- Red pepper
- 1/2 cup of chopped green onions.
- 1 tablespoon of chopped mint.
- 2 tablespoons of chopped cilantro.
- 2 tablespoons of dry bread crumbs.
- 1/8 teaspoon of salt to taste.
- 1/4 teaspoon of ground black pepper to taste.
- 5 hamburger buns.

Directions:
1. Preheat a Wood Pellet Smoker or Grill to 350-450 degrees F then grease it grates. Using a large mixing bowl, add in all the ingredients on the list aside from the buns then mix properly to combine with clean hands. Make about five patties out of the mixture then set aside.
2. Place the lamb patties on the preheated grill and cook for about seven to nine minutes turning only

once until an inserted thermometer reads 160 degrees F. Serve the lamb burgers on the hamburger, add your favorite toppings and enjoy.

Nutrition Info: Calories: 376 Cal Fat: 18.5 g Carbohydrates: 25.4 g Protein: 25.5 g Fiber: 1.6 g

Sweetheart Steak

Servings: 1
Cooking Time: 14 Minutes
Ingredients:
- 20 ounces boneless strip steak, butterflied
- 2 ounces pure sea salt
- 2 teaspoons black pepper
- 2 tablespoons raw dark chocolate, finely chopped
- ½ tablespoon extra-virgin olive oil

Directions:
1. On a cutting board, trim the meat into heart shape using a sharp knife. Set aside.
2. In a smaller bowl, combine the rest of the ingredients to create a spice rub mix.
3. Rub onto the steak and massage until well-seasoned.
4. When ready to cook, fire the Traeger Grill to 450F. Use desired wood pellets when cooking. Close the lid and preheat for 15 minutes.
5. Grill the steak for 7 minutes on each side.
6. Allow to rest for 5 minutes before slicing.

Nutrition Info: Calories per serving: 727 ; Protein: 132.7g; Carbs: 8.8 g; Fat: 18.5g Sugar: 5.2g

Traeger Beef Short Rib Lollipop

Servings: 4
Cooking Time: 3 Hours
Ingredients:
- 4 beef short rib lollipops
- BBQ Rub
- BBQ Sauce

Directions:
1. Preheat your Traeger to 275F.
2. Season the short ribs with BBQ rub and place them on the grill.
3. Cook for 4 hours while turning occasionally until the meat is tender.
4. Apply the sauce on the meat in the last 30 minutes of cooking.
5. Serve and enjoy.

Nutrition Info: Calories: 265 Cal Fat: 19 g Carbohydrates: 1 g Protein: 22 g Fiber: 0 g

Cowboy Steak

Servings: 4
Cooking Time: 1 Hour
Ingredients:
- 2.5 lb. cowboy cut steaks
- Salt to taste
- Beef rub
- 1/4 cup olive oil
- 2 tablespoons fresh mint leaves, chopped
- ½ cup parsley, chopped
- 1 clove garlic, crushed and minced
- 1 tablespoon lemon juice
- 1 tablespoon lemon zest
- Salt and pepper to taste

Directions:
1. Season the steak with the salt and dry rub.
2. Preheat the Traeger wood pellet grill to 225 degrees F for 10 minutes while the lid is closed.
3. Grill the steaks for 45 minutes, flipping once or twice.
4. Increase temperature to 450 degrees F.
5. Put the steaks back to the grill. Cook for 5 minutes per side.
6. In a bowl, mix the remaining ingredients.
7. Serve steaks with the parsley mixture.
8. Tips: Let steak rest for 10 minutes before putting it back to the grill for the second round of cooking.

Smoked Sausages

Servings: 4
Cooking Time: 3 Hours
Ingredients:
- 3 pounds ground pork
- 1 tablespoon onion powder
- 1 tablespoon garlic powder
- 1 teaspoon curing salt
- 4 teaspoon black pepper
- 1/2 tablespoon salt
- 1/2 tablespoon ground mustard
- Hog casings, soaked
- 1/2 cup ice water

Directions:
1. Switch on the Traeger grill, fill the grill hopper with flavored wood pellets, power the grill on by using the control panel, select 'smoke' on the temperature dial, or set the temperature to 225 degrees F and let it preheat for a minimum of 15 minutes.
2. Meanwhile, take a medium bowl, place all the ingredients in it except for water and hog casings, and stir until well mixed.

3. Pour in water, stir until incorporated, place the mixture in a sausage stuffer, then stuff the hog casings and tie the link to the desired length.
4. When the grill has preheated, open the lid, place the sausage links on the grill grate, shut the grill, and smoke for 2 to 3 hours until the internal temperature reaches 155 degrees F.
5. When done, transfer sausages to a dish, let them rest for 5 minutes, then slice and serve.
Nutrition Info: Calories: 230 Cal ;Fat: 22 g ;Carbs: 2 g ;Protein: 14 g ;Fiber: 0 g

Grilled Lamb Kabobs

Servings: 7
Cooking Time: 16 Minutes
Ingredients:
- ½ cup olive oil
- ½ tablespoon salt
- 2 teaspoons black pepper
- 2 tablespoons chopped mint
- ½ tablespoon cilantro, chopped
- 1 teaspoon cumin
- ½ cup lemon juice
- 3 pounds boneless leg of lamb, cut into 2-inch cubes
- 15 apricots, halved and seeded
- 5 onions, cut into wedges

Directions:
1. In a bowl, combine the oil, salt, pepper, mint, cilantro, cumin, and lemon juice.
2. Massage the mixture on to the lamb shoulder and allow to marinate in the fridge for at least 2 hours.
3. Remove the lamb from the marinade and thread the lamb, apricots, and red onion alternatingly on a skewer.
4. When ready to cook, fire the Traeger Grill to 400F. Use desired wood pellets when cooking. Close the lid and preheat for 15 minutes.
5. Place the skewers on the grill grate and cook for 8 minutes on each side.
6. Remove from the grill.
Nutrition Info: Calories per serving: 652;
Protein: 53.9g; Carbs: 38.1g; Fat: 31.8g Sugar: 29.4g

Wood Pellet Grilled Aussie Leg Of Lamb Roast

Servings: 8
Cooking Time: 2 Hours
Ingredients:
- 5 lb Aussie leg of lamb, boneless
- Smoked Paprika Rub

- 1 tbsp raw sugar
- 1 tbsp kosher salt
- 1 tbsp black pepper
- 1 tbsp smoked paprika
- 1 tbsp garlic powder
- 1 tbsp rosemary, dried
- 1 tbsp onion powder
- 1tbsp cumin
- 1/2 tbsp cayenne pepper
- Roasted Carrots
- 1 bunch rainbow carrots
- Olive oil
- Salt
- pepper

Directions:
1. Heat the wood pellet grill to 375 F.
2. Trim any excess fat from the lamb.
3. Combine all the rub ingredients and rub all over the lamb. Place the lamb on the grill and smoke for 2 hours.
4. Toss the carrots in oil, salt, and pepper then add to the grill after the lamb has cooked for 1-1/2 hour.
5. Cook until the roast internal temperature reaches 135 F. Remove the lamb from the grill and cover with foil. Let rest for 30 minutes.
6. Remove the carrots from the grill once soft and serve with the lamb. Enjoy.

Nutrition Info: Calories 257, Total fat 8g, Saturated fat 2g, Total Carbs 6g, Net Carbs 5g, Protein 37g, Sugar 3g, Fiber 1g, Sodium: 431mg, Potassium 666mg

Maple-smoked Pork Chops

Servings: 4
Cooking Time: 55 Minutes
Ingredients:
- 1 (12-pound) full packer brisket
- 2 tablespoons yellow mustard
- 1 batch Espresso Brisket Rub
- Worcestershire Mop and Spritz, for spritzing

Directions:
1. Supply your smoker with wood pellets and follow the manufacturer's specific start-up procedure. Preheat the grill, with the lid closed, to 180°F.
2. Season the pork chops on both sides with salt and pepper.
3. Place the chops directly on the grill grate and smoke for 30 minutes.
4. Increase the grill's temperature to 350°F. Continue to cook the chops until their internal temperature reaches 145°F.
5. Remove the pork chops from the grill and let them rest for 5 minutes before serving.

Smoked Apple Bbq Ribs

Servings: 6
Cooking Time: 2 Hours
Ingredients:
- 2 racks St. Louis-style ribs
- ¼ cup Traeger Big Game Rub
- 1 cup apple juice
- A bottle of Traeger BBQ Sauce

Directions:
1. Place the ribs on a working surface and remove the film of connective tissues covering it.
2. In another bowl, mix the Game Rub and apple juice until well-combined.
3. Massage the rub on to the ribs and allow to rest in the fridge for at least 2 hours.
4. When ready to cook, fire the Traeger Grill to 225F. Use apple wood pellets when cooking the ribs. Close the lid and preheat for 15 minutes.
5. Place the ribs on the grill grate and close the lid. Smoke for 1 hour and 30 minutes. Make sure to flip the ribs halfway through the cooking time.
6. Ten minutes before the cooking time ends, brush the ribs with BBQ sauce.
7. Remove from the grill and allow to rest before slicing.

Nutrition Info: Calories per serving: 337 ; Protein: 47.1g; Carbs: 4.7 g; Fat: 12.9g Sugar: 4g

Grilled Lamb Chops With Rosemary

Servings: 4
Cooking Time: 12 Minutes
Ingredients:
- ½ cup extra virgin olive oil
- ¼ cup coarsely chopped onion
- 2 cloves of garlic, minced
- 2 tablespoons soy sauce
- 2 tablespoons balsamic vinegar
- 1 tablespoon fresh rosemary
- 2 teaspoons Dijon mustard
- 1 teaspoon Worcestershire sauce
- Salt and pepper to taste
- 4 lamb chops (8 ounce each)

Directions:
1. Heat oil in a saucepan over medium flame and sauté the onion and garlic until fragrant. Place in food processor together with the soy sauce, vinegar, rosemary, mustard, Worcestershire sauce, salt, and pepper. Pulse until smooth. Set aside.
2. Fire the Traeger Grill to 500F. Use desired wood pellets when cooking. Close the lid and preheat for 15 minutes.
3. Brush the lamb chops on both sides with the paste.

4. Place on the grill grates and cook for 6 minutes per side or until the internal temperature reaches 135F for medium rare.

5. Serve with the paste if you have leftover.

Nutrition Info: Calories per serving: 442; Protein: 16.7g; Carbs: 6.1g; Fat:38.5 g Sugar: 3.7g

Slow Roasted Shawarma

Servings: 6-8
Cooking Time: 4 Hours 55 Minutes
Ingredients:
- Top sirloin - 5.5 lbs
- Lamb fat - 4.5 lbs
- Boneless, skinless chicken thighs- 5.5 lbs
- Pita bread
- Traeger rub - 4 tbsp
- Double skewer - 1
- Large yellow onions - 2
- Variety of topping options such as tomatoes, cucumbers, pickles, tahini, Israeli salad, fries, etc.
- Cast iron griddle

Directions:
1. Assemble the stack of shawarma the night before you wish to cook it.

2. Slice all the meat and fat into ½-inch slices. Place them into 3 bowls. If you partially freeze them, it will be much easier to slice them.

3. Season the bowl with the rub, massaging it thoroughly into the meat.

4. Place half a yellow onion on the bottom of the skewers to ensure a firm base. Add 2 layers at a time from each bowl. Try to make the entire stack symmetrical. Place the other 2 onions on top. Wrap them in plastic wrap and refrigerate overnight.

5. When the meat is ready to cook, preheat the pellet grill for about 15 minutes with the lid closed at a temperature of 275 degrees Fahrenheit.

6. Lay the shawarma directly on the grill grate and cook it for at least 3-4 hours. Rotate the skewers at least once.

7. Remove them from the grill and increase its temperature to 445 degrees Fahrenheit. When the grill is preheating, place a cast iron griddle directly on the grill grate and brush it with some olive oil.

8. Once the griddle is hot enough, place the shawarma directly on the cast iron. Sear it on each side for 5-10 minutes. Remove it from the grill and slice off the edges. Repeat the process with the remaining shawarma.

9. Serve in pita bread and favorite toppings, such as tomatoes, cucumbers, Israeli salad, fries, pickles, or tahini. Enjoy!

Nutrition Info: Carbohydrates: 4.6 g Protein: 30.3 g Fat: 26.3 g Sodium: 318.7 mg Cholesterol: 125.5 mg

Traeger Pulled Pork

Servings: 12
Cooking Time: 12 Hours
Ingredients:
- 8 lb. pork shoulder roast, bone-in
- BBQ Rub
- 3 cups dry hard apple cider vinegar

Directions:
1. Fire up your Traeger and set it at the smoke setting.

2. Rub the pork shoulder with the BBQ rub then place it on the grill grates. Smoke for 5 hours while turning it every hour.

3. Increase the heat o 225F and continue cooking for to 3 more hours.

4. Transfer the pork roast to a foil pan with apple cider vinegar at the bottom.

5. Continue cooking the roast until it reaches an internal temperature of 200F.

6. Remove the pork from the Traeger and remove the skin and any fat layer from the meat. shred it using 2 forks and serve

Nutrition Info: Calories 912, Total fat 65g, Saturated fat 24g, Total carbs 7g, Net carbs 7g Protein 70g, Sugars 6g, Fiber 0g, Sodium 208mg

Roasted Venison Tenderloin

Servings: 4
Cooking Time: 20 Minutes
Ingredients:
- 2 pounds venison
- ¼ cup dry red wine
- 2 cloves garlic, minced
- 2 tablespoons soy sauce
- 1 ½ tablespoons red wine vinegar
- 1 tablespoon rosemary
- 1 teaspoon black pepper
- ½ cup olive oil
- Salt to taste

Directions:
1. Remove the membrane covering the venison. Set aside.

2. Mix the rest of the ingredients in a bowl. Place the venison in the bowl and allow to marinate for at least 5 hours in the fridge.

3. Fire the Traeger Grill to 500F. Use desired wood pellets when cooking. Close the lid and preheat for 15 minutes.

4. Remove the venison from the marinade and pat dry using a paper towel.

5. Place on the grill grate and cook for 10 minutes on each side for medium rare.

Nutrition Info: Calories per serving: 611 ;
Protein: 68.4g; Carbs: 3.1g; Fat: 34.4g Sugar: 1.6g

Herby Lamb Chops

Servings: 4
Cooking Time: 2 Hours
Ingredients:
- 8 lamb chops, each about ¾-inch thick, fat trimmed
- For the Marinade:
- 1 teaspoon minced garlic
- Salt as needed
- 1 tablespoon dried rosemary
- Ground black pepper as needed
- ½ tablespoon dried thyme
- 3 tablespoons balsamic vinegar
- 1 tablespoon Dijon mustard
- ½ cup olive oil

Directions:
1. Prepare the marinade and for this, take a small bowl, place all of its ingredients in it and stir until well combined.
2. Place lamb chops in a large plastic bag, pour in marinade, seal the bag, turn it upside down to coat lamb chops with the marinade and let it marinate for a minimum of 4 hours in the refrigerator.
3. When ready to cook, switch on the Traeger grill, fill the grill hopper with flavored wood pellets, power the grill on by using the control panel, select 'smoke' on the temperature dial, or set the temperature to 450 degrees F and let it preheat for a minimum of 5 minutes.
4. Meanwhile, remove lamb chops from the refrigerator and bring them to room temperature.
5. When the grill has preheated, open the lid, place lamb chops on the grill grate, shut the grill and smoke for 5 minutes per side until seared.
6. When done, transfer lamb chops to a dish, let them rest for 5 minutes and then serve.

Nutrition Info: Calories: 280 Cal ;Fat: 12.3 g ;Carbs: 8.3 g ;Protein: 32.7 g ;Fiber: 1.2 g

Drunken Beef Jerky

Servings: 6
Cooking Time: 5 Hours
Ingredients:
- 1 (12-oz.) bottle dark beer
- 1 C. soy sauce
- ¼ C. Worcestershire sauce
- 2 tbsp. hot sauce
- 3 tbsp. brown sugar
- 2 tbsp. coarse ground black pepper, divided

- 1 tbsp. curing salt
- ½ tsp. garlic salt
- 2 lb. flank steak, trimmed and cut into ¼-inch thick slices

Directions:
1. In a bowl, add the beer, soy sauce, Worcestershire sauce, brown sugar, 2 tbsp. of black pepper, curing salt and garlic salt and mix well.
2. In a large resealable plastic bag, place the steak slices and marinade mixture.
3. Seal the bag, squeezing out the air and then shake to coat well.
4. Refrigerate to marinate overnight.
5. Set the temperature of Traeger Grill to 180 degrees F and preheat with closed lid for 15 minutes.
6. Remove the steak slices from the bag and discard the marinade.
7. With paper towels, pat dry the steak slices.
8. Sprinkle the steak slices with remaining black pepper generously.
9. Arrange the steak slices onto the grill in a single layer and cook for about 4-5 hours.

Nutrition Info: Calories per serving: 374; Carbohydrates: 13.3g; Protein: 45.3g; Fat: 12.7g; Sugar: 7.2g; Sodium: 2700mg; Fiber: 0.9g

Strip Steak

Servings: 2
Cooking Time: 10 Minutes
Ingredients:
- Salt and black pepper
- 1/4 teaspoon of garlic powder
- 1.25 pounds of bone-in New York steak
- Canola oil spray

Directions:
1. Insert grill grate inside the unit and preheat the unit for 10 minutes, at 510 degrees MAX.
2. Rub the steak with salt, black pepper, and garlic powder.
3. Spray canola oil on both sides of the steak.
4. Place steak inside the grill grate and lower the hood.
5. Set time to 10 minutes, at 500 degrees F.
6. After 4 minutes, open the lid and flip the steak to cook from the other side.
7. Cook it for the remaining minutes.
8. Once done, take out and serve.

Nutrition Info: Calories: 581 Total Fat: 38gSaturated Fat: 15.1gCholesterol: 188mg Sodium: 151mg Total Carbohydrate: 0.3g Dietary Fiber 0g Total Sugars: 0.1g Protein: 55.4g

Traeger Smoked Beef Roast

Servings: 6
Cooking Time: 6 Hours
Ingredients:
- 1-3/4 pounds beef sirloin tip roast
- 1/2 cup barbeque rub
- 2 bottles amber beer
- 1 bottle BBQ sauce

Directions:
1. Turn the Traeger onto the smoke setting.
2. Rub the beef with barbeque rub until well coated then place on the grill. Let smoke for 4 hours while flipping every 1 hour.
3. Transfer the beef to a pan and add the beer. The beef should be 1/2 way covered.
4. Braise the beef until fork tender. It will take 3 hours on the stovetop and 60 minutes on the instant pot.
5. Remove the beef from the ban and reserve 1 cup of the cooking liquid.
6. Use 2 forks to shred the beef into small pieces then return to the pan with the reserved braising liquid. Add BBQ sauce and stir well then keep warm until serving. You can also reheat if it gets cold.
Nutrition Info: Calories: 829 Cal Fat: 18 g Carbohydrates: 4 g   Protein: 86 g Fiber: 0 g

Greek-style Roast Leg Of Lamb

Servings: 12
Cooking Time: 1 Hour And 30 Minutes
Ingredients:
- 7 pounds leg of lamb, bone-in, fat trimmed
- 2 lemons, juiced
- 8 cloves of garlic, peeled, minced
- Salt as needed
- Ground black pepper as needed
- 1 teaspoon dried oregano
- 1 teaspoon dried rosemary
- 6 tablespoons olive oil

Directions:
1. Make a small cut into the meat of lamb by using a paring knife, then stir together garlic, oregano, and rosemary and stuff this paste into the slits of the lamb meat.
2. Take a roasting pan, place lamb in it, then rub with lemon juice and olive oil, cover with a plastic wrap and let marinate for a minimum of 8 hours in the refrigerator.
3. When ready to cook, switch on the Traeger grill, fill the grill hopper with oak flavored wood pellets, power the grill on by using the control panel, select 'smoke' on the temperature dial, or set the temperature to 400 degrees F and let it preheat for a minimum of 15 minutes.
4. Meanwhile, remove the lamb from the refrigerator, bring it to room temperature, uncover it and then season well with salt and black pepper.
5. When the grill has preheated, open the lid, place food on the grill grate, shut the grill, and smoke for 30 minutes.
6. Change the smoking temperature to 350 degrees F and then continue smoking for 1 hour until the internal temperature reaches 140 degrees F.
7. When done, transfer lamb to a cutting board, let it rest for 15 minutes, then cut it into slices and serve.
Nutrition Info: Calories: 168 Cal ;Fat: 10 g ;Carbs: 2 g ;Protein: 17 g ;Fiber: 0.7 g

Traeger Grilled Pork Tenderloin With Herb Sauce

Servings: 4
Cooking Time: 15 Minutes
Ingredients:
- 1 pork tenderloin
- Bbq seasoning
- Fresh Herb Sauce
- 1 handful basil, fresh
- 1/2 handful flat-leaf parsley, fresh
- 1/4 tbsp garlic powder
- 1/3 cup olive oil
- 1/2 tbsp kosher salt

Directions:
1. Preheat your Traeger to medium heat.
2. Remove silver skin from the pork tenderloin and pat it dry with a paper towel.
3. Generously rub the pork with the bbq seasoning then cook over indirect heat in the Traeger while turning occasionally.
4. Cook until the internal temperature reaches 145F. Remove the pork from the Traeger and let rest for 10 minutes.
5. Meanwhile, add all the fresh herb sauce ingredients in a food processor and pulse a few times.
6. Slice the pork tenderloin diagonally and spoon the sauce on top. Serve
Nutrition Info: Calories 300, Total fat 22g, Saturated fat 4g, Total carbs 13g, Net carbs 12g Protein 14g, Sugars 10g, Fiber 1g, Sodium 791mg

Baked Venison Meatloaf

Servings: 6
Cooking Time: 1 Hour And 30 Minutes
Ingredients:
- 2 pounds venison, ground
- 1-pound pork, ground
- 1 cup breadcrumbs

- 1 cup milk
- 2 tablespoons onion, diced
- 3 tablespoons salt
- 1 tablespoon black pepper
- ½ tablespoon thyme
- 1 ½ pounds parsnips, chopped
- 1 ½ pounds russet potatoes, chopped
- ¼ cup butter

Directions:
1.   Fire the Traeger Grill to 500F. Use desired wood pellets when cooking. Close the lid and preheat for 15 minutes.
2.   Combine all ingredients in a bowl. Place the mixture in a greased loaf pan.
3.   Place in the Traeger Grill and cook for 1 hour and 30 minutes or until the internal temperature reads at 160F.

Nutrition Info: Calories per serving: 668 ; Protein: 70.4g; Carbs: 45.7 g; Fat: 22g Sugar: 8.7g

Traditional Tomahawk Steak

Servings: 4 To 6
Cooking Time: 1 Or 2 Hours
Ingredients:
- 1 tomahawk ribeye steak (2 1/2 to 3 1/2 lbs)
- 5 garlic cloves, minced
- 2 tbsp kosher salt
- 1 bundle fresh thyme
- 2 tbsp ground black pepper
- 8 oz butter stick
- 1 tbsp garlic powder
- 1/8 cup olive oil

Directions:
1.   Mix rub ingredients (salt, black pepper, and garlic powder) in a small bowl. Use this mixture to season all sides of the ribeye steak generously. You can also substitute your favorite steak seasoning. After applying seasoning, let the steak rest at room temperature for at least 30 minutes.
2.   While the steak rests, preheat your pellet grill to 450°F - 550°F for searing
3.   Sear the steak for 5 minutes on each side. Halfway through each side (so after 2 1/2 minutes), rotate the steak 90° to form grill marks on the tomahawk
4.   After the tomahawk steak has seared for 5 minutes on each side (10 minutes total), move the steak to a raised rack
5.   Adjust your pellet grill's temperature to 250°F and turn up smoke setting if applicable. Leave the lid open for a moment to help allow some heat to escape
6.   Stick your probe meat thermometer into the very center of the cut to measure internal temperature.

7.   Place butter stick, garlic cloves, olive oil, and thyme in the aluminum pan. Then place the aluminum pan under the steak to catch drippings. After a few minutes, the steak drippings and ingredients will mix together
8.   Baste the steak with the aluminum pan mixture every 10 minutes until the tomahawk steak reaches your desired doneness
9.   Once the steak reaches its desired doneness, remove from the grill and place on a cutting board or serving dish. The steak should rest for 10-15 minutes before cutting/serving.

Spiced Rump Roast

Servings: 8
Cooking Time: 6 Hours
Ingredients:
- 1 tsp. smoked paprika
- 1 tsp. cayenne pepper
- 1 tsp. onion powder
- 1 tsp. garlic powder
- Salt and freshly ground black pepper, to taste
- 3 lb. beef rump roast
- ¼ C. Worcestershire sauce

Directions:
1.   Set the temperature of Traeger Grill to 200 degrees F and preheat with closed lid for 15 minutes, using charcoal.
2.   In a bowl, mix together all spices.
3.   Coat the rump roast with Worcestershire sauce evenly and then, rub with spice mixture generously.
4.   Place the rump roast onto the grill and cook for about 5-6 hours.
5.   Remove the roast from grill and place onto a cutting board for about 10-15 minutes before serving.
6.   With a sharp knife, cut the roast into desired-sized slices and serve.

Nutrition Info: Calories per serving: 252; Carbohydrates: 2.3g; Protein: 37.8g; Fat: 9.1g; Sugar: 1.8g; Sodium: 200mg; Fiber: 0.2g

Bbq Party Pork Ribs

Servings: 6
Cooking Time: 1 Hour 55 Minutes
Ingredients:
- 2 bone-in racks of pork ribs, silver skin removed
- 6 oz. BBQ rub
- 8 oz. apple juice
- ½ C. BBQ sauce

Directions:
1.   Coat each rack of ribs with BBQ rub generously.
2.   Arrange the racks onto a platter and set aside for about 30 minutes.

3.	Set the temperature of Traeger Grill to 225 degrees F and preheat with closed lid for 15 minutes.
4.	Arrange the racks onto the grill, bone side down and cook for about 1 hour.
5.	In a food-safe spray bottle, place apple juice.
6.	Spray the racks with vinegar mixture evenly.
7.	Cook for about 3½ hours, spraying with vinegar mixture after every 45 minutes.
8.	Now, coat the racks with a thin layer of BBQ sauce evenly and cook for about 10 minutes more.
9.	Remove the racks from grill and place onto a cutting board for about 10-15 minutes before slicing.
10.	With a sharp knife, cut each rack into individual ribs and serve.
Nutrition Info: Calories per serving: 801; Carbohydrates: 44.9g; Protein: 60.4g; Fat: 406g; Sugar: 37.4g; Sodium: 558mg; Fiber: 0.8g

Traeger Smoked Lamb Shoulder

Servings: 7
Cooking Time: 3 Hours
Ingredients:
- 5 lb. lamb shoulder
- 1 cup cider vinegar
- 2 tbsp. oil
- 2 tbsp. kosher salt
- 2 tbsp. black pepper, freshly ground
- 1 tbsp. dried rosemary
- For the Spritz
- 1 cup apple cider vinegar
- 1 cup apple juice

Directions:
1.	Preheat the Traeger to 225F with a pan of water for moisture.
2.	Trim any excess fat from the lamb and rinse the meat in cold water. Pat dry with a paper towel.
3.	Inject the cider vinegar in the meat then pat dry with a clean paper towel.
4.	Rub the meat with oil, salt, black pepper, and dried rosemary. Tie the lamb shoulder with a twine.
5.	Place in the smoker for an hour then spritz after every 15 minutes until the internal temperature reaches 165F.
6.	Remove from the Traeger and let rest for 1 hour before shredding and serving.
Nutrition Info: Calories 472, Total fat 37g, Saturated fat 19g, Total carbs 3g, Net carbs 3g Protein 31g, Sugars 0g, Fiber 0g, Sodium 458mg

Smoked Pork Tenderloin

Servings: 4-6
Cooking Time: 1 Hour And 30 Minutes
Ingredients:

- 2 (1½2 pounds) pork fillet
- ¼ Extra virgin olive oil with cup roasted garlic flavor
- ¼Cup Jan's Original Dry Rub or Pork Dry Rub

Directions:
1.	Configure a wood pellet smoker grill for indirect cooking and preheat to 230 ° F using hickory or apple pellets.
2.	Remove the wrap from the meat and insert a wood pellet smoker grill probe or remote meat probe into the thickest part of each tenderloin. If your grill does not have a meat probe or you do not have a remote meat probe, use an instant reading digital thermometer to read the internal temperature while cooking.
3.	Place the tenderloin directly on the grill and smoke at 230 ° F for 45 minutes.
4.	Raise the temperature of the pit to 350 ° F and finish cooking the tenderloin for about 45 minutes until the internal temperature of the thickest part reaches 145 ° F.
5.	Rest the pork tenderloin under a loose foil tent for 10 minutes before serving.
Nutrition Info: Calories: 115 Cal Fat: 3 g Carbohydrates: 0 g   Protein: 22 g Fiber: 0 g

Braised Short Ribs

Servings: 2 To 4
Cooking Time: 4 Hours
Ingredients:
- 4 beef short ribs
- Salt
- Freshly ground black pepper
- ½ cup beef broth

Directions:
1.	Supply your Traeger with wood pellets and follow the start-up procedure. Preheat the grill, with the lid closed, to 180°F.
2.	Season the ribs on both sides with salt and pepper.
3.	Place the ribs directly on the grill grate and smoke for 3 hours.
4.	Pull the ribs from the grill and place them on enough aluminum foil to wrap them completely.
5.	Increase the grill's temperature to 375°F.
6.	Fold in three sides of the foil around the ribs and add the beef broth. Fold in the last side, completely enclosing the ribs and liquid. Return the wrapped ribs to the grill and cook for 45 minutes more. Remove the short ribs from the grill, unwrap them, and serve immediately.

Wood Pellet Smoked Ribeye Steaks

Servings: 1
Cooking Time: 35 Minutes
Ingredients:
- 2-inch thick ribeye steaks
- Steak rub of choice

Directions:
1. Preheat your pellet grill to low smoke.
2. Sprinkle the steak with your favorite steak rub and place it on the grill. Let it smoke for 25 minutes.
3. Remove the steak from the grill and set the temperature to 400°F.
4. Return the steak to the grill and sear it for 5 minutes on each side.
5. Cook until the desired temperature is achieved; 125°F-rare, 145°F-Medium, and 165°F.-Well done.
6. Wrap the steak with foil and let rest for 10 minutes before serving. Enjoy.

Nutrition Info: Calories 225, Total fat 10.4g, Saturated fat 3.6g, Total Carbs 0.2g, Net Carbs 0.2g, Protein 32.5g, Sugar 0g, Fiber 0g, Sodium: 63mg, Potassium 463mg

Backyard Cookout Sausages

Servings: 6
Cooking Time: 23 Minutes
Ingredients:
- ½ C. apricot jam
- 1 tbsp. Dijon mustard
- 12 breakfast sausage links

Directions:
1. Set the temperature of Traeger Grill to 350 degrees F and preheat with closed lid for 15 minutes.
2. In a small pan, add jam and mustard over medium-low heat and cook until warmed.
3. Reduce the heat to low to keep the glaze warm.
4. Arrange the sausage links onto grill and cook for about 10-15 minutes, flipping twice.
5. Coat the sausage links with jam glaze evenly and cook for about 2-3 minutes.
6. Remove the sausage links from grill and serve alongside the remaining glaze.

Nutrition Info: Calories per serving: 575; Carbohydrates: 17.3g; Protein: 29.5g; Fat: 42.7g; Sugar: 11.6g; Sodium: 1164mg; Fiber: 0.2g

Traeger Smoked Lamb Meatballs

Servings: 20
Cooking Time: 1 Hour
Ingredients:
- 1 lb. lamb shoulder, ground
- 3 garlic cloves, finely diced
- 3 tbsp. shallot, diced
- 1 tbsp. salt
- 1 egg
- 1/2 tbsp. pepper
- 1/2 tbsp. cumin
- 1/2 tbsp. smoked paprika
- 1/4 tbsp. red pepper flakes
- 1/4 tbsp. cinnamon
- 1/4 cup panko breadcrumbs

Directions:
1. Set your Traeger to 250F .
2. Combine all the ingredients in a small bowl then mix thoroughly using your hands.
3. Form golf ball-sized meatballs and place them in a baking sheet.
4. Place the baking sheet in the smoker and smoke until the internal temperature reaches 160F.
5. Remove the meatballs from the smoker and serve when hot.

Nutrition Info: Calories 93, Total fat 5.9g, Saturated fat 2.5g, Total carbs 4.8g, Net carbs 4.5g Protein 5g, Sugars 0.3g, Fiber 0.3g, Sodium 174.1mg, Potassium 82.8mg

Traeger Grilled Lamb With Sugar Glaze

Servings: 4
Cooking Time: 20 Minutes
Ingredients:
- 1/4 cup sugar
- 2 tbsp ground ginger
- 2 tbsp dried tarragon
- 1/2 tbsp salt
- 1 tbsp black pepper, ground
- 1 tbsp ground cinnamon
- 1 tbsp garlic powder
- 4 lamb chops

Directions:
1. In a mixing bowl, mix sugar, ground ginger, tarragon, salt, pepper, cinnamon, and garlic.
2. Rub the lamb chops with the mixture and refrigerate for an hour.
3. Meanwhile, preheat your Traeger.
4. Brush the grill grates with oil and place the marinated lamb chops on it. Cook for 5 minutes on each side.
5. Serve and enjoy.

Nutrition Info: Calories 241, Total fat 13.1g, Saturated fat 5.6g, Total carbs 15.8g, Net carbs 15.1g Protein 14.6g, Sugars 13.6g, Fiber 0.7g, Sodium 339.2mg, Potassium 256.7mg

Elegant Lamb Chops

Servings: 4
Cooking Time: 30 Minutes
Ingredients:
- 4 lamb shoulder chops
- 4 C. buttermilk
- 1 C. cold water
- ¼ C. kosher salt
- 2 tbsp. olive oil
- 1 tbsp. Texas-style rub

Directions:
1. In a large bowl, add buttermilk, water and salt and stir until salt is dissolved.
2. Add chops and coat with mixture evenly.
3. Refrigerate for at least 4 hours.
4. Remove the chops from bowl and rinse under cold running water.
5. Coat the chops with olive oil and then sprinkle with rub evenly.
6. Set the temperature of Traeger Grill to 240 degrees F and preheat with closed lid for 15 minutes, using charcoal.
7. Arrange the chops onto grill and cook for about 25-30 minutes or until desired doneness.
8. Meanwhile, preheat the broiler of oven. Grease a broiler pan.
9. Remove the chops from grill and place onto the prepared broiler pan.
10. Transfer the broiler pan into the oven and broil for about 3-5 minutes or until browned.
11. Remove the chops from oven and serve hot.
Nutrition Info: Calories per serving: 414; Carbohydrates: 11.7g; Protein: 5.6g; Fat: 22.7g; Sugar: 11.7g; Sodium: 7000mg; Fiber: 0g

Braised Mediterranean Beef Brisket

Servings: 16
Cooking Time: 5 Hours
Ingredients:
- 3 tablespoons dried rosemary
- 2 tablespoons cumin seeds, ground
- 2 tablespoons dried coriander
- 1 tablespoon dried oregano
- 2 teaspoons ground cinnamon
- ½ teaspoon salt
- 8 pounds beef brisket, sliced into chunks
- 1 cup beef stock

Directions:
1. Mix the rosemary, cumin, coriander, oregano, cinnamon, and salt in a bowl.
2. Massage the spice mix into the beef brisket and allow to rest in the fridge for 12 hours.

3. When ready to cook, fire the Traeger Grill to 180F. Use desired wood pellets when cooking. Close the lid and preheat for 15 minutes.
4. Place the brisket fat side down on the grill grate and cook for 4 hours.
5. After 4 hours, turn up the heat to 250F.
6. Continue cooking the beef brisket until the internal temperature reaches 160F. Remove and place on a foil. Crimp the edges of the foil to create a sleeve. Pour in the beef stock.
7. Return the brisket in the foil sleeve and continue cooking for another hour.
Nutrition Info: Calories per serving: 453 ; Protein: 33.5g; Carbs: 1g; Fat: 34g Sugar: 0.1g

Pastrami

Servings: 6 To 8
Cooking Time: 12 To 16 Hours
Ingredients:
- 1 (8-pound) corned beef brisket
- 2 tablespoons yellow mustard
- 1 batch Espresso Brisket Rub
- Worcestershire Mop and Spritz, for spritzing

Directions:
1. Supply your Traeger with wood pellets and follow the start-up procedure. Preheat the grill, with the lid closed, to 225°F.
2. Coat the brisket all over with mustard and season it with the rub. Using your hands, work the rub into the meat. Pour the mop into a spray bottle.
3. Place the brisket directly on the grill grate and smoke until its internal temperature reaches 195°F, spritzing it every hour with the mop.
4. Pull the corned beef brisket from the grill and wrap it completely in aluminum foil or butcher paper. Place the wrapped brisket in a cooler, cover the cooler, and let it rest for 1 or 2 hours.
5. Remove the corned beef from the cooler and unwrap it. Slice the corned beef and serve.

Pork Steak

Servings: 4
Cooking Time: 20 Minutes
Ingredients:
- For the Brine:
- 2-inch piece of orange peel
- 2 sprigs of thyme
- 4 tablespoons salt
- 4 black peppercorns
- 1 sprig of rosemary
- 2 tablespoons brown sugar
- 2 bay leaves
- 10 cups water

- For Pork Steaks:
- 4 pork steaks, fat trimmed
- Game rub as needed

Directions:

1. Prepare the brine and for this, take a large container, place all of its ingredients in it and stir until sugar has dissolved.
2. Place steaks in it, add some weights to keep steak submerge into the brine and let soak for 24 hours in the refrigerator.
3. When ready to cook, switch on the Traeger grill, fill the grill hopper with hickory flavored wood pellets, power the grill on by using the control panel, select 'smoke' on the temperature dial, or set the temperature to 225 degrees F and let it preheat for a minimum of 15 minutes.
4. Meanwhile, remove steaks from the brine, rinse well, pat dry with paper towels and then season well with game rub until coated.
5. When the grill has preheated, open the lid, place steaks on the grill grate, shut the grill and smoke for 10 minutes per side until the internal temperature reaches the 140 degrees F.
6. When done, transfer steaks to a cutting board, let them rest for 10 minutes, then cut into slices and serve.

Nutrition Info: Calories: 260 Cal ;Fat: 21 g ;Carbs: 1 g ;Protein: 17 g ;Fiber: 0 g

Wood Pellet Grilled Tenderloin With Fresh Herb Sauce

Servings: 4
Cooking Time: 15 Minutes
Ingredients:
- Pork
- 1 pork tenderloin, silver skin removed and dried
- BBQ seasoning
- Fresh herb sauce
- 1 handful basil, fresh
- 1/4 tbsp garlic powder
- 1/3 cup olive oil
- 1/2 tbsp kosher salt

Directions:

1. Preheat the wood pellet grill to medium heat.
2. Coat the pork with BBQ seasoning then cook on semi-direct heat of the grill. Turn the pork regularly to ensure even cooking.
3. Cook until the internal temperature is 145°F. Remove from the grill and let it rest for 10 minutes.
4. Meanwhile, make the herb sauce by pulsing all the sauce ingredients in a food processor. Pulse for a few times or until well chopped.
5. Slice the pork diagonally and spoon the sauce on top. Serve and enjoy.

Nutrition Info: Calories 300, Total fat 22g, Saturated fat 4g, Total Carbs 13g, Net Carbs 12g, Protein 14g, Sugar 10g, Fiber 1g, Sodium: 791mg

Traeger Shredded Pork Tacos

Servings: 8
Cooking Time: 7 Hours
Ingredients:
- 5 lb pork shoulder, bone-in
- Dry Rub
- 3 tbsp. brown sugar
- 1 tbsp. salt
- 1 tbsp. garlic powder
- 1 tbsp. paprika
- 1 tbsp. onion powder
- 1/4 tbsp. cumin
- 1 tbsp. cayenne pepper

Directions:

1. Combine the dry rub ingredients in a mixing bowl then rub the pork roast.
2. Place the pork on the Traeger at 250F at indirect heat for 7 hours or until the internal temperature reaches 145F.
3. Remove the pork from the Traeger and let rest for 10 minutes before shredding.
4. Serve with tacos and enjoy

Nutrition Info: Calories 566, Total fat 41g, Saturated fat 0g, Total carbs 4g, Net carbs 4g Protein 44g, Sugars 3g, Fiber 0g, Sodium 659mg

Real Treat Chuck Roast

Servings: 8
Cooking Time: 4½ Hours
Ingredients:
- 2 tbsp. onion powder
- 2 tbsp. garlic powder
- 1 tbsp. red chili powder
- 1 tbsp. cayenne pepper
- Salt and freshly ground black pepper, to taste
- 1 (3 lb.) beef chuck roast
- 16 fluid oz. warm beef broth

Directions:

1. Set the temperature of Traeger Grill to 250 degrees F and preheat with closed lid for 15 minutes.
2. In a bowl, mix together spices, salt and black pepper.
3. Rub the chuck roast with spice mixture evenly.
4. Place the rump roast onto the grill and cook for about 1½ hours per side.
5. Now, arrange chuck roast in a steaming pan with beef broth.

6. With a piece of foil, cover the pan and cook for about 2-3 hours.
7. Remove the chuck roast from grill and place onto a cutting board for about 20 minutes before slicing.
8. With a sharp knife, cut the chuck roast into desired-sized slices and serve.
Nutrition Info: Calories per serving: 645; Carbohydrates: 4.2g; Protein: 46.4g; Fat: 48g; Sugar: 1.4g; Sodium: 329mg; Fiber: 1g

Barbecued Tenderloin

Servings: 4 To 6
Cooking Time: 30 Minutes
Ingredients:
- 2 (1-pound) pork tenderloins
- 1 batch Sweet and Spicy Cinnamon Rub
Directions:
1. Supply your smoker with wood pellets and follow the manufacturer's specific start-up procedure. Preheat the grill, with the lid closed, to 350°F.
2. Generously season the tenderloins with the rub. Using your hands, work the rub into the meat.
3. Place the tenderloins directly on the grill grate and smoke until their internal temperature reaches 145°F.
4. Remove the tenderloins from the grill and let them rest for 5 to 10 minutes, before thinly slicing and serving.

Favorite American Short Ribs

Servings: 6
Cooking Time: 3 Hours
Ingredients:
- For Mustard Sauce:
- 1 C. prepared yellow mustard
- ¼ C. red wine vinegar
- ¼ C. dill pickle juice
- 2 tbsp. soy sauce
- 2 tbsp. Worcestershire sauce
- 1 tsp. ground ginger
- 1 tsp. granulated garlic
- For Spice Rub:
- 2 tbsp. salt
- 2 tbsp. freshly ground black pepper
- 1 tbsp. white cane sugar
- 1 tbsp. granulated garlic
- For Ribs:
- 6 (14-oz.) (4-5-inch long) beef short ribs
Directions:

1. Set the temperature of Traeger Grill to 230-250 degrees F and preheat with closed lid for 15 minutes, using charcoal.
2. For sauce: in a bowl, add all the ingredients and with a wire whisk, bet until well combined.
3. For rub: in a small bowl, mix together all ingredients.
4. Coat the ribs with sauce generously and then sprinkle with spice rub evenly.
5. Place the ribs onto the grill over indirect heat, bone side down and cook for about 1-1½ hours.
6. Flip the side and cook for about 45 minutes.
7. Flip the side and cook for about 45 minutes more.
8. Remove the ribs from grill and place onto a cutting board for about 10 minutes before serving.
9. With a sharp knife, cut the ribs into equal-sized individual pieces and serve.
Nutrition Info: Calories per serving: 867; Carbohydrates: 7.7g; Protein: 117.1g; Fat: 37.5g; Sugar: 3.6g; Sodium: 3400mg; Fiber: 2.1g

Lamb Skewers

Servings: 6
Cooking Time: 8-12 Minutes
Ingredients:
- One lemon, juiced
- Two crushed garlic cloves
- Two chopped red onions
- One t. chopped thyme
- Pepper
- Salt
- One t. oregano
- 1/3 c. oil
- ½ t. cumin
- Two pounds cubed lamb leg
Directions:
1. Refrigerate the chunked lamb.
2. The remaining ingredients should be mixed together. Add in the meat. Refrigerate overnight.
3. Pat the meat dry and thread onto some metal or wooden skewers. Wooden skewers should be soaked in water.
4. Add wood pellets to your smoker and follow your cooker's startup procedure. Preheat your smoker, with your lid closed, until it reaches 450.
5. Grill, covered, for 4-6 minutes on each side.
6. Serve.
Nutrition Info: Calories: 201 Cal Fat: 9 g Carbohydrates: 3 g Protein: 24 g Fiber: 1 g

Smoked Texas Bbq Brisket

Servings: 4

Cooking Time: 5 Hours
Ingredients:
- 6 pounds whole packer brisket
- Commercial BBQ rub of your choice

Directions:
1. Trim the brisket from any membrane and loose fat. Trim the fat side to ¼ inch thick.
2. Season all sides of the brisket with the BBQ rub and allow to rest for 30 minutes inside the fridge.
3. When ready to cook, fire the Traeger Grill to 275F. Use mesquite wood pellets when cooking. Close the lid and preheat for 15 minutes.
4. Place the brisket fat side up on the grill grate and cook for 5 hours or until the internal temperature reaches 165F.
5. Once cooked, remove the brisket from the grill and allow to rest before slicing.

Nutrition Info: Calories per serving: 703; Protein: 93.9g; Carbs: 0 g; Fat: 33.4g Sugar: 0g

Lamb Chops With Rosemary And Olive Oil

Servings: 4
Cooking Time: 50 Minutes
Ingredients:
- 12 Lamb loin chops, fat trimmed
- 1 tablespoon chopped rosemary leaves
- Salt as needed for dry brining
- Jeff's original rub as needed
- ¼ cup olive oil

Directions:
1. Take a cookie sheet, place lamb chops on it, sprinkle with salt, and then refrigerate for 2 hours. Meanwhile, take a small bowl, place rosemary leaves in it, stir in oil and let the mixture stand for 1 hour.
2. When ready to cook, switch on the Traeger grill, fill the grill hopper with apple-flavored wood pellets, power the grill on by using the control panel, select 'smoke' on the temperature dial, or set the temperature to 225 degrees F and let it preheat for a minimum of 5 minutes.
3. Meanwhile, brush rosemary-oil mixture on all sides of lamb chops and then sprinkle with Jeff's original rub.
4. When the grill has preheated, open the lid, place lamb chops on the grill grate, shut the grill and smoke for 50 minutes until the internal temperature of lamb chops reach to 138 degrees F.
5. When done, wrap lamb chops in foil, let them rest for 7 minutes and then serve.

Nutrition Info: Calories: 171.5 Cal ;Fat: 7.8 g ;Carbs: 0.4 g ;Protein: 23.2 g ;Fiber: 0.1 g

Pickled-pepper Pork Chops

Servings: 4
Cooking Time: 45 To 50 Minutes
Ingredients:
- 4 (1-inch-thick) pork chops
- ½ cup pickled jalapeño juice or pickle juice
- ¼ cup chopped pickled (jarred) jalapeño pepper slices
- ¼ cup chopped roasted red peppers
- ¼ cup canned diced tomatoes, well-drained
- ¼ cup chopped scallions
- 2 teaspoons poultry seasoning
- 2 teaspoons salt
- 2 teaspoons freshly ground black pepper

Directions:
1. Pour the jalapeño juice into a large container with a lid. Add the pork chops, cover, and marinate in the refrigerator for at least 4 hours or overnight, supplementing with or substituting pickle juice as desired.
2. In a small bowl, combine the chopped pickled jalapeños, roasted red peppers, tomatoes, scallions, and poultry seasoning to make a relish. Set aside.
3. Remove the pork chops from the marinade and shake off any excess. Discard the marinade. Season both sides of the chops with the salt and pepper.
4. Supply your smoker with wood pellets and follow the manufacturer's specific start-up procedure. Preheat, with the lid closed, to 325°F.
5. To serve, divide the chops among plates and top with the pickled pepper relish.

Grilled Leg Of Lambs Steaks

Servings: 4
Cooking Time: 10 Minutes
Ingredients:
- 4 lamb steaks, bone-in
- 1/4 cup olive oil
- 4 garlic cloves, minced
- 1 tbsp rosemary, freshly chopped
- Salt and black pepper

Directions:
1. Place the lamb in a shallow dish in a single layer. Top with oil, garlic cloves, rosemary, salt, and black pepper then flip the steaks to cover on both sides.
2. Let sit for 30 minutes to marinate.
3. Preheat the wood pellet grill to high and brush the grill grate with oil.
4. Place the lamb steaks on the grill grate and cook until browned and the internal is slightly pink. The internal temperature should be 140 F.
5. Let rest for 5 minutes before serving. Enjoy.

Nutrition Info: Calories 327, Total Fat 21.9g, Saturated fat 5g, Total Carbs 1.7g, Net Carbs 1.5g,

Protein 29.6g, Sugar 0g, Fiber 0.2g, Sodium: 112mg, Potassium 410mg.

Nutrition Info: Calories 1073, Total fat 42g, Saturated fat 15g, Total Carbs 111g, Net Carbs 108g, Protein 61g, Sugar 99g, Fiber 3g, Sodium: 1663mg

Lamb Shank

Servings: 6
Cooking Time: 4 Hours
Ingredients:
- 8-ounce red wine
- 2-ounce whiskey
- 2 tablespoons minced fresh rosemary
- 1 tablespoon minced garlic
- Black pepper
- 6 (1¼-pound) lamb shanks

Directions:
1. In a bowl, add all ingredients except lamb shank and mix till well combined.
2. In a large resealable bag, add marinade and lamb shank.
3. Seal the bag and shake to coat completely.
4. Refrigerate for about 24 hours.
5. Preheat the pallet grill to 225 degrees F.
6. Arrange the leg of lamb in pallet grill and cook for about 4 hours.

Nutrition Info: Calories: 1507 Cal Fat: 62 g
Carbohydrates: 68.7 g Protein:163.3 g Fiber: 6 g

Wood Pellet Smoked Pork Ribs

Servings: 4
Cooking Time: 10 Hours
Ingredients:
- 2 racks baby back ribs
- 1 cup homemade BBQ rub
- 24 oz hard apple cider
- 1 cup dark brown sugar
- 2 batches homemade BBQ sauce

Directions:
1. Set your wood pellet to smoke.
2. Remove the membrane from the pork ribs then generously coat with bbq sauce.
3. Smoke at 175°F for 5 hours. Increase the grill temperature to 225°F.
4. Transfer the pork to a high sided pan that has been sprayed with cooking spray.
5. Pour over the apple cider and rub the pork with sugar. Cover the pan with foil and place it back to the grill. Cook for 4 more hours.
6. Transfer the ribs from the pan to the grill grate and increase the temperature to 300°F.
7. Brush the ribs with BBQ sauce 3 times in the next 1 hour. Remove the ribs from the grill and serve them. Enjoy.

Simple Grilled Lamb Chops

Servings: 6
Cooking Time: 6 Minutes
Ingredients:
- 1/4 cup distilled white vinegar
- 2 tbsp salt
- 1/2 tbsp black pepper
- 1 tbsp garlic, minced
- 1 onion, thinly sliced
- 2 tbsp olive oil
- 2lb lamb chops

Directions:
1. In a resealable bag, mix vinegar, salt, black pepper, garlic, sliced onion, and oil until all salt has dissolved.
2. Add the lamb chops and toss until well coated. Place in the fridge to marinate for 2 hours.
3. Preheat the wood pellet grill to high heat.
4. Remove the lamb from the fridge and discard the marinade. Wrap any exposed bones with foil.
5. Grill the lamb for 3 minutes per side. You can also broil in a broiler for more crispness.
6. Serve and enjoy

Nutrition Info: Calories 519, Total fat 44.8g, Saturated fat 18g, Total Carbs 2.3g, Net Carbs 1.9g, Protein 25g, Sugar1g, Fiber 0.4g, Sodium: 861mg, Potassium 359mg

Cajun Double-smoked Ham

Servings: 12 To 15
Cooking Time: 4 Or 5 Hours
Ingredients:
- 1 (5- or 6-pound) bone-in smoked ham
- 1 batch Cajun Rub
- 3 tablespoons honey

Directions:
1. Supply your smoker with wood pellets and follow the manufacturer's specific start-up procedure. Preheat the grill, with the lid closed, to 225°F.
2. Generously season the ham with the rub and place it either in a pan or directly on the grill grate. Smoke it for 1 hour.
3. Drizzle the honey over the ham and continue to smoke it until the ham's internal temperature reaches 145°F.
4. Remove the ham from the grill and let it rest for 5 to 10 minutes, before thinly slicing and serving.

Roasted Leg Of Lamb

Servings: 12
Cooking Time: 2 Hours
Ingredients:
- 8 pounds leg of lamb, bone-in, fat trimmed
- 2 lemons, juiced, zested
- 1 tablespoon minced garlic
- 4 sprigs of rosemary, 1-inch diced
- 4 cloves of garlic, peeled, sliced lengthwise
- Salt as needed
- Ground black pepper as needed
- 2 teaspoons olive oil

Directions:
1. Switch on the Traeger grill, fill the grill hopper with cherry flavored wood pellets, power the grill on by using the control panel, select 'smoke' on the temperature dial, or set the temperature to 450 degrees F and let it preheat for a minimum of 15 minutes.
2. Meanwhile, take a small bowl, place minced garlic in it, stir in oil and then rub this mixture on all sides of the lamb leg.
3. Then make ¾-inch deep cuts into the lamb meat, about two dozen, stuff each cut with garlic slices and rosemary, sprinkle with lemon zest, drizzle with lemon juice, and then season well with salt and black pepper.
4. When the grill has preheated, open the lid, place the leg of lamb on the grill grate, shut the grill, and smoke for 30 minutes.
5. Change the smoking temperature to 350 degrees F and then continue smoking for 1 hour and 30 minutes until the internal temperature reaches 130 degrees F.
6. When done, transfer lamb to a cutting board, let it rest for 15 minutes, then cut it into slices and serve.
Nutrition Info: Calories: 219 Cal ;Fat: 14 g ;Carbs: 1 g ;Protein: 22 g ;Fiber: 0 g

Jalapeño-bacon Pork Tenderloin

Servings: 4 To 6
Cooking Time: 2 Hours And 30 Minutes
Ingredients:
- ¼ cup yellow mustard
- 2 (1-pound) pork tenderloins
- ¼ cup Pork Rub
- 8 ounces cream cheese, softened
- 1 cup grated Cheddar cheese
- 1 tablespoon unsalted butter, melted
- 1 tablespoon minced garlic
- 2 jalapeño peppers, seeded and diced
- 1½ pounds bacon

Directions:
1. Slather the mustard all over the pork tenderloins, then sprinkle generously with the dry rub to coat the meat.
2. Supply your smoker with wood pellets and follow the manufacturer's specific start-up procedure. Preheat, with the lid closed, to 225°F.
3. Place the tenderloins directly on the grill, close the lid, and smoke for 2 hours.
4. Remove the pork from the grill and increase the temperature to 375°F.
5. In a small bowl, combine the cream cheese, Cheddar cheese, melted butter, garlic, and jalapeños.
6. Starting from the top, slice deeply along the center of each tenderloin end to end, creating a cavity.
7. Spread half of the cream cheese mixture in the cavity of one tenderloin. Repeat with the remaining mixture and the other piece of meat.
8. Securely wrap one tenderloin with half of the bacon. Repeat with the remaining bacon and the other piece of meat.
9. Transfer the bacon-wrapped tenderloins to the grill, close the lid, and smoke for about 30 minutes, or until a meat thermometer inserted in the thickest part of the meat reads 160°F and the bacon is browned and cooked through.
10. Let the tenderloins rest for 5 to 10 minutes before slicing and serving.

Grilled Hanger Steak

Servings: 6
Cooking Time: 50 Minutes
Ingredients:
- Hanger Steak - 1
- Salt
- Pepper
- For Bourbon Sauce
- Bourbon whiskey - ⅛ cup
- Honey - ⅛ cup
- Sriracha - 1 tbsp
- Garlic - ½ tbsp
- Salt - ¼ tbsp

Directions:
1. Preheat the grill to 225 degrees.
2. Use pepper and salt to season the steak liberally.
3. Place the steak on the grill and close the lid.
4. Let it cook until the temperature goes down to the finish.
5. Take an iron skillet and place it on the stove.
6. Add some butter to the pan and place the steak on it.
7. Cook on both sides for 2 minutes each.
8. Remove the steak from the stove.
9. Add the bourbon sauce ingredients to the pan.
10. Cook and whisk for 3-4 minutes. Pour it over your steak.

11. Serve with your favorite side dish or simply have it with the bourbon sauce.
Nutrition Info: Carbohydrates: 6 g Protein: 10 g Fat: 7 g Sodium: 180 mg Cholesterol: 36 mg

Cowboy Cut Steak

Servings: 4
Cooking Time: 1 Hour And 15 Minutes
Ingredients:
- 2 cowboy cut steak, each about 2 ½ pounds
- Salt as needed
- Beef rub as needed
- For the Gremolata:
- 2 tablespoons chopped mint
- 1 bunch of parsley, leaves separated
- 1 lemon, juiced
- 1 tablespoon lemon zest
- ½ teaspoon minced garlic
- ¼ teaspoon salt
- 1/8 teaspoon ground black pepper
- 1/4 cup olive oil

Directions:
1. Switch on the Traeger grill, fill the grill hopper with mesquite flavored wood pellets, power the grill on by using the control panel, select 'smoke' on the temperature dial, or set the temperature to 225 degrees F and let it preheat for a minimum of 5 minutes.
2. Meanwhile, prepare the steaks, and for this, season them with salt and BBQ rub until well coated.
3. When the grill has preheated, open the lid, place steaks on the grill grate, shut the grill and smoke for 45 minutes to 1 hour until thoroughly cooked, and internal temperature reaches 115 degrees F.
4. Meanwhile, prepare gremolata and for this, take a medium bowl, place all of its ingredients in it and then stir well until combined, set aside until combined.
5. When done, transfer steaks to a dish, let rest for 15 minutes, and meanwhile, change the smoking temperature of the grill to 450 degrees F and let it preheat for a minimum of 10 minutes.
6. Then return steaks to the grill grate and cook for 7 minutes per side until the internal temperature reaches 130 degrees F.
Nutrition Info: Calories: 361 Cal ;Fat: 31 g ;Carbs: 1 g ;Protein: 19 g ;Fiber: 0.2 g

Stuffed Pork Crown Roast

Servings: 2-4
Cooking Time: 3 Hours 30 Minutes
Ingredients:
- 12-14 ribs or 1 Snake River Pork Crown Roast

- Apple cider vinegar - 2 tbsp
- Apple juice - 1 cup
- Dijon mustard - 2 tbsp
- Salt - 1 tsp
- Brown sugar - 1 tbsp
- Freshly chopped thyme or rosemary - 2 tbsp
- Cloves of minced garlic - 2
- Olive oil - ½ cup
- Coarsely ground pepper - 1 tsp
- Your favorite stuffing - 8 cups

Directions:
1. Set the pork properly in a shallow roasting pan on a flat rack. Cover both ends of the bone with a piece of foil.
2. To make the marinade, boil the apple cider or apple juice on high heat until it reduces to about half its quantity. Remove the content from the heat and whisk in the mustard, vinegar, thyme, garlic, brown sugar, pepper, and salt. Once all that is properly blended, whisk in the oil slowly.
3. Use a pastry brush to apply the marinade to the roast. Ensure that you coat all the surfaces evenly. Cover it on all sides using plastic wrap. Allow it to sit for about 60 minutes until the meat has reached room temperature.
4. At this time, feel free to brush the marinade on the roast again. Cover it and return it to the refrigerator until it is time to cook it. When you are ready to cook it, allow the meat to reach room temperature, and put it in on the pellet grill. Ensure that the grill is preheated for about 15 minutes before you do.
5. Roast the meat for 30 minutes, then reduce the temperature of the grill. Fill the crown loosely with the stuffing and mound it at the top. Cover the stuffing properly with foil. You can also bake the stuffing separately alongside the roast in a pan.
6. Roast the pork thoroughly for 90 more minutes. Get rid of the foil and continue to roast the stuffing for 30-90 minutes until the pork reaches an internal temperature of 150 degrees Fahrenheit. Ensure that you do not touch the bone of the meat with the temperature probe, or you will get a false reading.
7. Remove the roast from the grill. Allow it to rest for around 15 minutes so that the meat soaks in all the juices. Remove the foil covering the bones. Leave the butcher's string on until you are ready to carve it. Now, transfer it to a warm platter, carve between the bones, and enjoy!
Nutrition Info: Carbohydrates: 5.5 g Protein: 107.9 g Fat: 58.9 g Sodium: 702 mg Cholesterol: 325.3 mg

Rosemary Lamb

Servings: 2
Cooking Time: 3 Hours

Ingredients:
- 1 rack of lamb rib, membrane removed
- 12 baby potatoes
- 1 bunch of asparagus, ends trimmed
- Ground black pepper, as needed
- Salt, as needed
- 1 teaspoon dried rosemary
- 2 tablespoons olive oil
- 1/2 cup butter, unsalted

Directions:
1. Switch on the Traeger grill, fill the grill hopper with flavored wood pellets, power the grill on by using the control panel, select 'smoke' on the temperature dial, or set the temperature to 225 degrees F and let it preheat for a minimum of 5 minutes.
2. Meanwhile, drizzle oil on both sides of lamb ribs and then sprinkle with rosemary.
3. Take a deep baking dish, place potatoes in it, add butter and mix until coated.
4. When the grill has preheated, open the lid, place lamb ribs on the grill grate along with potatoes in the baking dish, shut the grill and smoke for 3 hours until the internal temperature reaches 145 degrees F.
5. Add asparagus into the baking dish in the last 20 minutes and, when done, remove baking dish from the grill and transfer lamb to a cutting board.
6. Let lamb rest for 15 minutes, cut it into slices, and then serve with potatoes and asparagus.

Nutrition Info: Calories: 355 Cal ;Fat: 12.5 g ;Carbs: 25 g ;Protein: 35 g ;Fiber: 6 g

Texas-style Beef Ribs

Servings: 4
Cooking Time: 6 Hours 3 Minutes
Ingredients:
- 2 tbsp. butter
- 1 C. white vinegar
- 1 C. yellow mustard
- 2 tbsp. brown sugar
- 2 tbsp. Tabasco sauce
- 1 tsp. Worcestershire sauce
- 2 racks of beef ribs
- Salt and freshly ground black pepper, to taste

Directions:
1. For BBQ sauce: in a pan, melt butter over medium heat. Stir in vinegar, mustard, brown sugar, Tabasco and Worcestershire sauce and remove from heat.
2. Set aside to cool completely.
3. Set the temperature of Traeger Grill to 225 degrees F and preheat with closed lid for 15 minutes.
4. Season the rib racks with salt and black pepper evenly.
5. Coat rib rack with cooled sauce evenly.
6. Arrange the rib racks onto the grill and cook for about 5-6 hours, coating with sauce after every 2 hours.
7. Remove the rib racks from grill and place onto a cutting board for about 10-15 minutes before slicing.
8. With a sharp knife, cut the rib racks into equal-sized individual ribs and serve.

Nutrition Info: Calories per serving: 504; Carbohydrates: 5.7g; Protein: 70.7g; Fat: 19.7g; Sugar: 3.6g; Sodium: 719mg; Fiber: 1.4g

Wood Pellet Smoked Lamb Shoulder

Servings: 7
Cooking Time: 1hour 30 Minutes;
Ingredients:
- For Smoked Lamb Shoulder
- 5 lb lamb shoulder, boneless and excess fat trimmed
- 2 tbsp kosher salt
- 2 tbsp black pepper
- 1 tbsp rosemary, dried
- The Injection
- 1 cup apple cider vinegar
- The Spritz
- 1 cup apple cider vinegar
- 1 cup apple juice

Directions:
1. Preheat the wood pellet smoker with a water pan to 225 F.
2. Rinse the lamb in cold water then pat it dry with a paper towel. Inject vinegar to the lamb.
3. Pat the lamb dry again and rub with oil, salt black pepper and rosemary. Tie with kitchen twine.
4. Smoke uncovered for 1 hour then spritz after every 15 minutes until the internal temperature reaches 195 F.
5. Remove the lamb from the grill and place it on a platter. Let cool before shredding it and enjoying it with your favorite side.

Nutrition Info: Calories 243, Total fat 19g, Saturated fat 8g, Total Carbs 0g, Net Carbs 0g, Protein 17g, Sugar 0g, Fiber 1g, Sodium: 63mg, Potassium 234mg

Trager New York Strip

Servings: 6
Cooking Time: 15 Minutes
Ingredients:
- 3 New York strips
- Salt and pepper

Directions:
1. If the steak is in the fridge, remove it 30 minutes prior to cooking.

2. Preheat the Traeger to 450F.
3. Meanwhile, season the steak generously with salt and pepper. Place it on the grill and let it cook for 5 minutes per side or until the internal temperature reaches 1280F.
4. Remove the steak from the grill and let it rest for 10 minutes.

Nutrition Info: Calories 198, Total fat 14g, Saturated fat 6g, Total carbs 0g, Net carbs 0g Protein 17g, Sugars 0g, Fiber 0g, Sodium 115mg

Lamb Breast

Servings: 2
Cooking Time: 2 Hours And 40 Minutes
Ingredients:
- 1 (2-pound) trimmed bone-in lamb breast
- ½ cup white vinegar
- ¼ cup yellow mustard
- ½ cup BBQ rub

Directions:
1. Preheat the pallet grill to 225 degrees F.
2. Rinse the lamb breast with vinegar evenly.
3. Coat lamb breast with mustard and the, season with BBQ rub evenly.
4. Arrange lamb breast in pallet grill and cook for about 2-2½ hours.
5. Remove the lamb breast from the pallet grill and transfer onto a cutting board for about 10 minutes before slicing.
6. With a sharp knife, cut the lamb breast in desired sized slices and serve.

Nutrition Info: Calories: 877 Cal Fat: 34.5 g Carbohydrates: 2.2 g Protein: 128.7 g Fiber: 0 g

FISH AND SEAFOOD RECIPES

Traeger Salmon With Togarashi

Servings: 3
Cooking Time: 20 Minutes
Ingredients:
- 1 salmon fillet
- 1/4 cup olive oil
- 1/2 tbsp kosher salt
- 1 tbsp Togarashi seasoning

Directions:
1. Preheat your Traeger to 400F.
2. Place the salmon on a sheet lined with non-stick foil with the skin side down.
3. Rub the oil into the meat then sprinkle salt and Togarashi.
4. Place the salmon on the grill and cook for 20 minutes or until the internal temperature reaches 145F with the lid closed.
5. Remove from the Traeger and serve when hot.
Nutrition Info: Calories 119, Total fat 10g, Saturated fat 2g, Total carbs 0g, Net carbs 0g Protein 0g, Sugars 0g, Fiber 0g, Sodium 720mg

Bacon-wrapped Shrimp

Servings: 12
Cooking Time: 10 Minutes
Ingredients:
- 1 lb raw shrimp
- 1/2 tbsp salt
- 1/4 tbsp garlic powder
- 1 lb bacon, cut into halves

Directions:
1. Preheat your Traeger to 350F.
2. Remove the shells and tails from the shrimp then pat them dry with the paper towels.
3. Sprinkle salt and garlic on the shrimp then wrap with bacon and secure with a toothpick.
4. Place the shrimps on a baking rack greased with cooking spray.
5. Cook for 10 minutes, flip and cook for another 10 minutes or until the bacon is crisp enough.
6. Remove from the Traeger and serve.
Nutrition Info: Calories 204, Total fat 14g, Saturated fat 5g, Total carbs 1g, Net carbs 1g Protein 18g, Sugars 0g, Fiber 0g, Sodium 939mg

Lobster Tail

Servings: 2
Cooking Time: 25 Minutes
Ingredients:
- 2 lobster tails
- Salt
- Freshly ground black pepper
- 1 batch Lemon Butter Mop for Seafood

Directions:
1. Supply your smoker with wood pellets and follow the manufacturer's specific start-up procedure. Preheat the grill, with the lid closed, to 375°F.
2. Using kitchen shears, slit the top of the lobster shells, through the center, nearly to the tail. Once cut, expose as much meat as you can through the cut shell.
3. Season the lobster tails all over with salt and pepper.
4. Place the tails directly on the grill grate and grill until their internal temperature reaches 145°F. Remove the lobster from the grill and serve with the mop on the side for dipping.

Barbeque Shrimp

Servings: 6
Cooking Time: 8 Minutes
Ingredients:
- 2-pound raw shrimp (peeled and deveined)
- ¼ cup extra virgin olive oil
- ½ tsp paprika
- ½ tsp red pepper flakes
- 2 garlic cloves (minced)
- 1 tsp cumin
- 1 lemon (juiced)
- 1 tsp kosher salt
- 1 tbsp chili paste
- Bamboo or wooden skewers (soaked for 30 minutes, at least)

Directions:
1. Combine the pepper flakes, cumin, lemon, salt, chili, paprika, garlic and olive oil. Add the shrimp and toss to combine.
2. Transfer the shrimp and marinade into a ziplock bag and refrigerate for 4 hours.
3. Let shrimp rest in room temperature after pulling it out from marinade
4. Start your grill on smoke, leaving the lid opened for 5 minutes, or until fire starts. Use hickory wood pellet.
5. Keep lid unopened and preheat the grill to "high" for 15 minutes.
6. Thread shrimps onto skewers and arrange the skewers on the grill grate.
7. Smoke shrimps for 8 minutes, 4 minutes per side.
8. Serve and enjoy.
Nutrition Info: Calories: 267 Cal Fat: 11.6 g Carbohydrates: 4.9 g   Protein: 34.9 g Fiber:0.4 g

Grilled Tilapia

Servings: 6
Cooking Time: 2o Minutes
Ingredients:
- 2 tsp dried parsley
- ½ tsp garlic powder
- 1 tsp cayenne pepper
- ½ tsp ground black pepper
- ½ tsp thyme
- ½ tsp dried basil
- ½ tsp oregano
- 3 tbsp olive oil
- ½ tsp lemon pepper
- 1 tsp kosher salt
- 1 lemon (juiced)
- 6 tilapia fillets
- 1 ½ tsp creole seafood seasoning

Directions:
1. In a mixing bowl, combine spices
2. Brush the fillets with oil and lemon juice.
3. Liberally, season all sides of the tilapia fillets with the seasoning mix.
4. Preheat your grill to 325°F
5. Place a non-stick BBQ grilling try on the grill and arrange the tilapia fillets onto it.
6. Grill for 15 to 20 minutes
7. Remove fillets and cool down

Nutrition Info: Calories: 176 Cal Fat: 9.6 g Carbohydrates: 1.5 g Protein: 22.3 g Fiber: 0.5 g

Chilean Sea Bass

Servings: 6
Cooking Time: 40 Minutes
Ingredients:
- 4 sea bass fillets, skinless, each about 6 ounces
- Chicken rub as needed
- 8 tablespoons butter, unsalted
- 2 tablespoons chopped thyme leaves
- Lemon slices for serving
- For the Marinade:
- 1 lemon, juiced
- 4 teaspoons minced garlic
- 1 tablespoon chopped thyme
- 1 teaspoon blackened rub
- 1 tablespoon chopped oregano
- 1/4 cup oil

Directions:
1. Prepare the marinade and for this, take a small bowl, place all of its ingredients in it, stir until well combined, and then pour the mixture into a large plastic bag.

2. Add fillets in the bag, seal it, turn it upside down to coat fillets with the marinade and let it marinate for a minimum of 30 minutes in the refrigerator.
3. When ready to cook, switch on the Traeger grill, fill the grill hopper with apple-flavored wood pellets, power the grill on by using the control panel, select 'smoke' on the temperature dial, or set the temperature to 325 degrees F and let it preheat for a minimum of 15 minutes.
4. Meanwhile, take a large baking pan and place butter on it.
5. When the grill has preheated, open the lid, place baking pan on the grill grate, and wait until butter melts.
6. Remove fillets from the marinade, pour marinade into the pan with melted butter, then season fillets with chicken rubs until coated on all sides, then place them into the pan, shut the grill and cook for 30 minutes until internal temperature reaches 160 degrees F, frequently basting with the butter sauce.
7. When done, transfer fillets to a dish, sprinkle with thyme and then serve with lemon slices.

Nutrition Info: Calories: 232 Cal ;Fat: 12.2 g ;Carbs: 0.8 g ;Protein: 28.2 g ;Fiber: 0.1 g

Grilled Shrimp Kabobs

Servings: 4
Cooking Time: 10 Minutes
Ingredients:
- 1 lb. colossal shrimp, peeled and deveined
- 2 tbsp. oil
- 1/2 tbsp. garlic salt
- 1/2 tbsp. salt
- 1/8 tbsp. pepper
- 6 skewers

Directions:
1. Preheat your Traeger to 375F.
2. Pat the shrimp dry with a paper towel.
3. In a mixing bowl, mix oil, garlic salt, salt, and pepper
4. Toss the shrimp in the mixture until well coated.
5. Skewer the shrimps and cook in the Traeger with the lid closed for 4 minutes.
6. Open the lid, flip the skewers and cook for another 4 minutes or until the shrimp is pink and the flesh is opaque.
7. Serve.

Nutrition Info: Calories 325, Total fat 0g, Saturated fat 0g, Total carbs 0g, Net carbs 0g Protein 20g, Sugars 0g, Fiber 0g, Sodium 120mg

Cajun Smoked Catfish

Servings: 4
Cooking Time: 2 Hours
Ingredients:
- 4 catfish fillets (5 ounces each)
- ½ cup Cajun seasoning
- 1 tsp ground black pepper
- 1 tbsp smoked paprika
- 1 /4 tsp cayenne pepper
- 1 tsp hot sauce
- 1 tsp granulated garlic
- 1 tsp onion powder
- 1 tsp thyme
- 1 tsp salt or more to taste
- 2 tbsp chopped fresh parsley

Directions:
1. Pour water into the bottom of a square or rectangular dish. Add 4 tbsp salt. Arrange the catfish fillets into the dish. Cover the dish and refrigerate for 3 to 4 hours.
2. Combine the paprika, cayenne, hot sauce, onion, salt, thyme, garlic, pepper and Cajun seasoning in a mixing bowl.
3. Remove the fish from the dish and let it sit for a few minutes, or until it is at room temperature. Pat the fish fillets dry with a paper towel.
4. Rub the seasoning mixture over each fillet generously.
5. Start your grill on smoke, leaving the lid opened for 5 minutes, or until fire starts.
6. Keep lid unopened and preheat to 200°F, using mesquite hardwood pellets.
7. Arrange the fish fillets onto the grill grate and close the grill. Cook for about 2 hours, or until the fish is flaky.
8. Remove the fillets from the grill and let the fillets rest for a few minutes to cool.
9. Serve and garnish with chopped fresh parsley.
Nutrition Info: Calories: 204 Cal Fat: 11.1 g Carbohydrates: 2.7 g   Protein: 22.9 g Fiber: 0.6 g

Wood-fired Halibut

Servings: 4
Cooking Time: 20 Minutes
Ingredients:
- 1 pound halibut fillet
- 1 batch Dill Seafood Rub

Directions:
1. Supply your smoker with wood pellets and follow the manufacturer's specific start-up procedure. Preheat the grill, with the lid closed, to 325°F.
2. Sprinkle the halibut fillet on all sides with the rub. Using your hands, work the rub into the meat.

3. Place the halibut directly on the grill grate and grill until its internal temperature reaches 145°F. Remove the halibut from the grill and serve immediately.

Crab Stuffed Lingcod

Servings: 6
Cooking Time: 30 Minutes
Ingredients:
- Lemon cream sauce
- 4 garlic cloves
- 1 shallot
- 1 leek
- 2 tbsp olive oil
- 1 tbsp salt
- 1/4 tbsp black pepper
- 3 tbsp butter
- 1/4 cup white wine
- 1 cup whipping cream
- 2 tbsp lemon juice
- 1 tbsp lemon zest
- Crab mix
- 1 lb crab meat
- 1/3 cup mayo
- 1/3 cup sour cream
- 1/3 cup lemon cream sauce
- 1/4 green onion, chopped
- 1/4 tbsp black pepper
- 1/2 tbsp old bay seasoning
- Fish
- 2 lb lingcod
- 1 tbsp olive oil
- 1 tbsp salt
- 1 tbsp paprika
- 1 tbsp green onion, chopped
- 1 tbsp Italian parsley

Directions:
1. Lemon cream sauce
2. Chop garlic, shallot, and leeks then add to a saucepan with oil, salt, pepper, and butter.
3. Saute over medium heat until the shallot is translucent.
4. Deglaze with white wine then add whipping cream. Bring the sauce to boil, reduce heat and simmer for 3 minutes.
5. Remove from heat and add lemon juice and lemon zest. Transfer the sauce to a blender and blend until smooth.
6. Set aside 1/3 cup for the crab mix
7. Crab mix
8. Add all the ingredients in a mixing bowl and mix thoroughly until well combined.
9. Set aside
10. Fish

11. Fire up your Traeger to high heat then slice the fish into 6-ounce portions.
12. Lay the fish on its side on a cutting board and slice it 3/4 way through the middle leaving a 1/2 inch on each end so as to have a nice pouch.
13. Rub the oil into the fish then place them on a baking sheet. Sprinkle with salt.
14. Stuff crab mix into each fish then sprinkle paprika and place it on the grill.
15. Cook for 15 minutes or more if the fillets are more than 2 inches thick.
16. Remove the fish and transfer to serving platters. Pour the remaining lemon cream sauce on each fish and garnish with onions and parsley.
Nutrition Info: Calories 476, Total fat 33g, Saturated fat 14g, Total carbs 6g, Net carbs 5g Protein 38g, Sugars 3g, Fiber 1g, Sodium 1032mg

- Salt to taste
- 1/2 cup butter

Directions:
1. In a bowl, combine all the ingredients for the spice blend.
2. Sprinkle both sides of the fish with the salt and spice blend.
3. Set your wood pellet grill to 450 degrees F.
4. Heat your cast iron pan and add the butter. Add the fillets to the pan.
5. Cook for 5 minutes per side.
6. Serving Suggestion: Garnish with lemon wedges.
7. Tip: Smoke the catfish for 20 minutes before seasoning.
Nutrition Info: Calories: 181.5 Fat: 10.5 g Cholesterol: 65.8 mg Carbohydrates: 2.9 g Fiber: 1.8 g Sugars: 0.4 g Protein: 19.2 g

Seared Tuna Steaks

Servings: 2
Cooking Time: 10 Minutes
Ingredients:
- 2 (1½- to 2-inch-thick) tuna steaks
- 2 tablespoons olive oil
- Salt
- Freshly ground black pepper

Directions:
1. Supply your smoker with wood pellets and follow the manufacturer's specific start-up procedure. Preheat the grill, with the lid closed, to 500°F.
2. Rub the tuna steaks all over with olive oil and season both sides with salt and pepper.
3. Place the tuna steaks directly on the grill grate and grill for 3 to 5 minutes per side, leaving a pink center. Remove the tuna steaks from the grill and serve immediately.

Blackened Salmon

Servings: 4
Cooking Time: 30 Minutes
Ingredients:
- 2 lb. salmon, fillet, scaled and deboned
- 2 tablespoons olive oil
- 4 tablespoons sweet dry rub
- 1 tablespoon cayenne pepper
- 2 cloves garlic, minced

Directions:
1. Turn on your wood pellet grill.
2. Set it to 350 degrees F.
3. Brush the salmon with the olive oil.
4. Sprinkle it with the dry rub, cayenne pepper, and garlic.
5. Grill for 5 minutes per side.
Nutrition Info: Calories: 460Fat: 23 gCholesterol: 140 mgCarbohydrates: 7 g Fiber: 5 g Sugars: 2 g Protein: 50 g

Blackened Catfish

Servings: 4
Cooking Time: 40 Minutes
Ingredients:
- Spice blend
- 1teaspoon granulated garlic
- 1/4 teaspoon cayenne pepper
- 1/2 cup Cajun seasoning
- 1teaspoon ground thyme
- 1teaspoon ground oregano
- 1teaspoon onion powder
- 1tablespoon smoked paprika
- 1teaspoon pepper
- Fish
- 4 catfish fillets

Crazy Delicious Lobster Tails

Servings: 4
Cooking Time: 25 Minutes
Ingredients:
- ½ C. butter, melted
- 2 garlic cloves, minced
- 2 tsp. fresh lemon juice
- Salt and freshly ground black pepper, to taste
- 4 (8-oz.) lobster tails

Directions:
1. Set the temperature of Traeger Grill to 450 degrees F and preheat with closed lid for 15 minutes.
2. In a metal pan, add all ingredients except for lobster tails and mix well.

3. Place the pan onto the grill and cook for about 10 minutes.
4. Meanwhile, cut down the top of the shell and expose lobster meat.
5. Remove pan of butter mixture from grill.
6. Coat the lobster meat with butter mixture.
7. Place the lobster tails onto the grill and cook for about 15 minutes, coating with butter mixture once halfway through.
8. Remove from grill and serve hot.
Nutrition Info: Calories per serving: 409; Carbohydrates: 0.6g; Protein: 43.5g; Fat: 24.9g; Sugar: 0.1g; Sodium: 1305mg; Fiber: 0g

Wood Pellet Smoked Buffalo Shrimp

Servings: 6
Cooking Time: 5 Minutes
Ingredients:
- 1 lb raw shrimps peeled and deveined
- 1/2 tbsp salt
- 1/4 tbsp garlic salt
- 1/4 tbsp garlic powder
- 1/4 tbsp onion powder
- 1/2 cup buffalo sauce

Directions:
1. Preheat the wood pellet grill to 450°F.
2. Coat the shrimp with both salts, garlic and onion powders.
3. Place the shrimp in a grill and cook for 3 minutes on each side.
4. Remove from the grill and toss in buffalo sauce. Serve with cheese, celery and napkins. Enjoy.
Nutrition Info: Calories 57, Total fat 1g, Saturated fat 0g, Total Carbs 1g, Net Carbs 1g, Protein 10g, Sugar 0g, Fiber 0g, Sodium: 1106mg, Potassium 469mg.

Lively Flavored Shrimp

Servings: 6
Cooking Time: 30 Minutes
Ingredients:
- 8 oz. salted butter, melted
- ¼ C. Worcestershire sauce
- ¼ C. fresh parsley, chopped
- 1 lemon, quartered
- 2 lb. jumbo shrimp, peeled and deveined
- 3 tbsp. BBQ rub

Directions:
1. In a metal baking pan, add all ingredients except for shrimp and BBQ rub and mix well.
2. Season the shrimp with BBQ rub evenly.
3. Add the shrimp in the pan with butter mixture and coat well.

4. Set aside for about 20-30 minutes.
5. Set the temperature of Traeger Grill to 250 degrees F and preheat with closed lid for 15 minutes.
6. Place the pan onto the grill and cook for about 25-30 minutes.
7. Remove the pan from grill and serve hot.
Nutrition Info: Calories per serving: 462; Carbohydrates: 4.7g; Protein: 34.9g; Fat: 33.3g; Sugar: 2.1g; Sodium: 485mg; Fiber: 0.2g

Summer Paella

Servings: 6
Cooking Time: 45 Minutes
Ingredients:
- 6 tablespoons extra-virgin olive oil, divided, plus more for drizzling
- 2 green or red bell peppers, cored, seeded, and diced
- 2 medium onions, diced
- 2 garlic cloves, slivered
- 1 (29-ounce) can tomato purée
- 1½ pounds chicken thighs
- Kosher salt
- 1½ pounds tail-on shrimp, peeled and deveined
- 1 cup dried thinly sliced chorizo sausage
- 1 tablespoon smoked paprika
- 1½ teaspoons saffron threads
- 2 quarts chicken broth
- 3½ cups white rice
- 2 (7½-ounce) cans chipotle chiles in adobo sauce
- 1½ pounds fresh clams, soaked in cold water for 15 to 20 minutes2 tablespoons chopped fresh parsley
- 2 lemons, cut into wedges, for serving

Directions:
1. Make the sofrito: On the stove top, in a saucepan over medium-low heat, combine ¼ cup of olive oil, the bell peppers, onions, and garlic, and cook for 5 minutes, or until the onions are translucent.
2. Stir in the tomato purée, reduce the heat to low, and simmer, stirring frequently, until most of the liquid has evaporated, about 30 minutes. Set aside. (Note: The sofrito can be made in advance and refrigerated.)
3. Supply your smoker with wood pellets and follow the manufacturer's specific start-up procedure. Preheat, with the lid closed, to 450°F.
4. Heat a large paella pan on the smoker and add the remaining 2 tablespoons of olive oil.
5. Add the chicken thighs, season lightly with salt, and brown for 6 to 10 minutes, then push to the outer edge of the pan.

6. Add the shrimp, season with salt, close the lid, and smoke for 3 minutes.
7. Add the sofrito, chorizo, paprika, and saffron, and stir together.
8. In a separate bowl, combine the chicken broth, uncooked rice, and 1 tablespoon of salt, stirring until well combined.
9. Add the broth-rice mixture to the paella pan, spreading it evenly over the other ingredients.
10. Close the lid and smoke for 5 minutes, then add the chipotle chiles and clams on top of the rice.
11. Close the lid and continue to smoke the paella for about 30 minutes, or until all of the liquid is absorbed.
12. Remove the pan from the grill, cover tightly with aluminum foil, and let rest off the heat for 5 minutes.
13. Drizzle with olive oil, sprinkle with the fresh parsley, and serve with the lemon wedges.

Traeger Spot Prawn Skewers

Servings: 6
Cooking Time: 10 Minutes
Ingredients:
- 2 lb spot prawns
- 2 tbsp oil
- Salt and pepper to taste

Directions:
1. Preheat your Traeger to 400F.
2. Skewer your prawns with soaked skewers then generously sprinkle with oil, salt, and pepper.
3. Place the skewers on the grill and cook with the lid closed for 5 minutes on each side.
4. Remove the skewers and serve when hot.
Nutrition Info: Calories 221, Total fat 7g, Saturated fat 1g, Total carbs 2g, Net carbs 2g Protein 34g, Sugars 0g, Fiber 0g, Sodium 1481mg

Bacon-wrapped Scallops

Servings: 4
Cooking Time: 30 Minutes
Ingredients:
- 12 scallops
- 12 bacon slices
- 3 tablespoons lemon juice
- Pepper to taste

Directions:
1. Turn on your wood pellet grill.
2. Set it to smoke.
3. Let it burn for 5 minutes while the lid is open.
4. Set it to 400 degrees F.
5. Wrap the scallops with bacon.
6. Secure with a toothpick.

7. Drizzle with the lemon juice and season with pepper.
8. Add the scallops to a baking tray.
9. Place the tray on the grill.
10. Grill for 20 minutes.
11. Serving Suggestion: Serve with sweet chili sauce.
Nutrition Info: Calories: 180.3 Fat: 8 g Cholesterol: 590.2 mg Carbohydrates: 3 g Fiber: 0 g Sugars: 0 g Protein: 22 g

Salmon With Avocado Salsa

Servings: 6
Cooking Time: 20 Minutes
Ingredients:
- 3 lb. salmon fillet
- Garlic salt and pepper to taste
- 4 cups avocado, sliced into cubes
- 1 onion, chopped
- 1 jalapeño pepper, minced
- 1 tablespoon lime juice
- 1 tablespoon olive oil
- ¼ cup cilantro, chopped
- Salt to taste

Directions:
1. Sprinkle both sides of salmon with garlic salt and pepper.
2. Set the Traeger wood pellet grill to smoke.
3. Grill the salmon for 7 to 8 minutes per side.
4. While waiting, prepare the salsa by combining the remaining ingredients in a bowl.
5. Serve salmon with the avocado salsa.
6. Tips: You can also use tomato salsa for this recipe if you don't have avocados.

Wood Pellet Salt And Pepper Spot Prawn Skewers

Servings: 6
Cooking Time: 10 Minutes
Ingredients:
- 2 lb spot prawns, clean
- 2 tbsp oil
- Salt and pepper to taste

Directions:
1. Preheat your grill to 400°F.
2. Meanwhile, soak the skewers then skewer with the prawns.
3. Brush with oil then season with salt and pepper to taste.
4. Place the skewers in the grill, close the lid, and cook for 5 minutes on each side.
5. Remove from the grill and serve. Enjoy.

Nutrition Info: Calories 221, Total fat 7g, Saturated fat 1g, Total Carbs 2g, Net Carbs 2g, Protein 34g, Sugar 0g, Fiber 0g, Sodium: 1481mg, Potassium 239mg

Traeger Rockfish

Servings: 6
Cooking Time: 20 Minutes
Ingredients:
- 6 rockfish fillets
- 1 lemon, sliced
- 3/4 tbsp salt
- 2 tbsp fresh dill, chopped
- 1/2 tbsp garlic powder
- 1/2 tbsp onion powder
- 6 tbsp butter

Directions:
1. Preheat your Traeger to 400F.
2. Season the fish with salt, dill, garlic and onion powder on both sides then place it in a baking dish.
3. Place a pat of butter and a lemon slice on each fillet. Place the baking dish in the Traeger and close the lid.
4. Cook for 20 minutes or until the fish is no longer translucent and is flaky.
5. Remove from Traeger and let rest for 5 minutes before serving.
Nutrition Info: Calories 270, Total fat 17g, Saturated fat 9g, Total carbs 2g, Net carbs 2g Protein 28g, Sugars 0g, Fiber 0g, Sodium 381mg

Cod With Lemon Herb Butter

Servings: 4
Cooking Time: 15 Minutes
Ingredients:
- 4 tablespoons butter
- 1 clove garlic, minced
- 1 tablespoon tarragon, chopped
- 1 tablespoon lemon juice
- 1 teaspoon lemon zest
- Salt and pepper to taste
- 1 lb. cod fillet

Directions:
1. Preheat the Traeger wood pellet grill to high for 15 minutes while the lid is closed.
2. In a bowl, mix the butter, garlic, tarragon, lemon juice and lemon zest, salt and pepper.
3. Place the fish in a baking pan.
4. Spread the butter mixture on top.
5. Bake the fish for 15 minutes.
6. Tips: You can also use other white fish fillet for this recipe.

Lemon Garlic Scallops

Servings: 6
Cooking Time: 5 Minutes
Ingredients:
- 1 dozen scallops
- 2 tablespoons chopped parsley
- Salt as needed
- 1 tablespoon olive oil
- 1 tablespoon butter, unsalted
- 1 teaspoon lemon zest
- For the Garlic Butter:
- ½ teaspoon minced garlic
- 1 lemon, juiced
- 4 tablespoons butter, unsalted, melted

Directions:
1. Switch on the Traeger grill, fill the grill hopper with alder flavored wood pellets, power the grill on by using the control panel, select 'smoke' on the temperature dial, or set the temperature to 400 degrees F and let it preheat for a minimum of 15 minutes.
2. Meanwhile, remove frill from scallops, pat dry with paper towels and then season with salt and black pepper.
3. When the grill has preheated, open the lid, place a skillet on the grill grate, add butter and oil, and when the butter melts, place seasoned scallops on it and then cook for 2 minutes until seared.
4. Meanwhile, prepare the garlic butter and for this, take a small bowl, place all of its ingredients in it and then whisk until combined.
5. Flip the scallops, top with some of the prepared garlic butter, and cook for another minute.
6. When done, transfer scallops to a dish, top with remaining garlic butter, sprinkle with parsley and lemon zest, and then serve.
Nutrition Info: Calories: 184 Cal ;Fat: 10 g ;Carbs: 1 g ;Protein: 22 g ;Fiber: 0.2 g

Wood Pellet Togarashi Grilled Salmon

Servings: 6
Cooking Time: 20 Minutes
Ingredients:
- 1 salmon fillet
- 1/4 cup olive oil
- 1/2 tbsp kosher salt
- 1 tbsp Togarashi seasoning

Directions:
1. Preheat the wood pellet grill to 400°F.
2. Place the salmon fillet on a non-stick foil sheet with the skin side up.

3. Rub the olive oil on the salmon and sprinkle with salt and togarashi seasoning.
4. Place the salmon on the preheated grill and close the lid. Cook for 20 minutes or until the internal temperature reaches 145°F.
5. Remove from the grill and serve when hot. Enjoy.
Nutrition Info: Calories 119, Total fat 10g, Saturated fat 2g, Total Carbs 0g, Net Carbs 0g, Protein 6g, Sugar 0g, Fiber 0g, Sodium: 720mg

Lobster Tails

Servings: 4
Cooking Time: 35 Minutes
Ingredients:
- 2 lobster tails, each about 10 ounces
- For the Sauce:
- 2 tablespoons chopped parsley
- 1/4 teaspoon garlic salt
- 1 teaspoon paprika
- 1/4 teaspoon ground black pepper
- 1/4 teaspoon old bay seasoning
- 8 tablespoons butter, unsalted
- 2 tablespoons lemon juice

Directions:
1. Switch on the Traeger grill, fill the grill hopper with flavored wood pellets, power the grill on by using the control panel, select 'smoke' on the temperature dial, or set the temperature to 450 degrees F and let it preheat for a minimum of 15 minutes.
2. Meanwhile, prepare the sauce and for this, take a small saucepan, place it over medium-low heat, add butter in it and when it melts, add remaining ingredients for the sauce and stir until combined, set aside until required.
3. Prepare the lobster and for this, cut the shell from the middle to the tail by using kitchen shears and then take the meat from the shell, keeping it attached at the base of the crab tail.
4. Then butterfly the crab meat by making a slit down the middle, then place lobster tails on a baking sheet and pour 1 tablespoon of sauce over each lobster tail, reserve the remaining sauce.
5. When the grill has preheated, open the lid, place crab tails on the grill grate, shut the grill and smoke for 30 minutes until opaque.
6. When done, transfer lobster tails to a dish and then serve with the remaining sauce.
Nutrition Info: Calories: 290 Cal ;Fat: 22 g ;Carbs: 1 g ;Protein: 20 g ;Fiber: 0.3 g

Wood Pellet Teriyaki Smoked Shrimp

Servings: 6
Cooking Time: 10 Minutes
Ingredients:
- 1 lb tail-on shrimp, uncooked
- 1/2 tbsp onion powder
- 1/2 tbsp salt
- 1/2 tbsp Garlic powder
- 4 tbsp Teriyaki sauce
- 4 tbsp sriracha mayo
- 2 tbsp green onion, minced

Directions:
1. Peel the shrimps leaving the tails then wash them removing any vein left over. Drain and pat with a paper towel to drain.
2. Preheat the wood pellet to 450°F
3. Season the shrimp with onion, salt, and garlic then place it on the grill to cook for 5 minutes on each side.
4. Remove the shrimp from the grill and toss it with teriyaki sauce. Serve garnished with mayo and onions. Enjoy.
Nutrition Info: Calories 87, Total fat 0g, Saturated fat 0g, Total Carbs 2g, Net Carbs 2g, Protein 16g, Sugar 1g, Fiber 0g, Sodium: 1241mg

Jerk Shrimp

Servings: 12
Cooking Time: 6 Minutes
Ingredients:
- 2 pounds shrimp, peeled, deveined
- 3 tablespoons olive oil
- For the Spice Mix:
- 1 teaspoon garlic powder
- 1 teaspoon of sea salt
- 1/4 teaspoon ground cayenne
- 1 tablespoon brown sugar
- 1/8 teaspoon smoked paprika
- 1 tablespoon smoked paprika
- 1/4 teaspoon ground thyme
- 1 lime, zested

Directions:
1. Switch on the Traeger grill, fill the grill hopper with flavored wood pellets, power the grill on by using the control panel, select 'smoke' on the temperature dial, or set the temperature to 450 degrees F and let it preheat for a minimum of 5 minutes.
2. Meanwhile, prepare the spice mix and for this, take a small bowl, place all of its ingredients in it and stir until mixed.
3. Take a large bowl, place shrimps in it, sprinkle with prepared spice mix, drizzle with oil and toss until well coated.

4. When the grill has preheated, open the lid, place shrimps on the grill grate, shut the grill and smoke for 3 minutes per side until firm and thoroughly cooked.

5. When done, transfer shrimps to a dish and then serve.

Nutrition Info: Calories: 131 Cal ;Fat: 4.3 g ;Carbs: 0 g ;Protein: 22 g ;Fiber: 0 g

Grilled Rainbow Trout

Servings: 6
Cooking Time: 2 Hours
Ingredients:
- 6 rainbow trout, cleaned, butterfly
- For the Brine:
- 1/4 cup salt
- 1 tablespoon ground black pepper
- 1/2 cup brown sugar
- 2 tablespoons soy sauce
- 16 cups water

Directions:
1. Prepare the brine and for this, take a large container, add all of its ingredients in it, stir until sugar has dissolved, then add trout and let soak for 1 hour in the refrigerator.
2. When ready to cook, switch on the Traeger grill, fill the grill hopper with oak flavored wood pellets, power the grill on by using the control panel, select 'smoke' on the temperature dial, or set the temperature to 225 degrees F and let it preheat for a minimum of 15 minutes.
3. Meanwhile, remove trout from the brine and pat dry with paper towels.
4. When the grill has preheated, open the lid, place trout on the grill grate, shut the grill and smoke for 2 hours until thoroughly cooked and tender.
5. When done, transfer trout to a dish and then serve.

Nutrition Info: Calories: 250 Cal ;Fat: 12 g ;Carbs: 1.4 g ;Protein: 33 g ;Fiber: 0.3 g

Charleston Crab Cakes With Remoulade

Servings: 4
Cooking Time: 45 Minutes
Ingredients:
- 1¼ cups mayonnaise
- ¼ cup yellow mustard
- 2 tablespoons sweet pickle relish, with its juices
- 1 tablespoon smoked paprika
- 2 teaspoons Cajun seasoning
- 2 teaspoons prepared horseradish
- 1 teaspoon hot sauce
- 1 garlic clove, finely minced
- 2 pounds fresh lump crabmeat, picked clean
- 20 butter crackers (such as Ritz brand), crushed
- 2 tablespoons Dijon mustard
- 1 cup mayonnaise
- 2 tablespoons freshly squeezed lemon juice
- 1 tablespoon salted butter, melted
- 1 tablespoon Worcestershire sauce
- 1 tablespoon Old Bay seasoning
- 2 teaspoons chopped fresh parsley
- 1 teaspoon ground mustard
- 2 eggs, beaten
- ¼ cup extra-virgin olive oil, divided

Directions:
1. For the remoulade:
2. In a small bowl, combine the mayonnaise, mustard, pickle relish, paprika, Cajun seasoning, horseradish, hot sauce, and garlic.
3. Refrigerate until ready to serve.
4. For the crab cakes:
5. Supply your smoker with wood pellets and follow the manufacturer's specific start-up procedure. Preheat, with the lid closed, to 375°F.
6. Spread the crabmeat on a foil-lined baking sheet and place over indirect heat on the grill, with the lid closed, for 30 minutes.
7. Remove from the heat and let cool for 15 minutes.
8. While the crab cools, combine the crushed crackers, Dijon mustard, mayonnaise, lemon juice, melted butter, Worcestershire sauce, Old Bay, parsley, ground mustard, and eggs until well incorporated.
9. Fold in the smoked crabmeat, then shape the mixture into 8 (1-inch-thick) crab cakes.
10. In a large skillet or cast-iron pan on the grill, heat 2 tablespoons of olive oil. Add half of the crab cakes, close the lid, and smoke for 4 to 5 minutes on each side, or until crispy and golden brown.
11. Remove the crab cakes from the pan and transfer to a wire rack to drain. Pat them to remove any excess oil.
12. Repeat steps 6 and 7 with the remaining oil and crab cakes.
13. Serve the crab cakes with the remoulade.

Enticing Mahi-mahi

Servings: 4
Cooking Time: 10 Minutes
Ingredients:
- 4 (6-oz.) mahi-mahi fillets
- 2 tbsp. olive oil
- Salt and freshly ground black pepper, to taste

Directions:

1. Set the temperature of Traeger Grill to 350 degrees F and preheat with closed lid for 15 minutes.
2. Coat fish fillets with olive oil and season with salt and black pepper evenly.
3. Place the fish fillets onto the grill and cook for about 5 minutes per side.
4. Remove the fish fillets from grill and serve hot.
Nutrition Info: Calories per serving: 195; Carbohydrates: 0g; Protein: 31.6g; Fat: 7g; Sugar: 0g; Sodium: 182mg; Fiber: 0g

Grilled Lingcod

Servings: 6
Cooking Time: 15 Minutes
Ingredients:
- 2 lb lingcod fillets
- 1/2 tbsp salt
- 1/2 tbsp white pepper
- 1/4 tbsp cayenne
- Lemon wedges

Directions:
1. Preheat the wood pellet grill to 375°F.
2. Place the lingcod on a parchment paper and season it with salt, white pepper, cayenne pepper then top with the lemon.
3. Place the fish on the grill and cook for 15 minutes or until the internal temperature reaches 145°F.
4. Serve and enjoy.
Nutrition Info: Calories 245, Total fat 2g, Saturated fat 0g, Total Carbs 2g, Net Carbs 1g, Protein 52g, Sugar 1g, Fiber 1g, Sodium: 442mg, Potassium 649mg

Wood Pellet Garlic Dill Smoked Salmon

Servings: 12
Cooking Time: 4 Hours
Ingredients:
- 2 salmon fillets
- Brine
- 4 cups water
- 1 cup brown sugar
- 1/3 cup kosher salt
- Seasoning
- 3 tbsp minced garlic
- 1 tbsp fresh dill, chopped

Directions:
1. In a zip lock bag, combine the brine ingredients until all sugar has dissolved. Place the salmon in the bag and refrigerate overnight.
2. Remove the salmon from the brine, rinse with water and pat dry with a paper towel. Let it rest for 2-4 hours at room temperature.
3. Season the salmon with garlic and dill generously.
4. Fire up the wood pellet grill to smoke and place the salmon on a cooling rack that is coated with cooking spray.
5. Place the rack in the smoker and close the lid.
6. Smoke the salmon for 4 hours until the smoke is between 130-180°F.
7. Remove the salmon from the grill and serve with crackers. Enjoy
Nutrition Info: Calories 139, Total fat 5g, Saturated fat 1g, Total Carbs 16g, Net Carbs 16g, Protein 9g, Sugar 0g, Fiber 0g, Sodium: 3143mg

Cajun Catfish

Servings: 6
Cooking Time: 15 Minutes
Ingredients:
- 2½ pounds catfish fillets
- 2 tablespoons olive oil
- 1 batch Cajun Rub

Directions:
1. Supply your smoker with wood pellets and follow the manufacturer's specific start-up procedure. Preheat the grill, with the lid closed, to 300°F.
2. Coat the catfish fillets all over with olive oil and season with the rub. Using your hands, work the rub into the flesh.
3. Place the fillets directly on the grill grate and smoke until their internal temperature reaches 145°F. Remove the catfish from the grill and serve immediately

Smoked Scallops

Servings: 6
Cooking Time: 15 Minutes
Ingredients:
- 2 pounds sea scallops
- 4 tbsp salted butter
- 2 tbsp lemon juice
- ½ tsp ground black pepper
- 1 garlic clove (minced)
- 1 kosher tsp salt
- 1 tsp freshly chopped tarragon

Directions:
1. Let the scallops dry using paper towels and drizzle all sides with salt and pepper to season
2. Place you're a cast iron pan in your grill and preheat the grill to 400°F with lid closed for 15 minutes.
3. Combine the butter and garlic in hot cast iron pan. Add the scallops and stir. Close grill lid and cook

for 8 minutes. Flip the scallops and cook for an additional 7 minutes.

4.   Remove the scallop from heat and let it rest for a few minutes.

5.   Stir in the chopped tarragon. Serve and top with lemon juice.

Nutrition Info: Calories: 204 Cal Fat: 8.9 g Carbohydrates: 4 g   Protein: 25.6 g Fiber: 0.1 g

Wood Pellet Smoked Salmon

Servings: 8
Cooking Time: 4 Hours
Ingredients:
*   Brine
*   4 cups water
*   1 cup brown sugar
*   1/3 cup kosher salt
*   Salmon
*   Salmon fillet, skin in
*   Maple syrup

Directions:
1.   Combine all the brine ingredients until the sugar has fully dissolved.

2.   Add the brine to a ziplock bag with the salmon and refrigerate for 12 hours.

3.   Remove the salmon from the brine, wash it and rinse with water. Pat dry with paper towel then let sit at room temperature for 2 hours.

4.   Startup your wood pellet to smoke and place the salmon on a baking rack sprayed with cooking spray.

5.   After cooking for an hour, baste the salmon with maple syrup. Do not let the smoker get above 180°F for accurate results.

6.   Smoke for 3-4 hours or until the salmon flakes easily.

Nutrition Info: Calories 101, Total fat 2g, Saturated fat 0g, Total carbs 16g, Net carbs 16g, Protein 4g, Sugar 16g, Fiber 0g, Sodium: 3131mg

Hot-smoked Salmon

Servings: 4
Cooking Time: 4 To 6 Hours
Ingredients:
*   1 (2-pound) half salmon fillet
*   1 batch Dill Seafood Rub

Directions:
1.   Supply your smoker with wood pellets and follow the manufacturer's specific start-up procedure. Preheat the grill, with the lid closed, to 180°F.

2.   Season the salmon all over with the rub. Using your hands, work the rub into the flesh.

3.   Place the salmon directly on the grill grate, skin-side down, and smoke until its internal temperature

reaches 145°F. Remove the salmon from the grill and serve immediately.

Grilled Herbed Tuna

Servings: 6
Cooking Time: 10 Minutes
Ingredients:
*   6 tuna steaks
*   1 tablespoon lemon zest
*   1 tablespoon fresh thyme, chopped
*   1 tablespoon fresh parsley, chopped
*   Garlic salt to taste

Directions:
1.   Sprinkle the tuna steaks with lemon zest, herbs and garlic salt.

2.   Cover with foil.

3.   Refrigerate for 4 hours.

4.   Grill for 3 minutes per side.

5.   Tips: Take the fish out of the refrigerator 30 minutes before cooking.

Traeger Grilled Lingcod

Servings: 6
Cooking Time: 15 Minutes
Ingredients:
*   2 lb lingcod fillets
*   1/2 tbsp salt
*   1/2 tbsp white pepper
*   1/4 tbsp cayenne pepper
*   Lemon wedges

Directions:
1.   Preheat your Traeger to 375F.

2.   Place the lingcod on a parchment paper or on a grill mat

3.   Season the fish with salt, pepper, and top with lemon wedges.

4.   Cook the fish for 15 minutes or until the internal temperature reaches 145F.

Nutrition Info: Calories 245, Total fat 2g, Saturated fat 0g, Total carbs 2g, Net carbs 0g Protein 52g, Sugars 1g, Fiber 1g, Sodium 442mg

Traeger Bacon-wrapped Scallops

Servings: 8
Cooking Time: 20 Minutes
Ingredients:
*   1 lb sea scallops
*   1/2 lb bacon
*   Sea salt

Directions:
1.   Preheat your Traeger to 375F.

2. Pat dry the scallops with a paper towel then wrap them with a piece of bacon and secure with a toothpick.
3. Lay the scallops on the grill with the bacon side down. Close the lid and cook for 5 minutes on each side.
4. Keep the scallops on the bacon side so that you will not get grill marks on the scallops.
5. Serve and enjoy.
Nutrition Info: Calories 261, Total fat 14g, Saturated fat 5g, Total carbs 5g, Net carbs 5g Protein 28g, Sugars 0g, Fiber 0g, Sodium 1238mg

Barbecued Shrimp

Servings: 4
Cooking Time: 10 Minutes
Ingredients:
• 1 pound peeled and deveined shrimp, with tails on
• 2 tablespoons olive oil
• 1 batch Dill Seafood Rub
Directions:
1. Soak wooden skewers in water for 30 minutes.
2. Supply your smoker with wood pellets and follow the manufacturer's specific start-up procedure. Preheat the grill, with the lid closed, to 375°F.
3. Thread 4 or 5 shrimp per skewer.
4. Coat the shrimp all over with olive oil and season each side of the skewers with the rub.
5. Place the skewers directly on the grill grate and grill the shrimp for 5 minutes per side. Remove the skewers from the grill and serve immediately.

Cured Cold-smoked Lox

Servings: 6
Cooking Time: 6 Hours
Ingredients:
• ¼ cup salt
• ¼ cup sugar
• 1 tablespoon freshly ground black pepper
• 1 bunch dill, chopped
• 1 pound sashimi-grade salmon, skin removed
• 1 avocado, sliced
• 8 bagels
• 4 ounces cream cheese
• 1 bunch alfalfa sprouts
• 1 (5-ounce) jar capers
Directions:
1. In a small bowl, combine the salt, sugar, pepper, and fresh dill to make the curing mixture. Set aside.
2. On a smooth surface, lay out a large piece of plastic wrap and spread half of the curing salt

mixture in the middle, spreading it out to about the size of the salmon.
3. Place the salmon on top of the curing salt.
4. Top the fish with the remaining curing salt, covering it completely. Wrap the salmon, leaving the ends open to drain.
5. Place the wrapped fish in a rimmed baking pan or dish lined with paper towels to soak up liquid.
6. Place a weight on the salmon evenly, such as a pan with a couple of heavy jars of pickles on top.
7. Put the salmon pan with weights in the refrigerator. Place something (a dishtowel, for example) under the back of the pan in order to slightly tip it down so the liquid drains away from the fish.
8. Leave the salmon to cure in the refrigerator for 24 hours.
9. Place the wood pellets in the smoker, but do not follow the start-up procedure and do not preheat.
10. Remove the salmon from the refrigerator, unwrap it, rinse it off, and pat dry.
11. Put the salmon in the smoker while still cold from the refrigerator to slow down the cooking process. You'll need to use a cold-smoker attachment or enlist the help of a smoker tube to hold the temperature at 80°F and maintain that for 6 hours to absorb smoke and complete the cold-smoking process.
12. Remove the salmon from the smoker, place it in a sealed plastic bag, and refrigerate for 24 hours. The salmon will be translucent all the way through.
13. Thinly slice the lox and serve with sliced avocado, bagels, cream cheese, alfalfa sprouts, and capers.

Octopus With Lemon And Oregano

Servings: 4
Cooking Time: 1 Hour And 30 Minutes
Ingredients:
• 3 lemons
• 3 pounds cleaned octopus, thawed if frozen
• 6 cloves garlic, peeled
• 4 sprigs fresh oregano
• 2 bay leaves
• Salt and pepper
• 3 tablespoons good-quality olive oil
• Minced fresh oregano for garnish
Directions:
1. Halve one of the lemons. Put the octopus, garlic, oregano sprigs, bay leaves, a large pinch of salt, and lemon halves in a large pot with enough water to cover by a couple of inches. Bring to a boil, adjust the heat so the liquid bubbles gently but steadily, and cook, occasionally turning with tongs, until the octopus is tender 30 to 90 minutes. (Check with the

tip of a sharp knife; it should go in smoothly.) Drain; discard the seasonings. (You can cover and refrigerate the octopus for up to 24 hours.)

2. Start the coals or heat a gas grill for direct hot cooking. Make sure the grates are clean.
3. Squeeze the juice 1 of the remaining lemons and whisk it with the oil and salt and pepper to taste. Cut the octopus into large serving pieces and toss with the oil mixture.
4. Put the octopus on the grill directly over the fire. Cover the grill and cook until heated through and charred, 4 to 5 minutes per side. Cut the remaining lemon in wedges. Transfer the octopus to a platter, sprinkle with minced oregano, and serve with the lemon wedges.

Nutrition Info: Calories: 139 Fats: 1.8 g Cholesterol: 0 mg Carbohydrates: 3.7 g Fiber: 0 g Sugars: 0 g Proteins: 25.4 g

Smoked Shrimp

Servings: 4
Cooking Time: 10 Minutes
Ingredients:
- 4 tablespoons olive oil
- 1 tablespoon Cajun seasoning
- 2 cloves garlic, minced
- 1 tablespoon lemon juice
- Salt to taste
- 2 lb. shrimp, peeled and deveined

Directions:
1. Combine all the ingredients in a sealable plastic bag.
2. Toss to coat evenly.
3. Marinate in the refrigerator for 4 hours.
4. Set the Traeger wood pellet grill to high.
5. Preheat it for 15 minutes while the lid is closed.
6. Thread shrimp onto skewers.
7. Grill for 4 minutes per side.
8. Tips: Soak skewers first in water if you are using wooden skewers.

Grilled Lobster Tail

Servings: 4
Cooking Time: 15 Minutes
Ingredients:
- 2 (8 ounces each) lobster tails
- 1/4 tsp old bay seasoning
- ½ tsp oregano
- 1 tsp paprika
- Juice from one lemon
- 1/4 tsp Himalayan salt
- 1/4 tsp freshly ground black pepper

- 1/4 tsp onion powder
- 2 tbsp freshly chopped parsley
- ¼ cup melted butter

Directions:
1. Slice the tail in the middle with a kitchen shear. Pull the shell apart slightly and run your hand through the meat to separate the meat partially
2. Combine the seasonings
3. Drizzle lobster tail with lemon juice and season generously with the seasoning mixture.
4. Preheat your wood pellet smoker to 450°F, using apple wood pellets.
5. Place the lobster tail directly on the grill grate, meat side down. Cook for about 15 minutes.
6. The tails must be pulled off and it must cool down for a few minutes
7. Drizzle melted butter over the tails.
8. Serve and garnish with fresh chopped parsley.

Nutrition Info: Calories: 146 Cal Fat: 11.7 g Carbohydrates: 2.1 g   Protein: 9.3 g Fiber: 0.8 g

Wine Infused Salmon

Servings: 4
Cooking Time: 5 Hours
Ingredients:
- 2 C. low-sodium soy sauce
- 1 C. dry white wine
- 1 C. water
- ½ tsp. Tabasco sauce
- 1/3 C. sugar
- ¼ C. salt
- ½ tsp. garlic powder
- ½ tsp. onion powder
- Freshly ground black pepper, to taste
- 4 (6-oz.) salmon fillets

Directions:
1. In a large bowl, add all ingredients except salmon and stir until sugar is dissolved.
2. Add salmon fillets and coat with brine well.
3. Refrigerate, covered overnight.
4. Remove salmon from bowl and rinse under cold running water.
5. With paper towels, pat dry the salmon fillets.
6. Arrange a wire rack in a sheet pan.
7. Place the salmon fillets onto wire rack, skin side down and set aside to cool for about 1 hour.
8. Set the temperature of Traeger Grill to 165 degrees F and preheat with closed lid for 15 minutes, using charcoal.
9. Place the salmon fillets onto the grill, skin side down and cook for about 3-5 hours or until desired doneness.
10. Remove the salmon fillets from grill and serve hot.

Cajun-blackened Shrimp

Servings: 4
Cooking Time: 20 Minutes
Ingredients:
- 1 pound peeled and deveined shrimp, with tails on
- 1 batch Cajun Rub
- 8 tablespoons (1 stick) butter
- ¼ cup Worcestershire sauce

Directions:
1. Supply your smoker with wood pellets and follow the manufacturer's specific start-up procedure. Preheat the grill, with the lid closed, to 450°F and place a cast-iron skillet on the grill grate. Wait about 10 minutes after your grill has reached temperature, allowing the skillet to get hot.
2. Meanwhile, season the shrimp all over with the rub.
3. When the skillet is hot, place the butter in it to melt. Once the butter melts, stir in the Worcestershire sauce.
4. Add the shrimp and gently stir to coat. Smoke-braise the shrimp for about 10 minutes per side, until opaque and cooked through. Remove the shrimp from the grill and serve immediately.

Oysters In The Shell

Servings: 4
Cooking Time: 20 Minutes
Ingredients:
- 8 medium oysters, unopened, in the shell, rinsed and scrubbed
- 1 batch Lemon Butter Mop for Seafood

Directions:
1. Supply your smoker with wood pellets and follow the manufacturer's specific start-up procedure. Preheat the grill, with the lid closed, to 375°F.
2. Place the unopened oysters directly on the grill grate and grill for about 20 minutes, or until the oysters are done and their shells open.
3. Discard any oysters that do not open. Shuck the remaining oysters, transfer them to a bowl, and add the mop. Serve immediately.

Super-tasty Trout

Servings: 8
Cooking Time: 5 Hours

Ingredients:
- 1 (7-lb.) whole lake trout, butterflied
- ½ C. kosher salt
- ½ C. fresh rosemary, chopped
- 2 tsp. lemon zest, grated finely

Directions:
1. Rub the trout with salt generously and then, sprinkle with rosemary and lemon zest.
2. Arrange the trout in a large baking dish and refrigerate for about 7-8 hours.
3. Remove the trout from baking dish and rinse under cold running water to remove the salt.
4. With paper towels, pat dry the trout completely.
5. Arrange a wire rack in a sheet pan.
6. Place the trout onto the wire rack, skin side down and refrigerate for about 24 hours.
7. Set the temperature of Traeger Grill to 180 degrees F and preheat with closed lid for 15 minutes, using charcoal.
8. Place the trout onto the grill and cook for about 2-4 hours or until desired doneness.
9. Remove the trout from grill and place onto a cutting board for about 5 minutes before serving.

Nutrition Info: Calories per serving: 633; Carbohydrates: 2.4g; Protein: 85.2g; Fat: 31.8g; Sugar: 0g; Sodium: 5000mg; Fiber: 1.6g

Barbecued Scallops

Servings: 4
Cooking Time: 10 Minutes
Ingredients:
- 1 pound large scallops
- 2 tablespoons olive oil
- 1 batch Dill Seafood Rub

Directions:
1. Supply your smoker with wood pellets and follow the manufacturer's specific start-up procedure. Preheat the grill, with the lid closed, to 375°F.
2. Coat the scallops all over with olive oil and season all sides with the rub.
3. Place the scallops directly on the grill grate and grill for 5 minutes per side. Remove the scallops from the grill and serve immediately.

Juicy Smoked Salmon

Servings: 5
Cooking Time: 50 Minutes
Ingredients:
- ½ cup of sugar
- 2 tablespoon salt
- 2 tablespoons crushed red pepper flakes
- ½ cup fresh mint leaves, chopped
- ¼ cup brandy

- 1(4 pounds) salmon, bones removed
- 2cups alder wood pellets, soaked in water

Directions:
1. Take a medium-sized bowl and add brown sugar, crushed red pepper flakes, mint leaves, salt, and brandy until a paste forms
2. Rub the paste all over your salmon and wrap the salmon with a plastic wrap
3. Allow them to chill overnight
4. Preheat your smoker to 220 degrees Fahrenheit and add wood Pellets
5. Transfer the salmon to the smoker rack and cook smoke for 45 minutes
6. Once the salmon has turned red-brown and the flesh flakes off easily, take it out and serve!

Nutrition Info: Calories: 370 Fats: 28g Carbs: 1g Fiber: 0g

Flavor-bursting Prawn Skewers

Servings: 5
Cooking Time: 8 Minutes
Ingredients:
- ¼ C. fresh parsley leaves, minced
- 1 tbsp. garlic, crushed
- 2½ tbsp. olive oil
- 2 tbsp. Thai chili sauce
- 1 tbsp. fresh lime juice
- 1½ pounds prawns, peeled and deveined

Directions:
1. In a large bowl, add all ingredients except for prawns and mix well.
2. In a resealable plastic bag, add marinade and prawns.
3. Seal the bag and shake to coat well
4. Refrigerate for about 20-30 minutes.
5. Set the temperature of Traeger Grill to 450 degrees F and preheat with closed lid for 15 minutes.
6. Remove the prawns from marinade and thread onto metal skewers.
7. Arrange the skewers onto the grill and cook for about 4 minutes per side.
8. Remove the skewers from grill and serve hot.

Nutrition Info: Calories per serving: 234; Carbohydrates: 4.9g; Protein: 31.2g; Fat: 9.3g; Sugar: 1.7g; Sodium: 562mg; Fiber: 0.1g

Grilled Tuna

Servings: 4
Cooking Time: 4 Minutes
Ingredients:
- 4 (6 ounce each) tuna steaks (1 inch thick)
- 1 lemon (juiced)
- 1 clove garlic (minced)

- 1 tsp chili
- 2 tbsp extra virgin olive oil
- 1 cup white wine
- 3 tbsp brown sugar
- 1 tsp rosemary

Directions:
1. Combine lemon, chili, white wine, sugar, rosemary, olive oil and garlic. Add the tuna steaks and toss to combine.
2. Transfer the tuna and marinade to a zip-lock bag. Refrigerate for 3 hours.
3. Remove the tuna steaks from the marinade and let them rest for about 1 hour
4. Start your grill on smoke, leaving the lid opened for 5 minutes, or until fire starts.
5. Do not open lid to preheat until 15 minutes to the setting "HIGH"
6. Grease the grill grate with oil and place the tuna on the grill grate. Grill tuna steaks for 4 minutes, 2 minutes per side.
7. Remove the tuna from the grill and let them rest for a few minutes.

Nutrition Info: Calories: 137 Cal Fat: 17.8 g Carbohydrates: 10.2 g Protein: 51.2 g Fiber: 0.6 g

Mango Shrimp

Servings: 4
Cooking Time: 15 Minutes
Ingredients:
- 1lb. shrimp, peeled and deveined but tail intact
- 2tablespoons olive oil
- Mango seasoning

Directions:
1. Turn on your wood pellet grill.
2. Preheat it to 425 degrees F.
3. Coat the shrimp with the oil and season with the mango seasoning.
4. Thread the shrimp into skewers.
5. Grill for 3 minutes per side.
6. Serving Suggestion: Garnish with chopped parsley.

Nutrition Info: Calories: 223.1 Fat: 4.3 g Cholesterol: 129.2 mg Carbohydrates: 29.2 g Fiber: 4.4 g Sugars: 15. 6g Protein: 19.5 g

Wood Pellet Grilled Scallops

Servings: 4
Cooking Time: 15 Minutes
Ingredients:
- 2 lb sea scallops, dried with a paper towel
- 1/2 tbsp garlic salt
- 2 tbsp kosher salt
- 4 tbsp salted butter

- Squeeze lemon juice

Directions:

1. Preheat the wood pellet grill to 400°F with the cast pan inside.
2. Sprinkle with both salts, pepper on both sides of the scallops.
3. Place the butter on the cast iron then add the scallops. Close the lid and cook for 8 minutes.
4. Flip the scallops and close the lid once more. Cook for 8 more minutes.
5. Remove the scallops from the grill and give a lemon squeeze. Serve immediately and enjoy.

Nutrition Info: Calories 177, Total fat 7g, Saturated fat 4g, Total Carbs 6g, Net Carbs 6g, Protein 23g, Sugar 0g, Fiber 0g, Sodium: 1430mg, Potassium 359mg

Grilled Shrimp Scampi

Servings: 4
Cooking Time: 10 Minutes
Ingredients:

- 1 lb raw shrimp, tail on
- 1/2 cup salted butter, melted
- 1/4 cup white wine, dry
- 1/2 tbsp fresh garlic, chopped
- 1 tbsp lemon juice
- 1/2 tbsp garlic powder
- 1/2 tbsp salt

Directions:

1. Preheat your wood pellet grill to 400°F with a cast iron inside.
2. In a mixing bowl, mix butter, wine, garlic, and juice then pour in the cast iron. Let the mixture mix for 4 minutes.
3. Sprinkle garlic and salt on the shrimp then place it on the cast iron. Grill for 10 minutes with the lid closed.
4. Remove the shrimp from the grill and serve when hot. Enjoy.

Nutrition Info: Calories 298, Total fat 24g, Saturated fat 15g, Total Carbs 2g, Net Carbs 2g, Protein 16g, Sugar 0g, Fiber 0g, Sodium: 1091mg, Potassium 389mg

Oyster In Shells

Servings: 4
Cooking Time: 8 Minutes
Ingredients:

- 12 medium oysters
- 1 tsp oregano
- 1 lemon (juiced)
- 1 tsp freshly ground black pepper
- 6 tbsp unsalted butter (melted)

- 1 tsp salt or more to taste
- 2 garlic cloves (minced)
- 2 ½ tbsp grated parmesan cheese
- 2 tbsp freshly chopped parsley

Directions:

1. Remove dirt
2. Open the shell completely. Discard the top shell.
3. Gently run the knife under the oyster to loosen the oyster foot from the bottom shell.
4. Repeat step 2 and 3 for the remaining oysters.
5. Combine melted butter, lemon, pepper, salt, garlic and oregano in a mixing bowl.
6. Pour ½ to 1 tsp of the butter mixture on each oyster.
7. Start your wood pellet grill on smoke, leaving the lid opened for 5 minutes, or until fire starts.
8. Keep lid unopened to preheat in the set "HIGH" with lid closed for 15 minutes.
9. Gently arrange the oysters onto the grill grate.
10. Grill oyster for 6 to 8 minutes or until the oyster juice is bubbling and the oyster is plump.
11. Remove oysters from heat. Serve and top with grated parmesan and chopped parsley.

Nutrition Info: Calories: 200 Cal Fat: 19.2 g Carbohydrates: 3.9 g Protein: 4.6 g Fiber: 0.8 g

Peppercorn Tuna Steaks

Servings: 3
Cooking Time: 10 Minutes
Ingredients:

- ¼ cup of salt
- 2 pounds yellowfin tuna
- ¼ cup Dijon mustard
- Freshly ground black pepper
- 2 tablespoons peppercorn

Directions:

1. Take a large-sized container and dissolve salt in warm water (enough water to cover fish)
2. Transfer tuna to the brine and cover, refrigerate for 8 hours
3. Preheat your smoker to 250 degrees Fahrenheit with your preferred wood
4. Remove tuna from bring and pat it dry
5. Transfer to grill pan and spread Dijon mustard all over
6. Season with pepper and sprinkle peppercorn on top
7. Transfer tuna to smoker and smoker for 1 hour
8. Enjoy!

Nutrition Info: Calories: 707 Fats: 57g Carbs: 10g Fiber: 2g

Stuffed Shrimp Tilapia

Servings: 5
Cooking Time: 45 Minutes
Ingredients:
- 5 ounces fresh, farmed tilapia fillets
- 2 tablespoons extra virgin olive oil
- 1and ½ teaspoons smoked paprika
- 1and ½ teaspoons Old Bay seasoning
- Shrimp stuffing
- 1pound shrimp, cooked and deveined
- 1tablespoon salted butter
- 1cup red onion, diced
- 1cup Italian bread crumbs
- ½ cup mayonnaise
- 1large egg, beaten
- 2teaspoons fresh parsley, chopped
- 1and ½ teaspoons salt and pepper

Directions:
1. Take a food processor and add shrimp, chop them up
2. Take a skillet and place it over medium-high heat, add butter and allow it to melt
3. Sauté the onions for 3 minutes
4. Add chopped shrimp with cooled Sautéed onion alongside remaining ingredients listed under stuffing ingredients and transfer to a bowl
5. Cover the mixture and allow it to refrigerate for 60 minutes
6. Rub both sides of the fillet with olive oil
7. Spoon 1/3 cup of the stuffing to the fillet
8. Flatten out the stuffing onto the bottom half of the fillet and fold the Tilapia in half
9. Secure with 2 toothpicks
10. Dust each fillet with smoked paprika and Old Bay seasoning
11. Preheat your smoker to 400 degrees Fahrenheit
12. Add your preferred wood Pellets and transfer the fillets to a non-stick grill tray
13. Transfer to your smoker and smoker for 30-45 minutes until the internal temperature reaches 145 degrees Fahrenheit
14. Allow the fish to rest for 5 minutes and enjoy!
Nutrition Info: Calories: 620 Fats: 50g Carbs: 6g Fiber: 1g

Mussels With Pancetta Aïoli

Servings: 4
Cooking Time: 30 Minutes
Ingredients:
- ¾ cup mayonnaise (to make your own, see page 460)
- 1tablespoon minced garlic, or more to taste
- 1.4-ounce slice pancetta, chopped
- Salt and pepper
- 4 pounds mussels
- 8 thick slices Italian bread
- ¼ cup good-quality olive oil

Directions:
1. Whisk the mayonnaise and garlic together in a small bowl. Put the pancetta in a small cold skillet, turn the heat to low; cook, occasionally stir, until most of the fat is rendered and the meat turns golden and crisp about 5 minutes. Drain on a paper towel, then stir into the mayonnaise along with 1 teaspoon of the rendered fat from the pan. Taste and add more garlic and some salt if you like. Cover and refrigerate until you're ready to serve. (You can make the aïoli up to several days ahead; refrigerate in an airtight container.)
2. Start the coals or heat a gas grill for direct hot cooking. Make sure the grates are clean.
3. Rinse the mussels and pull off any beards. Discard any that are broken or don't close when tapped.
4. Brush both sides of the bread slices with the oil. Put the bread on the grill directly over the fire. Close the lid and toast, turning once, until it develops grill marks with some charring, 1 to 2 minutes per side. Remove from the grill and keep warm.
5. Scatter the mussels onto the grill directly over the fire, spreading them out, so they are in a single layer. Immediately close the lid and cook for 3 minutes. Transfer the open mussels to a large bowl with tongs. If any have not opened, leave them on the grill, close the lid, and cook for another minute or 2, checking frequently and removing open mussels until they are all off the grill.
6. Dollop the aïoli over the tops of the mussels and use a large spoon to turn them over to coat them. Serve the mussels drizzled with their juices, either over (or alongside) the bread.
Nutrition Info: Calories: 159 Fats: 6.1 g Cholesterol: 0 mg Carbohydrates: 14.95 g Fiber: 0 g Sugars: 0 g Proteins: 9.57 g

Pacific Northwest Salmon

Servings: 4
Cooking Time: 1 Hour, 15 Minutes
Ingredients:
- 1 (2-pound) half salmon fillet
- 1 batch Dill Seafood Rub
- 2 tablespoons butter, cut into 3 or 4 slices

Directions:
1. Supply your smoker with wood pellets and follow the manufacturer's specific start-up procedure. Preheat the grill, with the lid closed, to 180°F.
2. Season the salmon all over with the rub. Using your hands, work the rub into the flesh.

3. Place the salmon directly on the grill grate, skin-side down, and smoke for 1 hour.
4. Place the butter slices on the salmon, equally spaced. Increase the grill's temperature to 300°F and continue to cook until the salmon's internal temperature reaches 145°F. Remove the salmon from the grill and serve immediately.

Grilled Teriyaki Salmon

Servings: 4
Cooking Time: 30 Minutes
Ingredients:
- 1 salmon fillet
- 1/8 cup olive oil
- 1/2 tbsp salt
- 1/4 tbsp pepper
- 1/4 tbsp garlic salt
- 1/4 cup butter, sliced
- 1/4 teriyaki sauce
- 1 tbsp sesame seeds

Directions:
1. Preheat the grill to 400°F.
2. Place the salmon fillet on a non-stick foil sheet. Drizzle the salmon with oil, seasonings, and butter on top.
3. Pace the foil tray on the grill and close the lid. Cook for 8 minutes then open the lid.
4. Brush the salmon with teriyaki sauce and repeat after every 5 minutes until all sauce is finished. The internal temperature should be 145°F.
5. Remove the salmon from the grill and sprinkle with sesame seeds.
6. Serve and enjoy with your favorite side dish.
Nutrition Info: Calories 296, Total fat 25g, Saturated fat 10g, Total Carbs 3g, Net Carbs 3g, Protein 14g, Sugar 3g, Fiber 0g, Sodium: 1179mg, Potassium 459mg

Yummy Buttery Clams

Servings: 6
Cooking Time: 8 Minutes
Ingredients:
- 24 littleneck clams
- ½ C. cold butter, chopped
- 2 tbsp. fresh parsley, minced
- 3 garlic cloves, minced
- 1 tsp. fresh lemon juice

Directions:
1. Set the temperature of Traeger Grill to 450 degrees F and preheat with closed lid for 15 minutes.
2. Scrub the clams under cold running water.
3. In a large casserole dish, mix together remaining ingredients.

4. Place the casserole dish onto the grill.
5. Now, arrange the clams directly onto the grill and cook for about 5-8 minutes or until they are opened. (Discard any that fail to open).
6. With tongs, carefully transfer the opened clams into the casserole dish and remove from grill.
7. Serve immediately.
Nutrition Info: Calories per serving: 306; Carbohydrates: 6.4g; Protein: 29.3g; Fat: 7.6g; Sugar: 0.1g; Sodium: 237mg; Fiber: 0.1g

No-fuss Tuna Burgers

Servings: 6
Cooking Time: 15 Minutes
Ingredients:
- 2 lb. tuna steak
- 1 green bell pepper, seeded and chopped
- 1 white onion, chopped
- 2 eggs
- 1 tsp. soy sauce
- 1 tbsp. blackened Saskatchewan rub
- Salt and freshly ground black pepper, to taste

Directions:
1. Set the temperature of Traeger Grill to 500 degrees F and preheat with closed lid for 15 minutes.
2. In a bowl, add all the ingredients and mix until well combined.
3. With greased hands, make patties from mixture.
4. Place the patties onto the grill close to the edges and cook for about 10-15 minutes, flipping once halfway through.
5. Serve hot.
Nutrition Info: Calories per serving: 313; Carbohydrates: 3.4g; Protein: 47.5g; Fat: 11g; Sugar: 1.9g; Sodium: 174mg; Fiber: 0.7g

Traeger Smoked Shrimp

Servings: 6
Cooking Time: 10 Minutes
Ingredients:
- 1 lb tail-on shrimp, uncooked
- 1/2 tbsp onion powder
- 1/2 tbsp garlic powder
- 1/2 tbsp salt
- 4 tbsp teriyaki sauce
- 2 tbsp green onion, minced
- 4 tbsp sriracha mayo

Directions:
1. Peel the shrimp shells leaving the tail on then wash well and rise.
2. Drain well and pat dry with a paper towel.
3. Preheat your Traeger to 450F.

4. Season the shrimp with onion powder, garlic powder, and salt. Place the shrimp in the Traeger and cook for 6 minutes on each side.
5. Remove the shrimp from the Traeger and toss with teriyaki sauce then garnish with onions and mayo.
Nutrition Info: Calories 87, Total fat 0g, Saturated fat 0g, Total carbs 2g, Net carbs 2g Protein 16g, Sugars 0g, Fiber 0g, Sodium 1241mg

Cider Salmon

Servings: 4
Cooking Time: 1 Hour
Ingredients:
- 1 ½ pound salmon fillet, skin-on, center-cut, pin bone removed
- For the Brine:
- 4 juniper berries, crushed
- 1 bay leaf, crumbled
- 1 piece star anise, broken
- 1 1/2 cups apple cider
- For the Cure:
- 1/2 cup salt
- 1 teaspoon ground black pepper
- 1/4 cup brown sugar
- 2 teaspoons barbecue rub

Directions:
1. Prepare the brine and for this, take a large container, add all of its ingredients in it, stir until mixed, then add salmon and let soak for a minimum of 8 hours in the refrigerator.
2. Meanwhile, prepare the cure and for this, take a small bowl, place all of its ingredients in it and stir until combined.
3. After 8 hours, remove salmon from the brine, then take a baking dish, place half of the cure in it, top with salmon skin-side down, sprinkle remaining cure on top, cover with plastic wrap and let it rest for 1 hour in the refrigerator.
4. When ready to cook, switch on the Traeger grill, fill the grill hopper with oak flavored wood pellets, power the grill on by using the control panel, select 'smoke' on the temperature dial, or set the temperature to 200 degrees F and let it preheat for a minimum of 5 minutes.
5. Meanwhile, remove salmon from the cure, pat dry with paper towels, and then sprinkle with black pepper.
6. When the grill has preheated, open the lid, place salmon on the grill grate, shut the grill, and smoke for 1 hour until the internal temperature reaches 150 degrees F.
7. When done, transfer salmon to a cutting board, let it rest for 5 minutes, then remove the skin and serve.

Nutrition Info: Calories: 233 Cal ;Fat: 14 g ;Carbs: 0 g ;Protein: 25 g ;Fiber: 0 g

Citrus Salmon

Servings: 6
Cooking Time: 30 Minutes
Ingredients:
- 2 (1-lb.) salmon fillets
- Salt and freshly ground black pepper, to taste
- 1 tbsp. seafood seasoning
- 2 lemons, sliced
- 2 limes, sliced

Directions:
1. Set the temperature of Traeger Grill to 225 degrees F and preheat with closed lid for 15 minutes.
2. Season the salmon fillets with salt, black pepper and seafood seasoning evenly.
3. Place the salmon fillets onto the grill and top each with lemon and lime slices evenly.
4. Cook for about 30 minutes.
5. Remove the salmon fillets from grill and serve hot.

Nutrition Info: Calories per serving: 327; Carbohydrates: 1g; Protein: 36.1g; Fat: 19.8g; Sugar: 0.2g; Sodium: 237mg; Fiber: 0.3g

Spicy Shrimps Skewers

Servings: 4
Cooking Time: 6 Minutes
Ingredients:
- 2 pounds shrimp, peeled, and deveined
- For the Marinade:
- 6 ounces Thai chilies
- 6 cloves of garlic, peeled
- 1 ½ teaspoon sugar
- 2 tablespoons Napa Valley rub
- 1 ½ tablespoon white vinegar
- 3 tablespoons olive oil

Directions:
1. Prepare the marinade and for this, place all of its ingredients in a food processor and then pulse for 1 minute until smooth.
2. Take a large bowl, place shrimps on it, add prepared marinade, toss until well coated, and let marinate for a minimum of 30 minutes in the refrigerator.
3. When ready to cook, switch on the Traeger grill, fill the grill hopper with apple-flavored wood pellets, power the grill on by using the control panel, select 'smoke' on the temperature dial, or set the temperature to 450 degrees F and let it preheat for a minimum of 5 minutes.

4. Meanwhile, remove shrimps from the marinade and then thread onto skewers.
5. When the grill has preheated, open the lid, place shrimps' skewers on the grill grate, shut the grill and smoke for 3 minutes per side until firm.
6. When done, transfer shrimps' skewers to a dish and then serve.
Nutrition Info: Calories: 187.2 Cal ;Fat: 2.7 g ;Carbs: 2.7 g ;Protein: 23.2 g ;Fiber: 0.2 g

Togarashi Smoked Salmon

Servings: 10
Cooking Time: 20 Hours 15 Minutes
Ingredients:
- Salmon filet - 2 large
- Togarashi for seasoning
- For Brine:
- Brown sugar - 1 cup
- Water - 4 cups
- Kosher salt - ⅓ cup

Directions:
1. Remove all the thorns from the fish filet.
2. Mix all the brine ingredients until the brown sugar is dissolved completely.
3. Put the mix in a big bowl and add the filet to it.
4. Leave the bowl to refrigerate for 16 hours.
5. After 16 hours, remove the salmon from this mix. Wash and dry it.
6. Place the salmon in the refrigerator for another 2-4 hours. (This step is important. DO NOT SKIP IT.)
7. Season your salmon filet with Togarashi.
8. Start the wood pellet grill with the 'smoke' option and place the salmon on it.
9. Smoke for 4 hours.
10. Make sure the temperature does not go above 180 degrees or below 130 degrees.
11. Remove from the grill and serve it warm with a side dish of your choice.
Nutrition Info: Carbohydrates: 19 g Protein: 10 g Fat: 6 g Sodium: 3772 mg Cholesterol: 29 mg

Wood Pellet Rockfish

Servings: 6
Cooking Time: 20 Minutes
Ingredients:
- 6 rockfish fillets
- 1 lemon, sliced
- 3/4 tbsp Himalayan salt
- 2 tbsp fresh dill, chopped
- 1/2 tbsp garlic powder
- 1/2 tbsp onion powder
- 6 tbsp butter

Directions:

1. Preheat your wood pellet grill to 375°F.
2. Place the rockfish in a baking dish and season with salt, dill, garlic, and onion.
3. Place butter on top of the fish then close the lid. Cook for 20 minutes or until the fish is no longer translucent.
4. Remove from grill and let sit for 5 minutes before serving. enjoy.
Nutrition Info: Calories 270, Total fat 17g, Saturated fat 9g, Total Carbs 2g, Net Carbs 0g, Protein 28g, Sugar 0g, Fiber 0g, Sodium: 381mg

Dijon-smoked Halibut

Servings: 6
Cooking Time: 2 Hours
Ingredients:
- 4 (6-ounce) halibut steaks
- ¼ cup extra-virgin olive oil
- 2 teaspoons kosher salt
- 1 teaspoon freshly ground black pepper
- ½ cup mayonnaise
- ½ cup sweet pickle relish
- ¼ cup finely chopped sweet onion
- ¼ cup chopped roasted red pepper
- ¼ cup finely chopped tomato
- ¼ cup finely chopped cucumber
- 2 tablespoons Dijon mustard
- 1 teaspoon minced garlic

Directions:
1. Rub the halibut steaks with the olive oil and season on both sides with the salt and pepper. Transfer to a plate, cover with plastic wrap, and refrigerate for 4 hours.
2. Supply your smoker with wood pellets and follow the manufacturer's specific start-up procedure. Preheat, with the lid closed, to 200°F.
3. Remove the halibut from the refrigerator and rub with the mayonnaise.
4. Put the fish directly on the grill grate, close the lid, and smoke for 2 hours, or until opaque and an instant-read thermometer inserted in the fish reads 140°F.
5. While the fish is smoking, combine the pickle relish, onion, roasted red pepper, tomato, cucumber, Dijon mustard, and garlic in a medium bowl. Refrigerate the mustard relish until ready to serve.
6. Serve the halibut steaks hot with the mustard relish.

Grilled Salmon

Servings: 4
Cooking Time: 25 Minutes
Ingredients:

- 1 (2-pound) half salmon fillet
- 3 tablespoons mayonnaise
- 1 batch Dill Seafood Rub

Directions:
1. Supply your smoker with wood pellets and follow the manufacturer's specific start-up procedure. Preheat the grill, with the lid closed, to 325°F.
2. Using your hands, rub the salmon fillet all over with the mayonnaise and sprinkle it with the rub.
3. Place the salmon directly on the grill grate, skin-side down, and grill until its internal temperature reaches 145°F. Remove the salmon from the grill and serve immediately.

Sriracha Salmon

Servings: 4
Cooking Time: 25 Minutes
Ingredients:
- 3-pound salmon, skin on
- For the Marinade:
- 1 teaspoon lime zest
- 1 tablespoon minced garlic
- 1 tablespoon grated ginger
- Sea salt as needed
- Ground black pepper as needed
- 1/4 cup maple syrup
- 2 tablespoons soy sauce
- 2 tablespoons Sriracha sauce
- 1 tablespoon toasted sesame oil
- 1 tablespoon rice vinegar
- 1 teaspoon toasted sesame seeds

Directions:
1. Prepare the marinade and for this, take a small bowl, place all of its ingredients in it, stir until well combined, and then pour the mixture into a large plastic bag.
2. Add salmon in the bag, seal it, turn it upside down to coat salmon with the marinade and let it marinate for a minimum of 2 hours in the refrigerator.
3. When ready to cook, switch on the Traeger grill, fill the grill hopper with flavored wood pellets, power the grill on by using the control panel, select 'smoke' on the temperature dial, or set the temperature to 450 degrees F and let it preheat for a minimum of 5 minutes.
4. Meanwhile, take a large baking sheet, line it with parchment paper, place salmon on it skin-side down and then brush with the marinade.
5. When the grill has preheated, open the lid, place baking sheet containing salmon on the grill grate, shut the grill and smoke for 25 minutes until thoroughly cooked.

6. When done, transfer salmon to a dish and then serve.
Nutrition Info: Calories: 360 Cal ;Fat: 21 g ;Carbs: 28 g ;Protein: 16 g ;Fiber: 1.5 g

Fish Fillets With Pesto

Servings: 6
Cooking Time: 15 Minutes
Ingredients:
- 2 cups fresh basil
- 1 cup parsley, chopped
- 1/2 cup walnuts
- 1/2 cup olive oil
- 1 cup Parmesan cheese, grated
- Salt and pepper to taste
- 4 white fish fillets

Directions:
1. Preheat the Traeger wood pellet grill to high for 15 minutes while the lid is closed.
2. Add all the ingredients except fish to a food processor.
3. Pulse until smooth. Set aside.
4. Season fish with salt and pepper.
5. Grill for 6 to 7 minutes per side.
6. Serve with the pesto sauce.
7. Tips: You can also spread a little bit of the pesto on the fish before grilling.

Halibut In Parchment

Servings: 4
Cooking Time: 15 Minutes
Ingredients:
- 16 asparagus spears, trimmed, sliced into 1/2-inch pieces
- 2 ears of corn kernels
- 4 ounces halibut fillets, pin bones removed
- 2 lemons, cut into 12 slices
- Salt as needed
- Ground black pepper as needed
- 2 tablespoons olive oil
- 2 tablespoons chopped parsley

Directions:
1. Switch on the Traeger grill, fill the grill hopper with flavored wood pellets, power the grill on by using the control panel, select 'smoke' on the temperature dial, or set the temperature to 450 degrees F and let it preheat for a minimum of 5 minutes.
2. Meanwhile, cut out 18-inch long parchment paper, place a fillet in the center of each parchment, season with salt and black pepper, and then drizzle with oil.

3. Cover each fillet with three lemon slices, overlapping slightly, sprinkle one-fourth of asparagus and corn on each fillet, season with some salt and black pepper, and seal the fillets and vegetables tightly to prevent steam from escaping the packet.

4. When the grill has preheated, open the lid, place fillet packets on the grill grate, shut the grill and smoke for 15 minutes until packets have turned slightly brown and puffed up.

5. When done, transfer packets to a dish, let them stand for 5 minutes, then cut 'X' in the center of each packet, carefully uncover the fillets an vegetables, sprinkle with parsley, and then serve.

Nutrition Info: Calories: 186.6 Cal ;Fat: 2.8 g ;Carbs: 14.2 g ;Protein: 25.7 g ;Fiber: 4.1 g

Halibut

Servings: 4
Cooking Time: 3o Minutes
Ingredients:
- 1-pound fresh halibut filet (cut into 4 equal sizes)
- 1 tbsp fresh lemon juice
- 2 garlic cloves (minced)
- 2 tsp soy sauce
- ½ tsp ground black pepper
- ½ tsp onion powder
- 2 tbsp honey
- ½ tsp oregano
- 1 tsp dried basil
- 2 tbsp butter (melted)
- Maple syrup for serving

Directions:
1. Combine the lemon juice, honey, soy sauce, onion powder, oregano, dried basil, pepper and garlic.
2. Brush the halibut filets generously with the filet the mixture. Wrap the filets with aluminum foil and refrigerate for 4 hours.
3. Remove the filets from the refrigerator and let them sit for about 2 hours, or until they are at room temperature.
4. Activate your wood pellet grill on smoke, leaving the lid opened for 5 minutes or until fire starts.
5. The lid must not be opened for it to be preheated and reach 275°F 15 minutes, using fruit wood pellets.
6. Place the halibut filets directly on the grill grate and smoke for 30 minutes
7. Remove the filets from the grill and let them rest for 10 minutes.
8. Serve and top with maple syrup to taste

Nutrition Info: Calories: 180 Cal Fat: 6.3 g
Carbohydrates: 10 g   Protein: 20.6 g Fiber: 0.3 g

Wood Pellet Grilled Salmon Sandwich

Servings: 4
Cooking Time: 15 Minutes
Ingredients:
- Salmon Sandwiches
- 4 salmon fillets
- 1 tbsp olive oil
- Fin and feather rub
- 1 tbsp salt
- 4 toasted bun
- Butter lettuce
- Dill Aioli
- 1/2 cup mayonnaise
- 1/2 tbsp lemon zest
- 2 tbsp lemon juice
- 1/4 tbsp salt
- 1/2 tbsp fresh dill, minced

Directions:
1. Mix all the dill aioli ingredients and place them in the fridge.
2. Preheat the wood pellet grill to 450°F.
3. Brush the salmon fillets with oil, rub, and salt. Place the fillets on the grill and cook until the internal temperature reaches 135°F.
4. Remove the fillets from the grill and let rest for 5 minutes.
5. Spread the aioli on the buns then top with salmon, lettuce, and the top bun.
6. Serve when hot.

Nutrition Info: Calories 852, Total fat 54g, Saturated fat 10g, Total Carbs 30g, Net Carbs 28g, Protein 57g, Sugar 5g, Fiber 2g, Sodium: 1268mg, Potassium 379mg

Grilled Blackened Salmon

Servings: 4
Cooking Time: 30 Minutes
Ingredients:
- 4 salmon fillet
- Blackened dry rub
- Italian seasoning powder

Directions:
1. Season salmon fillets with dry rub and seasoning powder.
2. Grill in the Traeger wood pellet grill at 325 degrees F for 10 to 15 minutes per side.
3. Tips: You can also drizzle salmon with lemon juice

Buttered Crab Legs

Servings: 4
Cooking Time: 10 Minutes
Ingredients:
- 12 tablespoons butter
- 1 tablespoon parsley, chopped

- 1 tablespoon tarragon, chopped
- 1 tablespoon chives, chopped
- 1 tablespoon lemon juice
- 4 lb. king crab legs, split in the center

Directions:
1. Set the Traeger wood pellet grill to 375 degrees F.
2. Preheat it for 15 minutes while lid is closed.
3. In a pan over medium heat, simmer the butter, herbs and lemon juice for 2 minutes.
4. Place the crab legs on the grill.
5. Pour half of the sauce on top.
6. Grill for 10 minutes.
7. Serve with the reserved butter sauce.
8. Tips: You can also use shrimp for this recipe.

Omega-3 Rich Salmon

Servings: 6
Cooking Time: 20 Minutes
Ingredients:
- 6 (6-oz.) skinless salmon fillets
- 1/3 C. olive oil
- ¼ C. spice rub
- ¼ C. honey
- 2 tbsp. Sriracha
- 2 tbsp. fresh lime juice

Directions:
1. Set the temperature of Traeger Grill to 300 degrees F and preheat with closed lid for 15 minutes.
2. Coat salmon fillets with olive oil and season with rub evenly.
3. In a small bowl, mix together remaining ingredients.
4. Arrange salmon fillets onto the grill, flat-side up and cook for about 7-10 minutes per side, coating with honey mixture once halfway through.
5. Serve hot alongside remaining honey mixture.
Nutrition Info: Calories per serving: 384; Carbohydrates: 15.7g; Protein: 33g; Fat: 21.7g; Sugar: 11.6g; Sodium: 621mg; Fiber: 0g

Bbq Oysters

Servings: 4-6
Cooking Time: 16 Minutes
Ingredients:
- Shucked oysters - 12
- Unsalted butter - 1 lb.
- Chopped green onions - 1 bunch
- Honey Hog BBQ Rub or Meat Church "The Gospel" - 1 tbsp
- Minced green onions - ½ bunch
- Seasoned breadcrumbs - ½ cup
- Cloves of minced garlic - 2
- Shredded pepper jack cheese - 8 oz
- Traeger Heat and Sweet BBQ sauce

Directions:

1. Preheat the pellet grill for about 10-15 minutes with the lid closed.
2. To make the compound butter, wait for the butter to soften. Then combine the butter, onions, BBQ rub, and garlic thoroughly.
3. Lay the butter evenly on plastic wrap or parchment paper. Roll it up in a log shape and tie the ends with butcher's twine. Place these in the freezer to solidify for an hour. This butter can be used on any kind of grilled meat to enhance its flavor. Any other high-quality butter can also replace this compound butter.
4. Shuck the oysters, keeping the juice in the shell.
5. Sprinkle all the oysters with breadcrumbs and place them directly on the grill. Allow them to cook for 5 minutes. You will know they are cooked when the oysters begin to curl slightly at the edges.
6. Once they are cooked, put a spoonful of the compound butter on the oysters. Once the butter melts, you can add a little bit of pepper jack cheese to add more flavor to them.
7. The oysters must not be on the grill for longer than 6 minutes, or you risk overcooking them. Put a generous squirt of the BBQ sauce on all the oysters. Also, add a few chopped onions.
8. Allow them to cool for a few minutes and enjoy the taste of the sea!
Nutrition Info: Carbohydrates: 2.5 g Protein: 4.7 g Fat: 1.1 g Sodium: 53 mg Cholesterol: 25 mg

Teriyaki Smoked Shrimp

Servings: 6
Cooking Time: 20 Minutes
Ingredients:
- Uncooked shrimp - 1 lb.
- Onion powder - ½ tbsp
- Garlic powder - ½ tbsp
- Teriyaki sauce - 4 tbsp
- Mayo - 4 tbsp
- Minced green onion - 2 tbsp
- Salt - ½ tbsp

Directions:
1. Remove the shells from the shrimp and wash thoroughly.
2. Preheat the wood pellet grill to 450 degrees.
3. Season with garlic powder, onion powder, and salt.
4. Cook the shrimp for 5-6 minutes on each side.
5. Once cooked, remove the shrimp from the grill and garnish it with spring onion, teriyaki sauce, and mayo.
Nutrition Info: Carbohydrates: 2 g Protein: 16 g Sodium: 1241 mg Cholesterol: 190 mg

Halibut With Garlic Pesto

Servings: 4

Cooking Time: 10 Minutes
Ingredients:
- 4 halibut fillets
- 1 cup olive oil
- Salt and pepper to taste
- 1/4 cup garlic, chopped
- 1/4 cup pine nuts

Directions:
1. Set the Traeger wood pellet grill to smoke.
2. Establish fire for 5 minutes.
3. Set temperature to high.
4. Place a cast iron on a grill.
5. Season fish with salt and pepper.
6. Add fish to the pan.
7. Drizzle with a little oil.
8. Sear for 4 minutes per side.
9. Prepare the garlic pesto by pulsing the remaining ingredients in the food processor until smooth.
10. Serve fish with garlic pesto.
11. Tips: You can also use other white fish fillets for this recipe.

- Nonstick spray, oil, or butter, for greasing
- 1 tablespoon chopped fresh parsley
- 1 lemon, sliced

Directions:
1. Fillet the fish and pat dry with paper towels.
2. Pour the orange juice into a large container with a lid and stir in the brown sugar, salt, and pepper.
3. Place the trout in the brine, cover, and refrigerate for 1 hour.
4. Cover the grill grate with heavy-duty aluminum foil. Poke holes in the foil and spray with cooking spray (see Tip).
5. Supply your smoker with wood pellets and follow the manufacturer's specific start-up procedure. Preheat, with the lid closed, to 225°F.
6. Remove the trout from the brine and pat dry. Arrange the fish on the foil-covered grill grate, close the lid, and smoke for 1 hour 30 minutes to 2 hours, or until flaky.
7. Remove the fish from the heat. Serve garnished with the fresh parsley and lemon slices.

Wood Pellet Grilled Lobster Tail

Servings: 2
Cooking Time: 15 Minutes
Ingredients:
- 10 oz lobster tail
- 1/4 tbsp old bay seasoning
- 1/4 tbsp Himalayan sea salt
- 2 tbsp butter, melted
- 1 tbsp fresh parsley, chopped

Directions:
1. Preheat the wood pellet to 450°F.
2. Slice the tails down the middle using a knife.
3. Season with seasoning and salt then place the tails on the grill grate.
4. Grill for 15 minutes or until the internal temperature reaches 140°F..
5. Remove the tails and drizzle with butter and garnish with parsley.
6. Serve and enjoy.

Nutrition Info: Calories 305, Total fat 14g, Saturated fat 8g, Total Carbs 5g, Net Carbs 5g, Protein 18g, Sugar 0g, Fiber 0g, Sodium: 685mg, Potassium 159mg

Citrus-smoked Trout

Servings: 6
Cooking Time: 1 To 2 Hours
Ingredients:
- 6 to 8 skin-on rainbow trout, cleaned and scaled
- 1 gallon orange juice
- ½ cup packed light brown sugar
- ¼ cup salt
- 1 tablespoon freshly ground black pepper

Spicy Shrimp

Servings: 4
Cooking Time: 10 Minutes
Ingredients:
- 3 tablespoons olive oil
- 6 cloves garlic
- 2 tablespoons chicken dry rub
- 6 oz. chili
- 1 1/2 tablespoons white vinegar
- 1 1/2 teaspoons sugar
- 2 lb. shrimp, peeled and deveined

Directions:
1. Add olive oil, garlic, dry rub, chili, vinegar and sugar in a food processor.
2. Blend until smooth.
3. Transfer mixture to a bowl.
4. Stir in shrimp.
5. Cover and refrigerate for 30 minutes.
6. Preheat the Traeger wood pellet grill to hit for 15 minutes while the lid is closed.
7. Thread shrimp onto skewers.
8. Grill for 3 minute per side.
9. Tips: You can also add vegetables to the skewers.

Grilled King Crab Legs

Servings: 4
Cooking Time: 25 Minutes
Ingredients:
- 4 pounds king crab legs (split)
- 4 tbsp lemon juice
- 2 tbsp garlic powder
- 1 cup butter (melted)
- 2 tsp brown sugar
- 2 tsp paprika

- Black pepper (depends to your liking)

Directions:

1. In a mixing bowl, combine the lemon juice, butter, sugar, garlic, paprika and pepper.
2. Arrange the split crab on a baking sheet, split side up. Drizzle ¾ of the butter mixture over the crab legs. Configure your pellet grill for indirect cooking and preheat it to 225°F, using mesquite wood pellets.
3. Arrange the crab legs onto the grill grate, shell side down. Cover the grill and cook 25 minutes.
4. Remove the crab legs from the grill. Serve and top with the remaining butter mixture.

Nutrition Info: Calories: 480 Cal Fat: 53.2 g Carbohydrates: 6.1 g   Protein: 88.6 g Fiber: 1.2 g

Traeger Lobster Tail

Servings: 2

Cooking Time: 15 Minutes

Ingredients:

- 10 oz lobster tail
- 1/4 tbsp old bay seasoning
- 1/4 tbsp Himalayan salt
- 2 tbsp butter, melted
- 1 tbsp fresh parsley, chopped

Directions:

1. Preheat your Traeger to 450F.
2. Slice the tail down the middle then season it with bay seasoning and salt.
3. Place the tails directly on the grill with the meat side down. Grill for 15 minutes or until the internal temperature reaches 140F.
4. Remove from the Traeger and drizzle with butter.
5. Serve when hot garnished with parsley.

Nutrition Info: Calories 305, Total fat 14g, Saturated fat 8g, Total carbs 5g, Net carbs 5g Protein 38g, Sugars 0g, Fiber 0g, Sodium 684mg

Grilled Shrimp

Servings: 4

Cooking Time: 15 Minutes

Ingredients:

- Jumbo shrimp peeled and cleaned - 1 lb.

- Oil - 2 tbsp
- Salt - ½ tbsp
- Skewers - 4-5
- Pepper - ⅛ tbsp
- Garlic salt - ½ tbsp

Directions:

1. Preheat the wood pellet grill to 375 degrees.
2. Mix all the ingredients in a small bowl.
3. After washing and drying the shrimp, mix it well with the oil and seasonings.
4. Add skewers to the shrimp and set the bowl of shrimp aside.
5. Open the skewers and flip them.
6. Cook for 4 more minutes. Remove when the shrimp is opaque and pink.

Nutrition Info: Carbohydrates: 1.3 g Protein: 19 g Fat: 1.4 g Sodium: 805 mg Cholesterol: 179 mg

Cajun Seasoned Shrimp

Servings: 4

Cooking Time: 16-20 Minutes

Ingredients:

- 20 pieces of jumbo Shrimp
- 1/2 teaspoon of Cajun seasoning
- 1tablespoon of Canola oil
- 1teaspoon of magic shrimp seasoning

Directions:

1. Take a large bowl and add canola oil, shrimp, and seasonings.
2. Mix well for fine coating.
3. Now put the shrimp on skewers.
4. Put the grill grate inside the grill and set a timer to 8 minutes at high for preheating.
5. Once the grill is preheated, open the unit and place the shrimp skewers inside.
6. Cook the shrimp for 2 minutes.
7. Open the unit to flip the shrimp and cook for another 2 minutes at medium.
8. Own done, serve.

Nutrition Info: Calories: 382 Total Fat: 7.4g Saturated Fat: 0g Cholesterol: 350mg Sodium: 2208mg Total Carbohydrate: 23.9g Dietary Fiber 2.6g Total Sugars: 2.6g Protein: 50.2g

OTHER FAVORITE RECIPES

Smoked Hot Paprika Pork Tenderloin

Servings: 6
Cooking Time: 2 ½ To 3 Hours
Ingredients:
- 2-pound pork tenderloin
- 3/4 cup chicken stock
- 1/2 cup tomato-basil sauce
- 2 tbsp smoked hot paprika (or to taste)
- 1 tbsp oregano
- Salt and pepper to taste

Directions:
1. In a bowl, combine the chicken stock, tomato-basil sauce, paprika, oregano, salt, and pepper together.
2. Brush over tenderloin.
3. Smoke grill for 4-5 minutes. Pre head, lid closed for 10-14 minutes
4. Place pork for 2 ½ to 3 hours.
5. Rest for 10 minutes.
Nutrition Info: Calories: 360.71 Cal Fat: 14.32 g Carbohydrates: 3.21 g Protein: 52.09 g Fiber: 1.45 g

Keto Quiche

Servings: 6
Cooking Time: 45 Minutes
Ingredients:
- 12 tbsp unsalted butter (soften)
- 12 large eggs
- 8 ounces grated cheddar cheese (divided)
- 4 ounces cream cheese
- ½ tsp salt or to taste
- ½ tsp ground black pepper or to taste
- 1 yellow onion (diced)
- 1 green bell pepper (chopped)
- 3 cups broccoli florets (chopped)
- 1 tbsp olive oil

Directions:
1. Preheat the grill to 325°F with the lid closed for 15 minutes.
2. Heat up the olive oil in a skillet over high heat.
3. Add the chopped onion, broccoli, and green pepper. Cook for about 8 minutes, stirring constantly.
4. Remove the skillet from heat.
5. Process the egg and cheese in a food processor, adding the melted butter in a bit while processing.
6. Combine 4ounce grated cheddar cheese, salt, and pepper in a quiche pan.
7. Toss the cooked vegetable into the pan and mix.
8. Pour the egg mixture over the ingredients in the quiche pan.
9. Sprinkle the remaining grated cheese over it.

10. Place the pan in the preheated grill and bake for 45 minutes.
11. Remove and transfer the quiche to a rack to cool.
12. Slice and serve.
Nutrition Info: Calories: 615 Total Fat: 54.7 g Saturated Fat: 30.1 g Cholesterol: 494 mg Sodium: 804 mg Total Carbohydrate 8.1 g Dietary Fiber 1.9 g Total Sugars: 3.6 g Protein: 25.4 g

Compound Butter

Servings: 1/2 Cup
Cooking Time: 10 Minutes
Ingredients:
- 8 tablespoons unsalted butter
- 1 tablespoon herb leaves, minced
- 1 small shallot, peeled and minced
- 2 teaspoons freshly squeezed lemon or lime juice
- Splash Champagne or white-wine vinegar

Directions:
1. Put the butter on a cutting board and, using a fork, cut the other ingredients into it until the butter is creamy and smooth. Scrape the butter together with a chef's knife, and form it into a rough log. If making ahead of time, roll it tightly in a sheet of plastic wrap and refrigerate or freeze until ready to use.

Corned Beef Hash

Servings: 4
Cooking Time: 4 Hours
Ingredients:
- 2 lb. corned beef brisket
- Pepper to taste
- 2 cups chicken broth
- 1 lb. potatoes, peeled
- 6 slices bacon, chopped
- 1 red bell pepper, chopped
- 1 onion, chopped
- 1 teaspoon thyme, chopped
- 1-1/2 teaspoon hickory bacon rub
- 2 tablespoons parsley, chopped

Directions:
1. Season the corned beef with the seasoning packet from its package and with the pepper.
2. Let it rest for 30 minutes.
3. Set your wood pellet grill to smoke setting for 10 to 15 minutes.
4. Set it to 225 degrees F.
5. Place the corned beef on top of the grills.
6. Smoke for 3 hours.

7. Transfer the corned beef to a baking pan.
8. Add the chicken broth and potatoes to the pan.
9. Cover the pan with foil.
10. Cook for 30 minutes.
11. Let the corned beef and potatoes cool.
12. Refrigerate for 1 hour.
13. Slice the potatoes and corned beef.
14. Add a cast iron pan to the pellet grill.
15. Preheat it to 400 degrees F.
16. Cook the bacon until golden and crispy.
17. Transfer to a plate lined with a paper towel.
18. Add the red bell pepper and onion to the pan.
19. Cook for 3 minutes.
20. Stir in the corned beef.
21. Add the rest of the ingredients.
22. Serve while hot.

Nutrition Info: Calories: 380 Fat: 24 g Cholesterol: 80mg Carbohydrates: 22.1 g Fiber: 1.9 g Sugars: 1.1 g Protein: 20 g

Smoked Sausage & Potatoes

Servings: 4 To 6
Cooking Time: 50 Minutes
Ingredients:
- 2 Pound Hot Sausage Links
- 2 Pound Potatoes, fingerling
- 1 Tablespoon fresh thyme
- 4 Tablespoon butter

Directions:
1. When ready to cook, set the Traeger to 375°F and preheat, lid closed for 15 minutes.
2. Put your sausage links on the grill to get some color. This should take about 3 minutes on each side.
3. While sausage is cooking, cut the potatoes into bite size pieces all about the same size so they cook evenly. Chop the thyme and butter, then combine all the ingredients into a Traeger cast iron skillet.
4. Pull your sausage off the grill, slice into bite size pieces and add to your cast iron.
5. Turn grill down to 275°F and put the cast iron in the grill for 45 minutes to an hour or until the potatoes are fully cooked.
6. After 45 minutes, use a butter knife to test your potatoes by cutting into one to see if its done. To speed up cook time you can cover cast iron will a lid or foil. Serve. Enjoy!

Native Southern Cornbread

Servings: 8
Cooking Time: 20 Minutes
Ingredients:
- 2 tbsp. butter
- 1½ C. all-purpose flour

- 1½ C. yellow cornmeal
- 2 tbsp. sugar
- 3 tsp. baking powder
- ¾ tsp. baking soda
- ¾ tsp. salt
- 1 C. whole milk
- 1 C. buttermilk
- 3 large eggs
- 3 tbsp. butter, melted

Directions:
1. Set the temperature of Traeger Grill to 400 degrees F and preheat with closed lid for 15 minutes.
2. In a 13x9-inch baking dish, place 2 tbsp. of butter.
3. Place the baking dish onto grill to melt butter and heat up the pan.
4. In a large bowl, mix together flour, cornmeal, sugar, baking powder, baking soda and salt.
5. In another bowl, add milk, buttermilk, eggs and melted butter and beat until well combined.
6. Add the egg mixture into flour mixture and mix until just moistened.
7. Carefully, remove the heated baking dish from grill.
8. Place the bread mixture into heated baking dish evenly.
9. Place the pan onto the grill and cook for about 20 minutes or until a toothpick inserted in the center comes out clean.
10. Remove from grill and place the pan onto a wire rack to cool for about 10 minutes.
11. Carefully, invert the bread onto the wire rack to cool completely before slicing.
12. Cut the bread into desired-sized slices and sere.

Nutrition Info: Calories per serving: 302; Carbohydrates: 42.4g; Protein: 8.7g; Fat: 10.4g; Sugar: 6.4g; Sodium: 467mg; Fiber: 2.3g

Dinner Rolls

Servings: 12
Cooking Time: 10 Minutes
Ingredients:
- 2 tablespoon active dry yeast
- 1/3 cup vegetable oil
- 1 1/10 cup warm water (115 degrees F)
- 1/4 cup sugar
- 1 egg, beaten
- Pinch salt
- 3 1/2 cups all-purpose flour
- Cooking spray

Directions:
1. Set the Traeger wood pellet grill to 400 degrees F.
2. Preheat for 15 minutes while the lid is closed.

3. Use a stand mixer to mix dry yeast, oil, warm water, and sugar.
4. Let it rest for 10 minutes.
5. Stir in the egg, salt, and flour.
6. Spray cast iron pan with oil.
7. Knead the dough and shape into 12 balls.
8. Place the balls on the pan.
9. Let rest for 10 minutes.
10. Bake in the wood pellet grill for 10 minutes.
Nutrition Info: Calories: 77 Fats: 1.6 g Cholesterol: 1 mg Carbohydrates: 13 g Fiber: 0.5 g Sugar: 1.4 g Protein: 2.7 g

Traeger Steak Kabobs

Servings: 6
Cooking Time: 10 Minutes
Ingredients:
- 3 lb steak
- 2 small zucchini
- 1 onion
- 2 small yellow squash
- Salt and pepper
- 1 cup teriyaki sauce
- 3 tbsp sesame seeds, toasted

Directions:
1. Preheat your Traeger to 400F.
2. Cut the steak and veggies into skewable pieces.
3. Place the meat and veggies on the skewers then sprinkle with salt and pepper.
4. Place the skewers on the grill and cook for 5 minutes per side.
5. Remove the skewers, drizzle teriyaki sauce and top with sesame seeds.
6. Serve when hot. Enjoy.
Nutrition Info: Calories 727, Total fat 44g, Saturated fat 17g, Total carbs 15g, Net carbs 13g Protein 64g, Sugars 10g, Fiber 2g, Sodium 2011mg

Carne Asada Marinade

Servings: 5
Cooking Time: 2hours
Ingredients:
- cloves garlic, chopped
- tsp Lemon juice
- 1/2 cup extra virgin olive oil
- 1/2 tsp Salt
- 1/2 tsp Pepper

Directions:
1. Mix all your ingredients in a bowl.
2. Pour the beef into the bowl and allow to marinate for 2-3hours before grilling.
Nutrition Info: Per Serving: Calories: 465kcal, Carbs: 26g Fat: 15g, Protein: 28g

Scrambled Eggs

Servings: 3 To 4
Cooking Time: 10 Minutes
Ingredients:
- 1/4 cup Cheddar and Monterey Cheese Blend, shredded
- Sea Salt and Black Pepper, as needed
- 1 tbsp. Butter
- 6 Eggs
- 3 tbsp. Nut Milk or milk of your choice
- Green onion or fresh herbs of your choice, for garnish

Directions:
1. First, place eggs, milk, cheese blend, pepper, and salt in the blender pitcher.
2. Next, press the 'medium' button and blend the mixture for 25 to 30 seconds or until everything comes together and is frothy.
3. Then, heat the butter in a medium-sized saucepan over medium-low heat.
4. Once the skillet becomes hot and the butter has melted, swirl the pan so that the butter coats all the sides.
5. Pour the egg mixture into it and allow it to sit for 20 seconds.
6. With a spatula, break it down and continue cooking until the egg is set and cooked. Garnish with green onion.
7. Serve it along with toasted bread.
Nutrition Info: Calories: 70 Fat: 5.6 g Total Carbs: 0.3 g Fiber: 0 g Sugar: 0.3 g Protein: 4.7 g Cholesterol: 157.5 mg

Sweet Potato Spiced Fries

Servings: 4
Cooking Time: 30 Minutes
Ingredients:
- 1 tsp of kosher salt
- 2 Tbsp of olive oil
- 1 tsp of paprika
- 1/2 tsp of cumin, ground
- 2 pounds of sliced sweet potatoes
- 1 tsp of brown sugar, light
- 1 tsp of chili powder
- 1 tsp of garlic powder

Directions:
1. Mix the brown sugar, paprika, garlic powder, chili powder, salt, and cumin in a bowl.
2. Mix the sliced potatoes and oil in a separate bowl, then add the brown sugar mixture and toss well. Pour the coated potatoes into a roasting pan

and roast until it is brown and tender. This will take about 15-20 minutes.
3.   Serve as soon as possible.
Nutrition Info: Per Serving: Calories: 177.85kcal, Protein: 23.9g, Carbs: 21.9g, Fat: 39.8g.

Shepherd's Pie With Steak

Servings: 4
Cooking Time: 45 Minutes
Ingredients:
- 2 tablespoons flour
- 2 tablespoons butter
- 1 cup beef broth
- 2 tablespoons steak seasoning
- 2 cups of mixed frozen vegetables
- 2 cups steak, cooked and diced
- 1 cup cooked mashed potatoes

Directions:
1.   Preheat your wood pellet grill to 350 degrees F.
2.   In a pan over medium heat, add the flour and butter.
3.   Cook for 1 minute, stirring.
4.   Pour in the beef broth.
5.   Cook for 5 to 6 minutes.
6.   Stir in the steak seasoning. Set aside.
7.   Add the vegetables and diced steak into the mixture.
8.   Pour this mixture into a baking pan.
9.   Spread the mashed potatoes on top.
10.   Grill the pie for 15 minutes.
Nutrition Info: Calories: 272 Fat: 8.21 g Cholesterol: 34 mg Carbohydrates: 34.5 g Fiber: 3.4 g Sugars: 3.3 g Protein: 15.6 g

Soy Dipping Sauce

Servings: 4
Cooking Time: 10 Minutes
Ingredients:
- ¼ cup soy sauce
- ¼ cup sugar
- ¼ cup rice vinegar
- ½ cup scallions
- ½ cup cilantro

Directions:
1.   In a blender place all ingredients and blend until smooth
2.   Pour sauce in a bowl and serve

Red Chile And Lime Shortbread Cookies

Servings: 8
Cooking Time: 30 Minutes

Ingredients:
- 2 tsp lime zest
- 8 Tbsp unsalted butter
- 1 cup of all-purpose flour
- 1/2 tsp Salt
- 1 tsp Red Chile rub
- 1/4 cup of sugar

Directions:
1.   Set the wood pellet smoker-grill to indirect cooking at 300 F
2.   In a large bowl, combine all the ingredients (except flour). Mix thoroughly until the butter is creamy but not smooth. Gradually add the flour until it forms a ball.
3.   Transfer the dough onto a floured surface, roll until about 1/4-inches thick. Cut into eight equal parts, but do not cut through.
4.   Arrange in a cake pan, bake for 10 minutes. Allow to cool before serving.
Nutrition Info: Per Serving: Calories: 478kcal, Carbs: 46g, Fat: 8g, Protein: 2g

Roasted Snapper

Servings: 4
Cooking Time: 15 Minutes
Ingredients:
- 4 snapper fillets
- Salt and pepper to taste
- 2 teaspoons dried tarragon
- Olive oil
- 2 lemons, sliced

Directions:
1.   Set the Traeger wood pellet grill to high.
2.   Preheat it for 15 minutes while the lid is closed.
3.   Add 1 fish fillet on top of a foil sheet.
4.   Sprinkle with salt, pepper, and tarragon.
5.   Drizzle with oil.
6.   Place lemon slices on top.
7.   Fold and seal the packets.
8.   Put the foil packets on the grill.
9.   Bake for 15 minutes.
10.   Open carefully and serve.
Nutrition Info: Calories: 305.2 Fats: 9.8 g Cholesterol: 79.9 mg Carbohydrates: 6.6 g Fiber: 1 g Sugar: 0.7 g Protein: 45.8g

Smoking Burgers

Servings: 8
Cooking Time: 4o Minutes
Ingredients:
- For the topping:
- 3 apples, peeled and cut into slices

- 75g blueberries
- 25g salted butter
- 2 tablespoons maple syrup
- For the cake:
- 75g butter, cut into cubes
- 75g organic virgin coconut oil, cut into cubes
- 100g cane sugar
- 2 large free-range eggs, beaten
- 75g buckwheat flour
- 75g ground almonds
- ½ teaspoon bicarbonate of soda
- 1 teaspoon baking powder
- 1 teaspoon cinnamon

Directions:
1. Preheat oven to 180°C. Caramelize the apples.
2. Add the blueberries last. Set aside. Place the sugar, butter and coconut oil into a mixing bowl and cream until pale and fluffy.
3. Gradually add the beaten eggs, adding a bit of flour if the mixture begins to curdle. Continue to beat the mixture until fluffy. Fold in the remaining flour, ground almonds, baking powder and cinnamon.
4. Transfer the apple and blueberry mixture into the bottom of a greased Bundt cake mold, leveling well with the back of a spoon. Then pour the cake mixture over the top. Bake for about 40 minutes or until a skewer comes out clean. Leave to cool. Delicious served with Greek yogurt.

Nutrition Info: Calories: 275 Cal Fat: 10 g Carbohydrates: 31 g   Protein: 14 g Fiber: 4 g

Green Smoothie

Servings: 3 To 4
Cooking Time: 5 Minutes
Ingredients:
- 1/4 cup Baby Spinach
- 1/2 cup Ice
- 1/4 cup Kale
- 1/2 cup Pineapple Chunks
- 1/2 cup Coconut Water
- 1/2 cup mango, diced
- 1/2 banana, diced

Directions:
1. Begin by placing all the ingredients needed to make the smoothie in the blender pitcher.
2. Now, press the 'extract' button.
3. Transfer the smoothie into the serving glass.

Nutrition Info: Calories: 184 Fat: 1.3 g Total Carbs: 44.6 g Fiber: 4.5 g Sugar: 21.9 g Protein: 4.3 g Cholesterol: 0

Barbeque Sauce

Servings: 2
Cooking Time: 15 Minutes
Ingredients:
- 1/4 cup of water
- 1/4 cup red wine vinegar
- Tbsp Worcestershire sauce
- 1 tsp Paprika
- 1 tsp Salt
- Tbsp Dried mustard
- 1 tsp black pepper
- 1 cup ketchup
- 1 cup brown sugar

Directions:
1. Pour all the ingredients into a food processor, one after the other.
2. Process until they are evenly mixed.
3. Transfer sauce to a close lid jar. Store in the refrigerator.

Nutrition Info: Per Serving: Calories: 43kcal, Carbs: 10g Fat: 0.3g, Protein: 0.9g

Traditional English Mac N' Cheese

Servings: 12
Cooking Time: 1 Hour 20 Minutes
Ingredients:
- 2 lb. elbow macaroni
- ¾ C. butter
- ½ C. flour
- 1 tsp. dry mustard
- 1½ C. milk
- 2 lb. Velveeta cheese, cut into ½-inch cubes
- Salt and freshly ground black pepper, to taste
- 1½ C. cheddar cheese, shredded
- 2 C. plain dry breadcrumbs
- Paprika, to taste

Directions:
1. Set the temperature of Traeger Grill to 350 degrees F and preheat with closed lid for 15 minutes.
2. In a large pan of lightly salted boiling water, cook the macaroni for about 7-8 minutes.
3. Drain the macaroni well and transfer into a large bowl.
4. Meanwhile, in a medium pan, melt 8 tbsp. of butter over medium heat.
5. Slowly, add flour and mustard, beating continuously until smooth.
6. Cook for about 2 minutes, beating continuously.
7. Slowly, add milk, beating continuously until smooth.
8. Reduce the heat to medium-low and slowly, stir in Velveeta cheese until melted.
9. Stir in salt and black pepper and remove from heat.

10. Place cheese sauce over cooked macaroni and gently, stir to combine.
11. Place the macaroni mixture into greased casserole dish evenly and sprinkle with cheddar cheese.
12. In a small frying pan, melt remaining 4 tbsp. of butter.
13. Stir in breadcrumbs and remove from heat.
14. Place breadcrumbs mixture over cheddar cheese evenly and sprinkle with paprika lightly.
15. Arrange the casserole dish onto the grill and cook for about 45-60 minutes, rotating the pan once halfway through.
16. Serve hot.
Nutrition Info: Calories per serving: 914; Carbohydrates: 99.9g; Protein: 37.2g; Fat: 42.3g; Sugar: 12g; Sodium: 1600mg; Fiber: 4.1g

Garlic Butter Injectable

Servings: 2 Cups
Cooking Time: 5 Minutes
Ingredients:
- 16 tablespoons (2 sticks) salted butter
- 2 tablespoons salt
- 1½ tablespoons garlic powder

Directions:
1. In a small skillet over medium heat, melt the butter.
2. Stir in the salt and garlic powder until well mixed. Use immediately.

Sweet Sensation Pork Meat

Servings: 3
Cooking Time: 3 Hours
Ingredients:
- 2 tsp of nutmeg, ground
- 1/4 cup of allspice
- 2 tsp of thyme, dried
- 1/4 cup of brown sugar
- 2 pounds of pork
- 2 tsp of cinnamon, ground
- 2 Tbsp of salt, kosher or sea

Directions:
1. Preheat the grill for 15 minutes at 225°F. Use hickory wood pellets
2. Combine all the ingredients (except pork) in a bowl. Mix thoroughly.
3. Slice the sides of the pork meat in 4-5 places. Put some of the ingredients into the slices and rub the rest over the pork.
4. Place the pork on the preheated grill and smoke for 3 hours or until internal temperature reads 145°F.
5. Allow it to rest before serving.

Nutrition Info: Per Serving: Calories: 300kcal, Protein: 36g, Carbs: 45g, Fat: 31g

Traeger Apple Cake

Servings: 12
Cooking Time: 45 Minutes
Ingredients:
- Cake
- 1/2 cup canola oil
- 1-1/2 cup brown sugar
- 1 egg
- 1 cup sour cream
- 1 tbsp baking soda
- 1/2 tbsp baking soda
- 1/2 tbsp baking powder
- 1-1/2 tbsp vanilla
- 2-1/2 cups flour
- 2 apples, finely diced.
- Streusel
- 1 stick butter
- 1/2 cup brown sugar
- 1/2 cup flour
- 1/2 cup oats
- 1/2 tbsp cinnamon
- Glaze
- 2 cups powdered sugar
- 1 tbsp apple cinnamon blend
- 3 tbsp milk

Directions:
1. Preheat your Traeger to 325F.
2. Add the cake ingredients except for the apples in a blender and pulse until well-combined .fold in the diced apples.
3. Spread the mixture on a 9x13 baking pan.
4. Mix the streusel ingredients using hands until crumbly then pour the mixture over the cake mixture.
5. Place the baking pan at the top rack of your Traeger to create a space between the cake pan and the fire.
6. Bake for 45 minutes or until the tester comes out with moist crumbs only.
7. Let rest for 10 minutes before serving.

Nutrition Info: Calories 452, Total fat 21g, Saturated fat 8g, Total carbs 61g, Net carbs 59g Protein 5g, Sugars 34g, Fiber 2g, Sodium 207mg

Fennel And Almonds Sauce

Servings: 4
Cooking Time: 10 Minutes
Ingredients:
- 1 cup fennel bulb
- 1 cup olive oil

- 1 cup almonds
- 1 cup fennel fronds

Directions:
1. In a blender place all ingredients and blend until smooth
2. Pour sauce in a bowl and serve

Ancho-dusted Jícama Sticks With Lime

Servings: 8
Cooking Time: 30 Minutes
Ingredients:
- 1/2-pound jícama, trimmed and peeled
- 2tablespoons good-quality olive oil
- 2teaspoons ancho chile powder
- Salt
- 1lime, cut into wedges

Directions:
1. Start the coals or heat the gas grill for medium-high direct cooking. Make sure the grates are clean.
2. Cut the jícama into ½-inch slices. Brush the slices on both sides with the olive oil. Put the slices on the grill directly over the fire. Close the lid and cook, turning once, until they develop grill marks, 7 to 10 minutes per side.
3. Transfer the jícama to a cutting board and cut the slices into ½-inch-wide sticks. Put on a serving platter and sprinkle with the ancho powder and salt to taste, turning them to coat evenly. Squeeze the lime wedges over them, again turning to coat evenly, and serve.

Nutrition Info: Calories: 49 Fats: 0.1 g Cholesterol: 0 mg Carbohydrates: 12 g Fiber: 6.4 g Sugars: 0 g Proteins: 1 g

Rosemary-garlic Lamb Seasoning

Servings: 2
Cooking Time: 5 Minutes
Ingredients:
- 2 teaspoons dried rosemary leaves
- 2 teaspoons coarse kosher salt
- 1 teaspoon garlic powder
- 1 teaspoon freshly ground black pepper
- ½ teaspoon onion powder
- ½ teaspoon dried minced onion

Directions:
1. In a small airtight container or zip-top bag, combine the rosemary, salt, garlic powder, black pepper, onion powder, and minced onion.
2. Close the container and shake to mix. Unused seasoning will keep in an airtight container for months.

Sweet Brown Sugar Rub

Servings: 1/4 Cup
Cooking Time: 5 Minutes
Ingredients:
- 2 tablespoons light brown sugar
- 1 teaspoon coarse kosher salt
- 1 teaspoon garlic powder
- 1 teaspoon onion powder
- 1 teaspoon sweet paprika
- ½ teaspoon freshly ground black pepper
- ½ teaspoon cayenne pepper
- ½ teaspoon dried oregano leaves
- ¼ teaspoon smoked paprika

Directions:
1. In a small airtight container or zip-top bag, combine the brown sugar, salt, garlic powder, onion powder, sweet paprika, black pepper, cayenne, oregano, and smoked paprika.
2. Close the container and shake to mix. Unused rub will keep in an airtight container for months.

Black Bean Dipping Sauce

Servings: 4
Cooking Time: 10 Minutes
Ingredients:
- 2 tablespoons black bean paste
- 2 tablespoons peanut butter
- 1 tablespoon maple syrup
- 2 tablespoons olive oil

Directions:
1. In a blender place all ingredients and blend until smooth
2. Pour sauce in a bowl and serve

Smoked Christmas Crown Roast Of Lamb

Servings: 4
Cooking Time: 1 To 2 Hours
Ingredients:
- 2 racks of lamb, trimmed, frenched, and tied into a crown
- 1¼ cups extra-virgin olive oil, divided
- 2 tablespoons chopped fresh basil
- 2 tablespoons chopped fresh rosemary
- 2 tablespoons ground sage
- 2 tablespoons ground thyme
- 8 garlic cloves, minced
- 2 teaspoons salt
- 2 teaspoons freshly ground black pepper

Directions:
1. Set the lamb out on the counter to take the chill off, about an hour.

2.   In a small bowl, combine 1 cup of olive oil, the basil, rosemary, sage, thyme, garlic, salt, and pepper.

3.   Baste the entire crown with the herbed olive oil and wrap the exposed frenched bones in aluminum foil.

4.   Supply your smoker with wood pellets and follow the manufacturer's specific start-up procedure. Preheat, with the lid closed, to 275°F.

5.   Put the lamb directly on the grill, close the lid, and smoke for 1 hour 30 minutes to 2 hours, or until a meat thermometer inserted in the thickest part reads 140°F.

6.   Remove the lamb from the heat, tent with foil, and let rest for about 15 minutes before serving. The temperature will rise about 5°F during the rest period, for a finished temperature of 145°F.

Polish Kielbasa

Servings: 8
Cooking Time: 1 To 2 Hours
Ingredients:
- 4 pounds ground pork
- ½ cup water
- 2 garlic cloves, minced
- 4 teaspoons salt
- 1 teaspoon freshly ground black pepper
- 1 teaspoon dried marjoram
- ½ teaspoon ground allspice
- 14 feet natural hog casings, medium size

Directions:

1.   In a large bowl, combine the pork, water, garlic, salt, pepper, marjoram, and allspice.

2.   Stuff the casings according to the instructions on your sausage stuffing device, or use a funnel (see Tip).

3.   Twist the casings according to your desired length and prick each with a pin in several places so the kielbasa won't burst.

4.   Transfer the kielbasa to a plate, cover with plastic wrap, and refrigerate for at least 8 hours or overnight.

5.   Remove from the refrigerator and allow the links to come to room temperature.

6.   Supply your smoker with wood pellets and follow the manufacturer's specific start-up procedure. Preheat, with the lid closed, to 225°F.

7.   Place the kielbasa directly on the grill grate, close the lid, and smoke for 1 hour 30 minutes to 2 hours, or until a meat thermometer inserted in each link reads 155°F. (The internal temperature will rise about 5°F when resting, for a finished temp of 160°F.)

8.   Serve with buns and condiments of your choosing, or cut up the kielbasa and serve with smoked cabbage

Hot Sauce With Cilantro

Servings: 4
Cooking Time: 10 Minutes
Ingredients:
- ½ tsp coriander
- ½ tsp cumin seeds
- ¼ tsp black pepper
- 2 green cardamom pods
- 2 garlic cloves
- 1 tsp salt
- 1 oz. parsley
- 2 tablespoons olive oil

Directions:

1.   In a blender place all ingredients and blend until smooth

2.   Pour sauce in a bowl and serve

Grilled Carrots

Servings: 6
Cooking Time: 20 Minutes
Ingredients:
- 1 lb carrots, large
- 1/2 tbsp salt
- 6 oz butter
- 1/2 tbsp black pepper
- Fresh thyme

Directions:

1.   Thoroughly wash the carrots and do not peel. Pat them dry and coat with olive oil.

2.   Add salt to your carrots.

3.   Meanwhile, preheat a pellet grill to 350F.

4.   Now place your carrots directly on the grill or on a raised rack.

5.   Close and cook for about 20 minutes.

6.   While carrots cook, cook butter in a saucepan, small, over medium heat until browned. Stir constantly to avoid it from burning. Remove from heat.

7.   Remove carrots from the grill onto a plate then drizzle with browned butter.

8.   Add pepper and splash with thyme.

9.   Serve and enjoy.

Nutrition Info: Calories: 250 Total Fat: 25 g Saturated Fat: 15 g Total Carbs: 6 g Net Carbs: 4g Protein: 1 g Sugars: 3 g Fiber: 2 g Sodium: 402 mg

Jerk Seasoning

Servings: ¼ Cup
Cooking Time: 5 Minutes
Ingredients:
- 1 tablespoon allspice berries

- ¼ teaspoon nutmeg pieces (crack a whole nutmeg with a hammer)
- 1 teaspoon black peppercorns
- 2 teaspoons dried thyme
- 1 teaspoon cayenne, or to taste
- 1 tablespoon paprika
- 1 tablespoon sugar
- 1 tablespoon salt
- 2 teaspoons minced garlic
- 2 teaspoons minced ginger (or 2 teaspoons ground ginger)

Directions:
1. Put allspice, nutmeg, peppercorns and thyme in a spice or coffee grinder and grind to a fine powder.
2. Mix in remaining ingredients and use immediately. To use later, omit garlic and ginger and store in a tightly covered container; add garlic and ginger immediately before using.

Beef Tartare Burger

Servings: 4
Cooking Time: 30 Minutes
Ingredients:
- 1 Tbsp of capers
- 1 shallot, already peeled
- Salt with pepper
- 1 medium of clove garlic
- 1-1/2 pound of fatty chuck
- 2 anchovy fillets, optional
- 1 medium-cooked egg, chopped
- 2 tsp of Worcestershire sauce
- 1/2 cup of parsley, preferably freshly chopped
- 1/2 tsp of tabasco sauce
- White onion and peeled lemon slices

Directions:
1. Set the grill for direct cooking at 300°F. Use maple pellets for a strong, woody taste.
2. Pour garlic, beef, anchovies, shallot, and capers inside a food processor. Pulse until it is has a coarse texture (soother than chopped, but not by much).
3. Mix the parsley, Worcestershire sauce, salt, pepper, and tabasco in a bowl. Stir together with blended beef. Mold the mixture to form 4 patties.
4. Grill the meat for about 3-4 minutes (rare). Flip and grill until the other side is done.
5. Serve immediately with caper, onion, parsley with egg, lemon.
Nutrition Info: Per Serving: Calories: 216kcal, Protein: 20g, Fat: 16g, Carbs: 45g

Low Carb Almond Flour Bread

Servings: 24

Cooking Time: 1 Hour 15 Minutes
Ingredients:
- 1tsp sea salt or to taste
- 1tbsp apple cider vinegar
- ½ cup of warm water
- ¼ cup of coconut oil
- 4large eggs (beaten)
- 1tbsp gluten-free baking powder
- 2cup blanched almond flour
- ¼ cup Psyllium husk powder
- 1tsp ginger (optional)

Directions:
1. Preheat the grill to 350°F with the lid closed for 15 minutes.
2. Line a 9 by 5 inch loaf pan with parchment paper. Set aside.
3. Combine the ginger, Psyllium husk powder, almond flour, salt, baking powder in a large mixing bowl.
4. In another mixing bowl, mix the coconut oil, apple cider vinegar, eggs and warm water. Mix thoroughly.
5. Gradually pour the flour mixture into the egg mixture, stirring as you pour. Stir until it forms a smooth batter.
6. Fill the lined loaf pan with the batter and cover the batter with aluminum foil.
7. Place the loaf pan directly on the grill and bake for about 1 hour or until a toothpick or knife inserted in the middle of the bread comes out clean.
Nutrition Info: Calories: 93 Total Fat: 7.5 g Saturated Fat: 2.6 g Cholesterol: 31 mg Sodium: 139 mg Total Carbohydrate: 3.6 g Dietary Fiber: 2.2 g Total Sugars: 0.1 g Protein: 3.1 g

Cinnamon Almond Shortbread

Servings: 5
Cooking Time: 20 Minutes
Ingredients:
- 2tsp cinnamon
- ½ cup unsalted butter (softened)
- 1large egg (beaten)
- ½ tsp salt or to taste
- 2cups almond flour
- ¼ cup sugar
- 1tsp ginger (optional)

Directions:
1. Preheat the grill to 300°F with the lid closed for 5 minutes.
2. Grease a cookie sheet with oil.
3. In a large bowl, combine the cinnamon, almond flour, sugar, ginger, and salt. Mix thoroughly to combine.

4. In another mixing bowl, whisk the egg and softened butter together.
5. Pour the egg mixture into the flour mixture and mix until the mixture forms a smooth batter.
6. Use a tablespoon to measure out equal amounts of the mixture and roll into balls.
7. Arrange the balls into the cookie sheet in a single layer.
8. Now, use the flat bottom of a clean glass cup to press each ball into a flat round cookie. Grease the bottom of the cup before using it to press the balls.
9. Place the cookie sheet on the grill and bake until browned. This will take about 20 to 25 minutes.
10. Remove the cookie sheet from the grill and let the shortbreads cool for a few minutes.
11. Serve and enjoy.
Nutrition Info: Calories: 152 Total Fat: 12.7 g Saturated Fat: 4.2 g Cholesterol: 27 mg Sodium: 124 mg Total Carbohydrate: 6.5 g Dietary Fiber: 1.7 g Total Sugars: 3.2 g Protein: 3.5 g

Smoked Spicy Pork Medallions

Servings: 6
Cooking Time: 1 Hour And 45 Minutes
Ingredients:
- 2 pounds pork medallions
- 3/4 cup chicken stock
- 1/2 cup tomato sauce (organic)
- 2 Tbs of smoked hot paprika (or to taste)
- 2 Tbsp of fresh basil finely chopped
- 1 Tbsp oregano
- Salt and pepper to taste

Directions:
1. Combine the chicken stock, tomato sauce, paprika, oregano, salt, and pepper.
2. Brush on tenderloin. Smoke grill for 4-5 minutes
3. Temperature must rise to 250 degrees Fahrenheit until 15 to 15 minutes at most
4. Place the pork on the grill grate and smoke until the internal temperature of the pork is at least medium-rare (about 145°F), for 1 1/2 hours.
Nutrition Info: Calories: 364.2 Cal Fat: 14.4 g Carbohydrates: 4 g Protein: 52.4 g Fiber: 2 g

Smoked Tuna

Servings: 6
Cooking Time: 3 Hours
Ingredients:
- 2 cups water
- 1 cup brown sugar
- 1 cup salt
- 1 tablespoon lemon zest
- 6 tuna fillets

Directions:
1. Mix water, brown sugar, salt and lemon zest in a bowl.
2. Coat the tuna fillets with the mixture.
3. Refrigerate for 6 hours.
4. Rinse the tuna and pat dry with paper towels.
5. Preheat the Traeger wood pellet grill to 180 degrees F for 15 minutes while the lid is closed.
6. Smoke the tuna for 3 hours.
7. Tips: You can also soak tuna in the brine for 24 hours.

Hickory Smoked Green Beans

Servings: 10
Cooking Time: 3 Hours
Ingredients:
- 6 cups fresh green beans, halved and ends cut off
- 2 cups chicken broth
- 1 tbsp pepper, ground
- 1/4 tbsp salt
- 2 tbsp apple cider vinegar
- 1/4 cup diced onion
- 6-8 bite-size bacon slices
- Optional: sliced almonds

Directions:
1. Add green beans to a colander then rinse thoroughly. Set aside.
2. Place chicken broth, pepper, salt, and apple cider in a pan, large. Add green beans.
3. Blanch over medium heat for about 3-4 minutes then remove from heat.
4. Transfer the mixture into an aluminum pan, disposable. Make sure all mixture goes into the pan, so do not drain them.
5. Place bacon slices over the beans and place the pan into the wood pellet smoker,
6. Smoke for about 3 hours uncovered.
7. Remove from the smoker and top with almonds slices.
8. Serve immediately.
Nutrition Info: Calories: 57 Total Fat: 3 g Saturated Fat: 1 g Total Carbs: 6 g Net Carbs: 4 g Protein: 4 g Sugars: 2 g Fiber: 2 g Sodium: 484 mg

Cajun Shrimp

Servings: 4
Cooking Time: 10 Minutes
Ingredients:
- 4 tablespoon olive oil
- 1 tablespoon lemon juice
- 2 cloves garlic, minced
- 1 tablespoon Cajun rub
- Salt to taste

- 2 lb. shrimp, peeled and deveined

Directions:
1. Mix all the ingredients in a bowl.
2. Cover the bowl and refrigerate for 3 hours.
3. Set the Traeger grill to high and preheat for 15 minutes while the lid is closed.
4. Thread the shrimp onto skewers.
5. Grill the shrimp for 4 minutes per side.
6. Tips: If using wooden skewers, soak first in water for 15 minutes before using.

Braised Lamb

Servings: 4
Cooking Time: 3 Hours And 20 Minutes
Ingredients:
- 4 lamb shanks
- Prime rib rub
- 1 cup red wine
- 1 cup beef broth
- 2 sprigs thyme
- 2 sprigs rosemary

Directions:
1. Sprinkle all sides of lamb shanks with prime rib rub.
2. Set temperature of the wood pellet grill to high.
3. Preheat it for 15 minutes while the lid is closed.
4. Add the lamb to the grill and cook for 20 minutes.
5. Transfer the lamb to a Dutch oven.
6. Stir in the rest of the ingredients.
7. Transfer back to the grill.
8. Reduce temperature to 325 degrees F.
9. Braise the lamb for 3 hours.
Nutrition Info: Calories: 207 Fats: 11 g Cholesterol: 90 mg Carbohydrates: 0 g Fiber: 0 g Sugar: 0 g Protein: 24 g

Smoked Bacon

Servings: 6
Cooking Time: 30 Minutes
Ingredients:
- 1-pound thick cut bacon

Directions:
1. Preheat your wood pellet grill to 375 degrees.
2. Line a huge baking sheet. Place a single layer of thick-cut bacon on it.
3. Bake for 20 minutes and then flip it to the other side.
4. Cook for another 10 minutes or until the bacon is crispy.
5. Take it out and enjoy your tasty grilled bacon.
Nutrition Info: Calories: 80 Cal Fat: 10 g Carbohydrates: 18 g Protein: 9 g Fiber: 0 g

Grilled Cocoa Steak

Servings: 8
Cooking Time: 10 Minutes
Ingredients:
- 1 tablespoon cocoa powder
- 1 1/2 tablespoons brown sugar
- 1 teaspoon chipotle chili powder
- 2 teaspoons chili powder
- 1/2 teaspoon onion powder
- 1/2 teaspoon garlic powder
- 1 tablespoon smoked paprika
- 1 tablespoon ground cumin
- Salt and pepper to taste
- 2 lb. flank steak
- Olive oil

Directions:
1. Make the dry rub by mixing the cocoa powder, sugar, spices, salt and pepper.
2. Coat the flank steak with olive oil.
3. Sprinkle dry rub on both sides.
4. Preheat your Traeger wood pellet grill to high for 15 minutes while the lid is closed.
5. Grill the steak for 5 minutes per side.
6. Let rest for 10 minutes before slicing and serving.
7. Tips: Slice against the grain after a few minutes of resting.

Grilled Pineapple With Chocolate Sauce

Servings: 6 To 8
Cooking Time: 25 Minutes
Ingredients:
- 1pineapple
- 8 oz bittersweet chocolate chips
- 1/2 cup spiced rum
- 1/2 cup whipping cream
- 2tbsp light brown sugar

Directions:
1. Preheat pellet grill to 400°F.
2. De-skin the pineapple and slice pineapple into 1 in cubes.
3. In a saucepan, combine chocolate chips. When chips begin to melt, add rum to the saucepan. Continue to stir until combined, then add a splash of the pineapple's juice.
4. Add in whipping cream and continue to stir the mixture. Once the sauce is smooth and thickening, lower heat to simmer to keep warm.
5. Thread pineapple cubes onto skewers. Sprinkle skewers with brown sugar.

6.	Place skewers on the grill grate. Grill for about 5 minutes per side, or until grill marks begin to develop.
7.	Remove skewers from grill and allow to rest on a plate for about 5 minutes. Serve alongside warm chocolate sauce for dipping.
Nutrition Info: Calories: 112.6 Fat: 0.5 g Cholesterol: 0 Carbohydrate: 28.8 g Fiber: 1.6 g Sugar: 0.1 g Protein: 0.4 g

Grilled Bacon Dog

Servings: 4 To 6
Cooking Time: 25 Minutes
Ingredients:
- 16 Hot Dogs
- 16 Slices Bacon, sliced
- 2 Onion, sliced
- 16 hot dog buns
- As Needed The Ultimate BBQ Sauce
- As Needed Cheese

Directions:
1.	When ready to cook, set the Traeger to 375°F and preheat, lid closed for 15 minutes.
2.	Wrap bacon strips around the hot dogs, and grill directly on the grill grate for 10 minutes each side. Grill onions at the same time as the hot dogs, and cook for 10 -15 minutes.
3.	Open hot dog buns and spread BBQ sauce, the grilled hot dogs, cheese sauce and grilled onions. Top with vegetables. Serve, enjoy!

Thanksgiving Turkey Brine

Servings: 1
Cooking Time: 5 Minutes
Ingredients:
- 2 gallons water
- 2 cups coarse kosher salt
- 2 cups packed light brown sugar

Directions:
1.	In a clean 5-gallon bucket, stir together the water, salt, and brown sugar until the salt and sugar dissolve completely.

Smoked Irish Bacon

Servings: 7
Cooking Time: 3 Hours
Ingredients:
- 1 bay leaf
- 2/4 cup of water
- 2/3 cup of sugar
- 6 star anise, whole

- 1 cup of fresh fennel, preferably bulb and fronds
- 2 spring thyme, fresh
- 1 clove of garlic
- 2 tsp of curing salt
- 2-1/2 pound of pork loin
- 1-1/2 tsp of peppercorns, black
- 1-1/2 tsp of fennel seed

Directions:
1.	In a big stockpot, mix the fennel seeds, peppercorn, star anise, and pork roast for about 3 minutes. Also, mix the sugar, water, thyme, garlic, curing salt, coarse salt, and bay leaves in a pot and, boil for 3 minutes until the salt and sugar dissolves.
2.	Place the pork loin in a Ziploc bag, seal it, and put it in a roasting pan. Keep refrigerated for 4 days.
3.	Preheat the grill for 15 minutes at 250°F. Use pecan wood pellets.
4.	Remove the pork from the brine and place on the grates of the grill. Smoke it for 2 hours 30 minutes or until internal temperature reads 145°F.
5.	Serves immediately or when it is cool.
Nutrition Info: Per Serving: Calories: 309kcal, Fat: 7g, Protein: 30.6g, Carbs: 40g

Pork And Portobello Burgers

Servings: 4
Cooking Time: 30 Minutes
Ingredients:
- 1 pound ground pork
- 1 tablespoon minced garlic
- 1 teaspoon minced fresh rosemary, fennel seed or parsley
- Salt and ground black pepper
- 4 large portobello mushroom caps, stems removed
- Olive oil
- 4 burger buns
- Any burger fixings you like

Directions:
1.	Combine the ground pork, garlic, rosemary and a sprinkle of salt and pepper. Use a spoon to lightly scrape away the gills of the mushrooms and hollow them slightly. Drizzle the mushrooms (inside and out) with olive oil and sprinkle with salt and pepper. Press 1/4 of the mixture into each of the hollow sides of the mushrooms; you want the meat to spread all the way across the width of the mushrooms. They should look like burgers.
2.	Grill the burgers, meat side down, until the pork is well browned, 4 to 6 minutes. Flip and cook until the top side of the mushrooms are browned and the mushrooms are tender, another 6 to 8 minutes. If you like, use an instant-read thermometer to check the

interior temperature of the pork, which should be a minimum of 145 degrees.
3. Serve the burgers on buns (toasted, if you like) with any fixings you like.

Veggie Lover's Burgers

Servings: 6
Cooking Time: 51 Minutes
Ingredients:
- ¾ C. lentils
- 1 tbsp. ground flaxseed
- 2 tbsp. extra-virgin olive oil
- 1 onion, chopped
- 2 garlic cloves, minced
- Salt and freshly ground black pepper, to taste
- 1 C. walnuts, toasted
- ¾ C. breadcrumbs
- 1 tsp. ground cumin
- 1 tsp. paprika

Directions:
1. In a pan of boiling water, add the lentils and cook for about 15 minutes or until soft.
2. Drain the lentils completely and set aside.
3. In a small bowl, mix together the flaxseed with 4 tbsp. of water. Set aside for about 5 minutes.
4. In a medium skillet, heat the oil over medium heat and sauté the onion for about 4-6 minutes.
5. Add the garlic and a pinch of salt and pepper and sauté for about 30 seconds.
6. Remove from the heat and place the onion mixture into a food processor.
7. Add the ¾ of the lentils, flaxseed mixture, walnuts, breadcrumbs and spices and pulse until smooth.
8. Transfer the mixture into a bowl and gently, fold in the remaining lentils.
9. Make 6 patties from the mixture.
10. Place the patties onto a parchment paper-lined plate and refrigerate for at least 30 minutes.
11. Set the temperature of Traeger Grill to 425 degrees F and preheat with closed lid for 15 minutes, using charcoal.
12. Place the burgers onto the grill and cook for about 8-10 minutes flipping once halfway through.
13. Serve hot.
Nutrition Info: Calories per serving: 324; Carbohydrates: 28.9g; Protein: 13.6g; Fat: 18.5g; Sugar: 13.6g; Sodium: 130mg; Fiber: 10.3g

Grilled Flank Steak

Servings: 6
Cooking Time: 2 Hours 15 Minutes
Ingredients:

- 1/2 cup of soy sauce
- 1-1/2 pound of flank steak.
- 1/2 cup of bourbon
- 1/2 cup of water

Directions:
1. Set the grill for direct cooking at 300°F. Use hickory wood pellets for a strong taste and aroma.
2. Pour the soy sauce, 1/2 cup of water, and bourbon in a bowl. Whisk together to make a marinade. Pour the marinade inside a food storage bag and add the steak to the bag. Keep in the refrigerator for 2 hours to allow flavors to combine and penetrate steak.
3. Remove from the refrigerator and dry with a paper towel.
4. Grill the steak for about 30 minutes, flipping every five minutes to ensure both sides are equally cooked.
5. Cover the steak with foil paper and allow it to rest for about 5 minutes.
6. Serve.
Nutrition Info: Per Serving: Calories: 370kcal, Carbs: 45g, Protein: 25.5g, Fat: 32 g.

Cinnamon Sugar Donut Holes

Servings: 4
Cooking Time: 35 Minutes
Ingredients:
- 1/2 cup flour
- 1tbsp cornstarch
- 1/2 tsp baking powder
- 1/8 tsp baking soda
- 1/8 tsp ground cinnamon
- 1/2 tsp kosher salt
- 1/4 cup buttermilk
- 1/4 cup sugar
- 11/2 tbsp butter, melted
- 1egg
- 1/2 tsp vanilla
- Topping
- 2tbsp sugar
- 1tbsp sugar
- 1tsp ground cinnamon

Directions:
1. Preheat pellet grill to 350°F.
2. In a medium bowl, combine flour, cornstarch, baking powder, baking soda, ground cinnamon, and kosher salt. Whisk to combine.
3. In a separate bowl, combine buttermilk, sugar, melted butter, egg, and vanilla. Whisk until the egg is thoroughly combined.
4. Pour wet mixture into the flour mixture and stir. Stir just until combined, careful not to overwork the mixture.

5. Spray mini muffin tin with cooking spray.
6. Spoon 1 tbsp of donut mixture into each mini muffin hole.
7. Place the tin on the pellet grill grate and bake for about 18 minutes, or until a toothpick can come out clean.
8. Remove muffin tin from the grill and let rest for about 5 minutes.
9. In a small bowl, combine 1 tbsp sugar and 1 tsp ground cinnamon.
10. Melt 2 tbsp of butter in a glass dish. Dip each donut hole in the melted butter, then mix and toss with cinnamon sugar. Place completed donut holes on a plate to serve.

Nutrition Info: Calories: 190 Fat: 17 g Cholesterol: 0 Carbohydrate: 21 g Fiber: 1 g Sugar: 8 g Protein: 3 g

Chicken Rub

Servings: 1/4 Cup
Cooking Time: 5 Minutes
Ingredients:
- 2 tablespoons packed light brown sugar
- 1½ teaspoons coarse kosher salt
- 1¼ teaspoons garlic powder
- ½ teaspoon onion powder
- ½ teaspoon freshly ground black pepper
- ½ teaspoon ground chipotle chile pepper
- ½ teaspoon smoked paprika
- ¼ teaspoon dried oregano leaves
- ¼ teaspoon mustard powder
- ¼ teaspoon cayenne pepper

Directions:
1. In a small airtight container or zip-top bag, combine the brown sugar, salt, garlic powder, onion powder, black pepper, chipotle pepper, paprika, oregano, mustard, and cayenne.
2. Close the container and shake to mix. Unused rub will keep in an airtight container for months.

Sweet And Spicy Cinnamon Rub

Servings: 1/4 Cup
Cooking Time: 5 Minutes
Ingredients:
- 2 tablespoons light brown sugar
- 1 teaspoon coarse kosher salt
- 1 teaspoon garlic powder
- 1 teaspoon onion powder
- 1 teaspoon sweet paprika
- ½ teaspoon freshly ground black pepper
- ½ teaspoon cayenne pepper
- ½ teaspoon dried oregano leaves
- ½ teaspoon ground ginger

- ½ teaspoon ground cumin
- ¼ teaspoon smoked paprika
- ¼ teaspoon ground cinnamon
- ¼ teaspoon ground coriander
- ¼ teaspoon chili powder

Directions:
1. In a small airtight container or zip-top bag, combine the brown sugar, salt, garlic powder, onion powder, sweet paprika, black pepper, cayenne, oregano, ginger, cumin, smoked paprika, cinnamon, coriander, and chili powder.
2. Close the container and shake to mix. Unused rub will keep in an airtight container for months.

Banana Walnut Bread

Servings: 1
Cooking Time: 1 Hour 15 Minutes
Ingredients:
- 2-1/2 cup of all-purpose flour
- 1 cup of sugar
- 2 eggs
- 1 cup ripe banana, mashed
- 1/4 cup whole milk
- 1/4 cup walnut, finely chopped
- 1 tsp salt
- 3 Tbsp of Vegetable oil
- 3 tsp baking powder

Directions:
1. Set the wood pellet smoker-grill for indirect cooking at 350 F.
2. Combine all the ingredients in a large bowl. Using a mixer (electric or manual), mix the ingredients. Grease and flour the loaf pan. Pour the mixture into the loaf pan.
3. Transfer loaf pan to the grill and cover with steel construction. Bake for 60-75 minutes. Remove and allow to cool.

Nutrition Info: Per Serving: Calories: 548kcal, Carbs: 69g, Fat: 36g, Protein: 14g

Smoked Pork Loin In Sweet-beer Marinade

Servings: 6
Cooking Time: 3 Hours
Ingredients:
- Marinade
- 1 onion finely diced
- 1/4 cup honey (preferably a darker honey)
- 1 1/2 cups of dark beer
- 4 Tbs of mustard
- 1 Tbs fresh thyme finely chopped
- Salt and pepper

- Pork 3 1/2 pounds of pork loin

Directions:

1. Combine all ingredients for the marinade in a bowl.
2. Place the pork along with marinade mixture in a container and refrigerate overnight. Remove the pork from marinade and dry on kitchen towel.
3. Prepare the grill on Smoke with the lid open until the fire is established (4 to 5 minutes).
4. The temperature must reach 250 degrees Fahrenheit and preheat, lid closed, for 10 to 15 minutes.
5. Place the pork on the grill rack and smoke until the internal temperature of the pork is at least 145-150 °F (medium-rare), 2-1/2 to 3 hours.
6. Remove meat from the smoker and let rest for 15 minutes before slicing.
7. Serve hot or cold.

Nutrition Info: Calories: 444.6 Cal Fat: 12.7 g Carbohydrates: 17 g Protein: 60.5 g Fiber: 0.8 g

Veal Kidney On Skewer

Servings: 4
Cooking Time: 30 Minutes
Ingredients:
- Salt with ground pepper, preferably fresh
- 8 slices of bacon
- Bearnaise Sauce
- 2 veal of kidney, fat removed
- 2 Tbsp of peanuts or vegetable oil

Directions:

1. Set the grill for direct cooking at 300°F. Use hickory wood pellets to give scallions a robust taste.
2. Dice kidney to obtain about 46 pieces. Also, cut the bacon into 2-inch pieces
3. Arrange kidney and bacon on a skewer. Prepare as many shewer as possible with the materials available, then brush the skewers with oil.
4. Carefully arrange the skewers on the preheated grill and let it cook for about 10 minutes. Flip, season with salt and pepper on it, then cook for another 10 minutes.
5. Serve immediately with béarnaise sauce if available.

Nutrition Info: Per Serving: Calories: 233.4kcal, Fat: 38g, Carbs: 39g, Protein: 22.3g

Espresso Brisket Rub

Servings: 1/2 Cup
Cooking Time: 5 Minutes
Ingredients:
- 3 tablespoons coarse kosher salt
- 2 tablespoons ground espresso coffee

- 2 tablespoons freshly ground black pepper
- 1 tablespoon garlic powder
- 1 tablespoon light brown sugar
- 1½ teaspoons dried minced onion
- 1 teaspoon ground cumin

Directions:

1. In a small airtight container or zip-top bag, combine the salt, espresso, black pepper, garlic powder, brown sugar, minced onion, and cumin.
2. Close the container and shake to mix. Unused rub will keep in an airtight container for months.

Baked Asparagus & Bacon

Servings: 8
Cooking Time: 20 Minutes
Ingredients:
- 3 eggs
- 1 cup heavy cream
- 1 tablespoon chopped fresh chives
- 1/4 cup goat cheese
- 4 tablespoons Parmesan cheese
- 8 oz. fresh asparagus, trimmed
- 8 oz. bacon, cooked crispy and chopped
- ¼ teaspoon lemon zest

Directions:

1. Preheat the Traeger wood pellet grill to 375 degrees F for 15 minutes while the lid is closed.
2. In a bowl, beat the eggs and stir in cream, chives, goat cheese and Parmesan cheese.
3. Arrange the asparagus in a baking pan.
4. Spread cream mixture on top.
5. Sprinkle bacon bits and lemon zest on top.
6. Bake for 20 minutes.
7. Tips: You can also use this recipe for other vegetables like broccoli.

Empanadas

Servings: 4
Cooking Time: 20 Minutes
Ingredients:
- 3/4 cup + 1 tbsp all-purpose flour
- ½ tsp baking powder
- 1tbsp sugar
- ¼ tsp salt or to taste
- 2tbsp cold water
- 1/3 cups butter
- 1small egg (beaten)
- Filling:
- ½ small onion (chopped)
- 57 g ground beef (1/8 pound)
- 2tbsp marinara sauce
- 1small carrot peeled and diced)

- 1/8 small potato (peeled and diced) 35 grams
- 2tbsp water
- 1garlic clove (minced)
- 1tbsp olive oil
- 1tbsp raisin
- 2tbsp green peas
- ½ tsp salt or taste
- 1/2 tsp ground black pepper or to taste
- 1hard-boiled egg (sliced)

Directions:

1. Start your grill on smoke mode and leave the lid open for 5 minutes, or until fire starts.
2. Close the grill and preheat grill to 400°F with the lid closed for 15 minutes, using hickory hardwood pellets.
3. For the fillet, place a cast iron skillet on the grill and add the oil.
4. Once the oil is hot, add the onion and garlic and sauté until the onion is tender and translucent.
5. Add the ground beef and sauté until it is tender, stirring often.
6. Stir in the marinara, salt, water, and pepper.
7. Bring to a boil and reduce the heat. Cook for 30 seconds.
8. Stir in the carrot, raisin, and potatoes and cook for 3 minutes.
9. Stir in the green peas and sliced egg. Cook for additional 2 minutes, stirring often.
10. Spray a baking dish with a non-stick spray.
11. For the dough, combine the flour, baking powder salt and sugar in a large mixing bowl. Mix until well combined.
12. Add butter and mix until it is well incorporated.
13. Add egg and mix until you form the dough.
14. Put the dough on a floured surface and knead the dough for a few minutes. Add more flour if the dough is not thick enough.
15. Roll the dough flat with a rolling pin. The flat dough should be ¼ inch thick.
16. Cut the flat dough into circles.
17. Add equal amounts of the beef mixture to the middle of each flat circular dough slice. Fold the dough slice and close the edges by pressing with your fingers or a fork.
18. Arrange the empanadas into the baking sheet in a single layer.
19. Place the baking sheet on the grill and bake for 10 minutes.
20. Remove the baking sheet from the grill and flip the empanadas.
21. Bake for another 10 minutes on the grill or until empanadas are golden brown.

Nutrition Info: Calories: 353 Total Fat: 22.3 g Saturated Fat: 11.3 g Cholesterol: 129 mg Sodium: 481 mg Total Carbohydrate 28.9 g Dietary Fiber 1.9 g Total Sugars: 6.6 g Protein: 10.4 g

Smoked Bananas Foster Bread Pudding

Servings: 8 To 10
Cooking Time: 2 Hours 15 Minutes
Ingredients:
- 1loaf (about 4 cups) brioche or challah, cubed to 1 inch cubes
- 3eggs, lightly beaten
- 2cups of milk
- 2/3 cups sugar
- 2large bananas, peeled and smashed
- 1tbsp vanilla extract
- 1tbsp cinnamon
- 1/4 tsp nutmeg
- 1/2 cup pecans
- Rum Sauce Ingredients:
- 1/2 cup spiced rum
- 1/4 cup unsalted butter
- 1cup dark brown sugar
- 1tsp cinnamon
- 5large bananas, peeled and quartered

Directions:

1. Place pecans on a skillet over medium heat and lightly toast for about 5 minutes, until you can smell them.
2. Remove from heat and allow to cool. Once cooled, chop pecans.
3. Lightly butter a 9" x 13" baking dish and evenly layer bread cubes in the dish.
4. In a large bowl, whisk eggs, milk, sugar, mashed bananas, vanilla extract, cinnamon, and nutmeg until combined.
5. Pour egg mixture over the bread in the baking dish evenly. Sprinkle with chopped pecans. Cover with aluminum foil and refrigerate for about 30 minutes.
6. Preheat pellet grill to 180°F. Turn your smoke setting to high, if applicable.
7. Remove foil from dish and place on the smoker for 5 minutes with the lid closed, allowing bread to absorb smoky flavor.
8. Remove dish from the grill and cover with foil again. Increase your pellet grill's temperature to 350°F.
9. Place dish on the grill grate and cook for 50-60 minutes until everything is cooked through and the bread pudding is bubbling.
10. In a saucepan, while pudding cooks heat up butter for rum sauce over medium heat. When the butter begins to melt, add the brown sugar, cinnamon, and bananas. Sauté until bananas begin to soften.
11. Add rum and watch. When the liquid begins to bubble, light a match, and tilt the pan. Slowly and

carefully move the match towards the liquid until the sauce lights. When the flames go away, remove skillet from heat.

12.   If you're uncomfortable lighting the liquid with a match, just cook it for 3-4 minutes over medium heat after the rum has been added.

13.   Keep rum sauce on a simmer or reheat once it's time to serve.

14.   Remove bread pudding from the grill and allow it to cool for about 5 minutes.

15.   Cut into squares, put each square on a plate and add a piece of banana then drizzle rum sauce over the top. Serve on its own or a la mode and enjoy it!

Nutrition Info: Calories: 274.7 Fat: 7.9 g Cholesterol: 10 mg Carbohydrate: 35.5 g Fiber: 0.9 g Sugar: 24.7 g Protein: 4 g

Amazing Irish Soda Bread

Servings: 10
Cooking Time: 1½ Hours
Ingredients:
- 4 C. flour
- 1 C. raisins
- ½ C. sugar
- 1 tbsp. caraway seeds
- 2 tsp. baking powder
- 1 tsp. baking soda
- ¾ tsp. salt
- 1¼ C. buttermilk
- 1 C. sour cream
- 2 eggs

Directions:
1.   Set the temperature of Traeger Grill to 350 degrees F and preheat with closed lid for 15 minutes.
2.   Grease a 9-inch round cake pan.
3.   Reserve 1 tbsp. of flour in a bowl.
4.   In a large bowl, mix together remaining flour, raisins, sugar, caraway seeds, baking powder, baking soda and salt.
5.   In another small bowl, add buttermilk, sour cream and eggs and beat until well combined.
6.   Add egg mixture into flour mixture and mix until just moistened.
7.   With your hands, knead the dough until sticky.
8.   Place the dough into the prepared pan evenly and cut a 4x¾-inch deep slit in the top.
9.   Dust the top with reserved flour.
10.   Place the pan onto the grill and cook for about 1½ hours or until a toothpick inserted in the center comes out clean.
11.   Remove from grill and place the pan onto a wire rack to cool for about 10 minutes.
12.   Carefully, invert the bread onto the wire rack to cool completely before slicing.
13.   Cut the bread into desired-sized slices and sere.

Nutrition Info: Calories per serving: 340; Carbohydrates: 63g; Protein: 8.6g; Fat: 6.6g; Sugar: 20.3g; Sodium: 361mg; Fiber: 2.2g

Baked Apple Crisp

Servings: 7
Cooking Time: 30 Minutes
Ingredients:
- Butter for greasing
- 1/2 cup flour
- 1/2 cup rolled oats
- 1 stick butter, sliced into cubes
- 1 cup brown sugar
- 1 1/2 teaspoon ground cinnamon
- 1/4 cup walnuts, chopped
- 3 lb. apples, sliced thinly
- ½ cup dried cranberries
- 2 1/2 tablespoons bourbon
- 1/2 cup brown sugar
- 1 tablespoon lemon juice
- 1/4 cup honey
- 1 teaspoon vanilla
- 1 1/2 teaspoons ground cinnamon
- Pinch salt

Directions:
1.   Grease cast iron pan with butter.
2.   Add flour, oats, butter cubes, 1 cup sugar, cinnamon and walnuts to a food processor. Pulse until crumbly.
3.   In a bowl, mix the apples with the rest of the ingredients.
4.   Pour apple mixture into the greased pan.
5.   Spread flour mixture on top.
6.   Bake in the Traeger wood pellet grill at 350 degrees F for 1 hour.
7.   Tips: Use freshly squeezed lemon juice.

Simplest Grilled Asparagus

Servings: 4
Cooking Time: 25 Minutes
Ingredients:
- 1½–2 pounds asparagus
- 1–2 tablespoons good-quality olive oil or melted butter
- Salt

Directions:
1.   Start the coals or heat a gas grill for direct hot cooking. Make sure the grates are clean.
2.   Cut the tough bottoms from the asparagus. If they're thick, trim the ends with a vegetable peeler. Toss with the oil and sprinkle with salt.

3. Put the asparagus on the grill directly over the fire, perpendicular to the grates, so they don't fall through. Close the lid and cook, turning once, until the thick part of the stalks can barely be pierced with a skewer or thin knife, 5 to 10 minutes total. Transfer to a platter and serve.

Nutrition Info: Calories: 225 Fats: 20.6 g Cholesterol: 0 mg Carbohydrates: 9.1 g Fiber: 4.2 g Sugars: 0 g Proteins: 4.6 g

Garlic Aioli And Smoked Salmon Sliders

Servings: 12
Cooking Time: 1 Hour And 30 Minutes
Ingredients:
- For Brine:
- Water as needed
- ½ a cup of salt
- 1 tablespoon of dried tarragon
- 1 and a ½ pound of salmon fillets
- For Aioli:
- 1 cup of mayonnaise
- 3 tablespoon of fresh lemon juice
- 3 minced garlic cloves
- 1 and a ½ teaspoon of ground black pepper
- ½ a teaspoon of lemon zest
- Salt as needed
- ½ a cup of apple wood chips
- 12 slide burger buns

Directions:
1. Take a large sized baking dish and add ½ a cup of salt alongside about half water
2. Add tarragon, salmon in the brine mix and keep adding more water
3. Cover up the dish and freeze for 2-12 hours. Take a small bowl and add lemon juice, mayonnaise, pepper, garlic, 1 pinch of salt and lemon zest.
4. Mix and chill for 30 minutes
5. Remove your Salmon from the brine and place it on a wire rack and let it sit for about 30 minutes.
6. Smoke them over low heat for 1 and a ½ to 2 hours. Assemble sliders by dividing the salmon among 12 individual buns.
7. Top each of the pieces with a spoonful of aioli and place another bun on top

Nutrition Info: Calories: 320 Cal Fat: 22 g Carbohydrates: 13 g Protein: 22 g Fiber: 0 g

Mouthwatering Cauliflower

Servings: 8
Cooking Time: 30 Minutes
Ingredients:

- 2 large heads cauliflower head, stem removed and cut into 2-inch florets
- 3 tbsp. olive oil
- Salt and freshly ground black pepper, to taste
- ¼ C. fresh parsley, chopped finely

Directions:
1. Set the temperature of Traeger Grill to 500 degrees F and preheat with closed lid for 15 minutes.
2. In a large bowl, add cauliflower florets, oil, salt and black pepper and toss to coat well.
3. Divide the cauliflower florets onto 2 baking sheets and spread in an even layer.
4. Place the baking sheets onto the grill and cook for about 20-30 minutes, stirring once after 15 minutes.
5. Remove the vegetables from grill and transfer into a large bowl.
6. Immediately, add the parsley and toss to coat well.
7. Serve immediately.

Nutrition Info: Calories per serving: 62; Carbohydrates: 3.6g; Protein: 1.4g; Fat: 5.3g; Sugar: 1.6g; Sodium: 40mg; Fiber: 1.7g

Pork Carnitas

Servings: 6
Cooking Time: 3 Hours
Ingredients:
- Lime wedges
- 3 jalapeno pepper, minced
- A handful of cilantro, chopped
- 1 cup of chicken broth
- 2 Tbsp olive oil
- Corn tortilla
- 3lb pork shoulder, cut into cubes
- Queso Fresco, crumbled
- 2 Tbsp pork rubs

Directions:
1. Preheat wood pellet smoker-grill to 300°F.
2. Mop the rub over the pork shoulder. Place pork shoulder in a cast-iron Dutch oven and pour in chicken broth. Transfer pot to grill grate and cook 2½ hours, until fork tender.
3. Remove the cover, bring to a boil then reduce the liquid in pot by half. All this happens within 15 minutes.
4. Place a tablespoon of bacon fat on the skillet and fry the pork for about 10 minutes, until crisp.
5. Take out pork and serve with cilantro, jalapeno, lime, queso fresco, and corn tortillas.

Nutrition Info: Per Serving: Calories: 254kcal, Carbs: 6g, Fat: 6g, Protein: 41g

Grilled Scallion Salad

Servings: 4-6
Cooking Time: 20 Minutes
Ingredients:
- 1/3 cup of rice vinegar
- 2 tsp of sugar
- 1 Tbsp of sesame oil
- 1 Tbsp of gochugaru
- 1 pound of scallion, untrimmed
- 1 Tbsp of sesame seeds

Directions:
1. Set the grill for indirect cooking at 250°F. Use hickory wood pellets to give scallions a robust taste.
2. Brush sesame oil on scallions, then arrange it on the cooking grid. Grill with for about 8 minutes.
3. Remove scallions from heat and rub with sugar, vinegar, sesame seeds, and vinegar. Serve immediately.

Nutrition Info: Per Serving: Calories: 56kcal, Carbs: 13g, Fat: 7g, Protein: -g

Curried Chicken Roast With Tarragon And Custard

Servings: 4
Cooking Time: 1 Hour 45 Minutes
Ingredients:
- 3 Tbsp of olive oil
- 1 Tbsp of salt, kosher
- 1 4pounds chicken
- 1/2 cup of grain mustard, whole
- 3 Tbsp of tarragon, freshly chopped
- 1 tsp of black pepper, freshly ground
- 1 Tbsp of curry powder

Directions:
1. Preheat the grill for direct cooking at 420°F (High). Use hickory wood pellets for a robust taste.
2. Mix the salt, olive oil, mustard, tarragon, pepper, and curry powder in a bowl. Coat the prepared rub all over the chicken with a grill brush. Put the chicken inside a Ziploc bag and refrigerate for an hour.
3. Roast the chicken on the preheated grill for 35 minutes. With a tong, flip the chicken and roast for another 15 minutes, or until the internal temperature of the thigh reads between 168-1690F.
4. Allow cooling for about 10 minutes before slicing and serving.

Nutrition Info: Per Serving: Calories: 330kcal, Protein: 34.1g, Carbs: 48g, Fat: 39g

Rib Roast And Yorkshire Pudding With Bacon And Rosemary Jus

Servings: 10

Cooking Time: 45 Minutes
Ingredients:
- 1 Tbsp of black pepper
- 1 bacon with rosemary jus
- 3 Tbsp of thyme, preferably fresh leaves
- 6 cloves of garlic, already peeled
- 2-1/2 Tbsp of salt
- 2-1/2 Tbsp of olive oil
- 1 of 5-bone of rib-eye roast, standing
- 1 scallion with parmesan Yorkshire pudding

Directions:
1. Put garlic inside a running food processor. Scrape it into a bowl, mix with pepper, salt, thyme, and oil until a paste is formed.
2. Preheat the grill for direct cooking at 350°F. Use mesquite wood pellets for a distinctive, strong woody taste.
3. Press the herb mixture into the sliced ribs. Put the ribs in the roasting pan and roast both sides for 20 minutes or until internal temperature reads 145°F.
4. Allow the ribs to rest for 10 minutes before serving. After then, serve with Yorkshire pudding.

Nutrition Info: Per Serving: Calories: 250kcal, Protein: 25.6g, Carbs: 33g, Fat: 25.5g.

Smoked Mushroom Sauce

Servings: 4
Cooking Time: 1 Hour
Ingredients:
- 1-quart chef mix mushrooms
- 2 tbsp canola oil
- 1/4 cup julienned shallots
- 2 tbsp chopped garlic
- Salt and pepper to taste
- 1/4 cup alfasi cabernet sauvignon
- 1 cup beef stock
- 2 tbsp margarine

Directions:
1. Crumple four foil sheets into balls. Puncture multiple places in the foil pan then place mushrooms in the foil pan. Smoke in a pellet grill for about 30 minutes. Remove and cool.
2. Heat canola oil in a pan, sauté, add shallots and sauté until translucent.
3. Add mushrooms and cook until supple and rendered down.
4. Add garlic and season with pepper and salt. Cook until fragrant.
5. Add beef stock and wine then cook for about 6-8 minutes over low heat. Adjust seasoning.
6. Add margarine and stir until sauce is thickened and a nice sheen.
7. Serve and enjoy!

Nutrition Info: Calories 300, Total fat 30g, Saturated fat 2g, Total carbs 10g, Net carbs 10g, Protein 4g, Sugar 0g, Fiber 0g, Sodium: 514mg

Lamb Shanks, Smoke-braised

Servings: 2
Cooking Time: 5 Hours 20 Minutes
Ingredients:
- 1/2 cup of brown sugar
- 2 cups of water
- 4 strips of orange
- 2 cinnamon sticks
- 3 whole of star anise
- 1/2 cup of soy sauce
- 2 shank of lamb
- 1/2 cup of rice wine
- 3 Tbsp of sesame oil, Asian

Directions:
1. Put the lamb shank on an aluminum foil paper.
2. In a bowl, mix the sesame oil, water, soy sauce, and brown sugar in a bowl until the sugar dissolves. Add the cinnamon stick, orange zest, and star anise to the bowl. Pour the mixture on the lamb.
3. Preheat the grill for 15 minutes at 250°F. Use alder wood pellets
4. Place the lamb shank on the cooking grates with the foil. Smoke the lamb for 5 hours, until it is brown.
5. Remove the lamb from the smoker and place it on a board to trim off excess fat. Serve immediately.
Nutrition Info: Per Serving: Calories: 255kcal, Carbs: 46g, Fat: 36g, Protein: 34.1g.

Twice-baked Spaghetti Squash

Servings: 2
Cooking Time: 1 Hour 15 Minutes
Ingredients:
- 1 medium spaghetti squash
- 1/2 cup of parmesan cheese (grated and divided)
- 1/2 cup of mozzarella cheese (shredded and divided)
- 1 tsp Salt
- Tbsp Extra-virgin olive oil
- 1/2 tsp Pepper

Directions:
1. Set the wood pellet smoker-grill to indirect cooking at 375 F
2. Using a knife, cut the squash into half lengthwise and remove the seed and pulp. Rub the inside of the squash with olive oil, salt, and pepper. Place on the hot grill with the open part facing up and bake for 45 minutes or until the squash can be easily pierced with a fork. Remove and allow to cool.
3. Place on a cutting board. Using a fork, scrape across the surface in a lengthwise direction to remove the flesh-in strand (to look like spaghetti). Transfer to a bowl, add parmesan and mozzarella cheese, then stir well. Stuff back into the shell, sprinkle cheese on the toppings.
4. Increase the pellet smoker-grill to 425 F, place the stuffed squash on the hot grill and bake for 15 minutes or until cheese starts to brown.
5. Remove and allow to cool, serve.
Nutrition Info: Per Serving: Calories: 294kcal, Carbs: 10.1g, Fat:12g, Protein: 16g

Smoked Porterhouse Steak

Servings: 2-4
Cooking Time: 1 Hour
Ingredients:
- 2 porterhouse steaks (1 inch thick) (20 oz. or 1.25 lb.).
- Melted butter – 4 tbsp.
- Worcestershire Sauce – 2 tsp.
- Dijon Mustard – 1 tbsp.
- Coffee rub – 1 tsp.

Directions:
1. Start your wood pellet smoker on grill instructions when you are ready to cook.
2. Set the temperature to smoke setting. Preheat for 5 minutes while keeping the lid closed.
3. Mix the butter, Worcestershire sauce, and mustard until it is smooth. Brush the mixture on both sides of the steaks. Season the porterhouse steaks with coffee rub.
4. Arrange the steaks on the grill grate and smoke them for about 30 minutes. Remove the steaks using tongs.
5. Increase the heat to 450° F. Brush the steaks again with the butter sauce mixture that was prepared earlier.
6. When the grill comes up to the temperature, place the steaks back on the grill grate and cook until it is done according to your choice. Whichever doneness you prefer i.e. rare, medium rare or well done.
7. In case of medium rare, cook until the internal temperature is about 135° F. Before serving, let the steaks rest for 5 minutes.
Nutrition Info: Calories: 346 Cal Fat: 11 g Carbohydrates: 3 g Protein: 28 g Fiber: 1 g

Barbecue Hot Dog

Servings: 6
Cooking Time: 10 Minutes
Ingredients:

- 6 hot dogs
- ½ cup barbecue sauce
- 6 hot dog buns
- 1 onion, chopped
- ½ cup cheddar cheese, shredded

Directions:
1. Set the Traeger grill to 450 degrees F.
2. Preheat while the lid is closed for 10 minutes.
3. Grill the hot dogs for 5 minutes per side.
4. Brush the hot dogs with the barbecue sauce.
5. Serve in the hot dog buns topped with the onion and cheese.
6. Tips: Use whole-wheat hot dog buns.

Grilled Brussels Sprouts

Servings: 8
Cooking Time: 20 Minutes
Ingredients:
- 1/2 lb bacon, grease reserved
- 1 b Brussels Sprouts
- 1/2 tbsp pepper
- 1/2 tbsp salt

Directions:
1. Cook bacon until crispy on a stovetop, reserve its grease then chop into small pieces.
2. Meanwhile, wash the Brussels sprouts, trim off the dry end and remove dried leaves, if any. Half them and set aside.
3. Place 1/4 cup reserved grease in a pan, cast-iron, over medium-high heat.
4. Season the Brussels sprouts with pepper and salt.
5. Brown the sprouts on the pan with the cut side down for about 3-4 minutes.
6. In the meantime, preheat your pellet grill to 350-375F.
7. Place bacon pieces and browned sprouts into your grill-safe pan.
8. Cook for about 20 minutes.
9. Serve immediately.

Nutrition Info: Calories: 153 Total Fat: 10 g Saturated Fat: 3 g Total Carbs: 5 g Net Carbs: 3 g Protein: 11 g Sugars: 1 g Fiber: 2 g Sodium: 622mg

Savory Applesauce On The Grill

Servings: 2
Cooking Time: 45 Minutes
Ingredients:
- 1½ pounds whole apples
- Salt

Directions:
1. Start the coals or heat a gas grill for medium direct cooking. Make sure the grates are clean.

2. Put the apples on the grill directly over the fire. Close the lid and cook until the fruit feels soft when gently squeezed with tongs, 10 to 20 minutes total, depending on their size. Transfer to a cutting board and let sit until cool enough to touch.
3. Cut the flesh from around the core of each apple; discard the cores. Put the chunks in a blender or food processor and process until smooth, or put them in a bowl and purée with an immersion blender until as chunky or smooth as you like. Add a generous pinch of salt, then taste and adjust the seasoning. Serve or refrigerate in an airtight container for up to 3 days.

Nutrition Info: Calories: 15 Fats: 0 g Cholesterol: 0 mg Carbohydrates: 3 g Fiber: 0 g Sugars: 3 g Proteins: 0 g

Pellet Grill Apple Crisp

Servings: 15
Cooking Time: 1 Hour
Ingredients:
- Apples
- 10 large apples
- 1/2 cup flour
- 1cup sugar, dark brown
- 1/2 tbsp cinnamon
- 1/2 cup butter slices
- Crisp
- 3cups oatmeal, old-fashioned
- 1-1/2 cups softened butter, salted
- 1-1/2 tbsp cinnamon
- 2cups brown sugar

Directions:
1. Preheat your grill to 350 F.
2. Wash, peel, core, and dice the apples into cubes, medium-size
3. Mix flour, dark brown sugar, and cinnamon, then toss with your apple cubes.
4. Spray a baking pan, 10x13", with cooking spray then place apples inside. Top with butter slices.
5. Mix all crisp ingredients in a medium bowl until well combined. Place the mixture over the apples.
6. Place on the grill and cook for about 1-hour checking after every 15-20 minutes to ensure cooking is even. Do not place it on the hottest grill part.
7. Remove and let sit for about 20-25 minutes
8. It's very warm.

Nutrition Info: Calories: 528 Total Fat: 26g Saturated Fat: 16g Total Carbs: 75g Net Carbs: 70g Protein: 4g Sugars: 51g Fiber: 5g Sodium: 209mg

Smoked Rib Eye With Bourbon Butter

Servings: 4-6

Cooking Time: 1 Hour And 30 Minutes
Ingredients:
- 4 Ribeye steaks (1 inch thick).
- Fresh ground pepper – 1/2 tsp.
- Garlic (minced) – 1-2 cloves.
- Green Onion (finely minced) – 1 tbsp.
- Parsley (finely minced) – 1 tbsp.
- Salt– 1/2 tsp.
- Bourbon – 2 tbsp.
- Butter – 1/2 cup.
- Traeger prime rub.

Directions:
1. In a mixing bowl, add butter, parsley, chives, bourbon, garlic, salt, and pepper. Stir all of the ingredients with a wooden spoon. Put the smoker on.
2. Until the fire is established, keep the lid open. The fire should be established in about 4-5 minutes.
3. Season the rib eye steaks with a prime rub. Arrange the steaks on the grill and smoke them for about an hour.
4. Then temporarily remove the steaks from the smoker and set your smoker's temperature up to 450F. Place the steaks back on the grill. Give one side about 6-8 minutes and then turn it over.
5. Keep the other side for the same amount of time. Otherwise, if you like your steak medium rare then keep cooking and turning over until the internal temperature is 135 F.
6. Take the steak out of the smoker after they are cooked to your liking and immediately pat them with the bourbon butter sauce you made earlier.
7. Let the meat rest for about 3 minutes before serving it.

Nutrition Info: Calories: 230 Cal Fat: 16 g Carbohydrates: 0 g Protein: 21 g Fiber: 0 g

Pork Dry Rub

Servings: 1
Cooking Time: 15 Minutes
Ingredients:
- Tbsp Kosher salt
- 2 Tbsp Powered onions
- Tbsp Cayenne pepper
- 1tsp Dried mustard
- 1/4 cup brown sugar
- Tbsp Powdered garlic
- Tbsp Powdered chili pepper
- 1/4 cup smoked paprika
- 2 Tbsp Black pepper

Directions:
1. Combine all the ingredients in a small bowl.
2. Transfer to an airtight jar or container.
3. Keep stored in a cool, dry place.

Nutrition Info: Per Serving: Calories: 16kcal, Carbs: 3g, Fat:0.9g, Protein: 0.8g

Grilled Pepper Steak With Mushroom Sauce

Servings: 4
Cooking Time: 30 Minutes
Ingredients:
- 2 cloves garlic, minced
- 1 tablespoon Worcestershire sauce
- 1/2 cup Dijon mustard
- 2 tablespoons bourbon
- 4 tenderloin steaks
- Salt and tri-color peppercorns to taste
- 1 tablespoon olive oil
- 1 onion, diced
- 1/2 cup white wine
- 1/2 cup chicken broth
- 16 oz. mushrooms, sliced
- ½ cup cream
- Salt and pepper to taste

Directions:
1. In a bowl, mix the garlic, Worcestershire sauce, Dijon mustard, and bourbon.
2. Spread the mixture on both sides of the steak and wrap with foil.
3. Marinate at room temperature for 1 hour.
4. Unwrap and season the steak with salt and peppercorns.
5. Press the peppercorns into the steak.
6. Preheat your Traeger wood pellet grill to 180 degrees F for 15 minutes while the lid is closed.
7. Grill the steaks for 30 minutes, flipping once or twice.
8. Make the mushroom gravy by cooking onion in olive oil in a pan over medium heat.
9. Add mushrooms.
10. Pour in the broth and white wine.
11. Simmer for 5 minutes.
12. Stir in the cream.
13. Season with salt and pepper.
14. Serve steaks with sauce.

Nutrition Info: Calories: 148.7 Fats: 5.6 g Cholesterol: 44 mg Carbohydrates: 5.5 g Fiber: 0.9 g Sugar: 0.4 g Protein: 18.7 g

Seafood On Skewers

Servings: 4
Cooking Time: 40 Minutes
Ingredients:
- 2 Tbsp of peanuts or corn oil
- 16 cubes of swordfish

146

- 8 sea scallops, big
- Salt and ground pepper, fresh
- 16 cubes of monkfish
- 12 jumbo shrimp
- Sauce Bearnaise

Directions:
1. Set the grill for direct cooking at 200°F. Use oak wood pellets for rich, woody taste.
2. Arrange four pieces of alternating swordfish and monkfish pieces, shrimps, and scallops on a metal skewer. Repeat this for the other three skewers. Rub oil on the skewers.
3. Place the skewers on the preheated grill, and cook for 10 minutes. Flip to the other side and season with salt and pepper. Allow the other side to cook for another 10 minutes. Serve it with béarnaise sauce.

Nutrition Info: Per Serving: Calories: 82kcal, Protein: 20.5g, Fat: 15g, Carb: 16g

Monster Smoked Pork Chops

Servings: 4
Cooking Time: 2 Hours 30 Minutes
Ingredients:
- 1/3 cup of sugar
- 4 tsp of pink curing salt
- Vegetable oil
- 1 cup of kosher or sea salt
- 1-1/4 pound pork chops
- 1/4 hot water
- 1/4 cold water

Directions:
1. Put the pork on a big baking pan. Mix the salt, curing salt, sugar, and hot water in a bowl. Add the pork to the mixture, and refrigerate for 12 hours.
2. Preheat the grill for 15 minutes at 250°F. Use pecan wood pellets
3. Bring the pork out and remove the brine from the pork.
4. Smoke the pork for about two and a half hours until it is done or until the internal temperature reads 145°F.
5. Brush olive oil all over the sides of the pork. Then increase the temperature of the cooker to 300°F and grill the pork chop for another 5 minutes until it is done.

Nutrition Info: Per Serving: Calories: 350kcal, Protein: 35g, Carbs: 45g, Fat: 40g.

Smoked Garlic Sauce

Servings: 2
Cooking Time: 30 Minutes
Ingredients:
- 3 whole garlic heads

- 1/2 cup mayonnaise
- 1/4 cup sour cream
- 2 tbsp lemon juice
- 2 tbsp cider vinegar
- Salt to taste

Directions:
1. Cut the garlic heads off then place in a microwave-safe bowl, add 2 tbsp water and cover. Microwave for about 5-6 minutes on medium.
2. Heat your grill on medium.
3. Place the garlic heads in a shallow 'boat' foil and smoke for about 20-25 minutes until soft.
4. Transfer the garlic heads into a blender. Process for a few minutes until smooth.
5. Add remaining ingredients and process until everything is combined.
6. Enjoy!

Nutrition Info: Calories 20, Total fat 0g, Saturated fat 0g, Total carbs 10g, Net carbs 9g, Protein 0g, Sugar 0g, Fiber 1g, Sodium: 0mg

Venison Meatloaf

Servings: 6
Cooking Time: 1 Hour And 15 Minutes
Ingredients:
- For the Meatloaf:
- 1 medium white onion, peeled, diced
- 2 pounds ground venison
- 1 cup bread crumbs
- 1 teaspoon salt
- 1 tablespoon Worcestershire sauce
- ½ teaspoon ground black pepper
- 2 tablespoons onion soup mix
- 1 egg, beaten
- 1 cup milk, unsweetened
- For the Glaze:
- 1/4 cup brown sugar
- 1/4 cup ketchup
- 1/4 cup apple cider vinegar

Directions:
1. Switch on the Traeger grill, fill the grill hopper with big game blend wood pellets, power the grill on by using the control panel, select 'smoke' on the temperature dial, or set the temperature to 350 degrees F and let it preheat for a minimum of 15 minutes.
2. Meanwhile, take a large bowl, place all the ingredients for the meatloaf in it, and stir until just combined; don't overmix.
3. Take a loaf pan, grease it with oil, place meatloaf mixture in it, and spread evenly.
4. Prepare the glaze and for this, take a small bowl, place all of its ingredients in it, stir until combined, and then spread evenly on top of meatloaf.

5.   When the grill has preheated, open the lid, place loaf pan on the grill grate, shut the grill and smoke for 1 hour and 15 minutes until the internal temperature reaches 165 degrees F.
6.   Serve straight away.
Nutrition Info: Calories: 186.5 Cal ;Fat: 7.2 g ;Carbs: 7.7 g ;Protein: 21.6 g ;Fiber: 0.4 g

Texas Barbeque Rub

Servings: 1/2 Cup
Cooking Time: 15 Minutes
Ingredients:
- 1 tsp Sugar
- Tbsp Seasoned salt
- Tbsp Black pepper
- tsp Chilli powder
- Tbsp Powdered onions
- Tbsp Smoked paprika
- 1 tsp Sugar
- Tbsp Powdered garlic

Directions:
1.   Pour all the ingredients into a small bowl and mix thoroughly.
2.   Keep stored in an airtight jar or container.
Nutrition Info: Per Serving: Calories: 22kcal, Carbs: 2g, Fat: 0.2g, Protein: 0.6g

Traeger Smoked Italian Meatballs

Servings: 6
Cooking Time: 1 Hour 5 Minutes;
Ingredients:
- 2 lb beef, ground
- 2 slices white bread
- 1/2 cup whole milk
- 1 tbsp salt
- 1/2 tbsp onion powder
- 1/2 tbsp minced garlic
- 2 tbsp Italian seasoning
- 1/4 tbsp black pepper

Directions:
1.   In a mixing bowl, mix all the ingredients until well combined using your hands. Turn on your Traeger and set it to smoke then line a baking sheet with parchment paper.
2.   Roll golf size meatballs using your hands .and place them on the baking dish. Place the baking dish in the Traeger and smoke for 35 minutes.
3.   Increase the Traeger heat to 325F and cook for 30 more minutes or until the internal temperature reaches 160F.
4.   Serve when hot
Nutrition Info: Calories 453, Total fat 27g, Saturated fat 10g, Total carbs 7g, Net carbs 7g Protein 0g, Sugars 2g, Fiber 0g, Sodium 550mg

Appendix : Recipes Index

Traeger Smoked Italian Meatballs 148
Traeger Smoked Lamb Meatballs 90
Traeger Smoked Lamb Shoulder 89
Traeger Smoked Leg 69
Traeger Smoked Mushrooms 26
Traeger Smoked Pork Ribs 79
Traeger Smoked Shrimp 117
Traeger Spot Prawn Skewers 105
Traeger Steak Kabobs 127
Traeger Tri-tip Roast 73
Trager New York Strip 98
Trager Smoked Spatchcock Turkey 51
Turkey Breast 38
Turkey Legs 48
Turkey Meatballs 41
Turkey With Apricot Barbecue Glaze 46
Twice-baked Spaghetti Squash 144
Twice-smoked Potatoes 27

U

Ultimate Tasty Chicken 42

V

Veal Kidney On Skewer 139
Vegan Smoked Carrot Dogs 27
Vegetable Sandwich 17
Vegetable Skewers 13
Veggie Lover's Burgers 137
Venison Meatloaf 147

W

Whole Roasted Cauliflower With Garlic
Parmesan Butter 16
Whole Smoked Chicken 64
Wild Turkey Egg Rolls 63
Wild West Wings 59
Wine Infused Salmon 112
Wood Pellet Bacon Wrapped Jalapeno Poppers
21
Wood Pellet Chicken Breasts 67
Wood Pellet Chicken Wings With Spicy Miso 46
Wood Pellet Chile Lime Chicken 49
Wood Pellet Cold Smoked Cheese 34
Wood Pellet Garlic Dill Smoked Salmon 109
Wood Pellet Grill Spicy Sweet Potatoes 29
Wood Pellet Grilled Asparagus And Honey
Glazed Carrots 25

Wood Pellet Grilled Aussie Leg Of Lamb Roast
83
Wood Pellet Grilled Buffalo Chicken 37
Wood Pellet Grilled Buffalo Chicken 47
Wood Pellet Grilled Buffalo Chicken Leg 50
Wood Pellet Grilled Chicken 43
Wood Pellet Grilled Chicken Kabobs 48
Wood Pellet Grilled Lobster Tail 123
Wood Pellet Grilled Mexican Street Corn 7
Wood Pellet Grilled Salmon Sandwich 121
Wood Pellet Grilled Scallops 114
Wood Pellet Grilled Stuffed Zucchini 35
Wood Pellet Grilled Tenderloin With Fresh
Herb Sauce 92
Wood Pellet Grilled Vegetables 9
Wood Pellet Grilled Zucchini Squash Spears 10
Wood Pellet Pulled Pork 71
Wood Pellet Rockfish 119
Wood Pellet Salt And Pepper Spot Prawn
Skewers 105
Wood Pellet Sheet Pan Chicken Fajitas 42
Wood Pellet Smoked Acorn Squash 33
Wood Pellet Smoked Asparagus 35
Wood Pellet Smoked Beef Jerky 76
Wood Pellet Smoked Buffalo Shrimp 104
Wood Pellet Smoked Cornish Hens 44
Wood Pellet Smoked Lamb Shoulder 98
Wood Pellet Smoked Mushrooms 29
Wood Pellet Smoked Pork Ribs 95
Wood Pellet Smoked Ribeye Steaks 90
Wood Pellet Smoked Salmon 110
Wood Pellet Smoked Spatchcock Turkey 38
Wood Pellet Smoked Spatchcock Turkey 52
Wood Pellet Smoked Vegetables 20
Wood Pellet Teriyaki Smoked Shrimp 107
Wood Pellet Togarashi Grilled Salmon 106
Wood-fired Chicken Breasts 66
Wood-fired Halibut 102

Y

Yummy Buttery Clams 117

Z

Zucchini Soup 26
Zucchini With Red Potatoes 7

CPSIA information can be obtained
at www.ICGtesting.com
Printed in the USA
LVHW011531160721
692882LV00018B/1133